Thalassemia

Editor

ALI T. TAHER

HEMATOLOGY/ONCOLOGY CLINICS OF NORTH AMERICA

www.hemonc.theclinics.com

Consulting Editors
GEORGE P. CANELLOS
H. FRANKLIN BUNN

April 2018 • Volume 32 • Number 2

ELSEVIER

1600 John F. Kennedy Boulevard • Suite 1800 • Philadelphia, Pennsylvania, 19103-2899

http://www.theclinics.com

HEMATOLOGY/ONCOLOGY CLINICS OF NORTH AMERICA Volume 32, Number 2
April 2018 ISSN 0889-8588, ISBN 13: 978-0-323-58308-4

Editor: Stacy Eastman
Developmental Editor: Kristen Helm

Hematology/Oncology Clinics (ISSN 0889-8588) is published bimonthly by Elsevier Inc., 360 Park Avenue South, New York, NY 10010-1710. Months of issue are February, April, June, August, October, and December. Business and Editorial Offices: 1600 John F. Kennedy Blvd., Ste. 1800, Philadelphia, PA 19103-2899. Customer Service Office: 3251 Riverport Lane, Maryland Heights, MO 63043. Periodicals postage paid at New York, NY and at additional mailing offices. Subscription prices are $413.00 per year (domestic individuals), $787.00 per year (domestic institutions), $100.00 per year (domestic students/residents), $471.00 per year (Canadian individuals), $974.00 per year (Canadian institutions) $536.00 per year (international individuals), $974.00 per year (international institutions), and $255.00 per year (international and Canadian students/residents). International air speed delivery is included in all *Clinics* subscription prices. All prices are subject to change without notice. **POSTMASTER:** Send address changes to *Hematology/Oncology Clinics of North America*, Elsevier Health Sciences Division, Subscription Customer Service, 3251 Riverport Lane, Maryland Heights, MO 63043. Customer Service (orders, claims, online, change of address): Elsevier Health Sciences Division, Subscription **Customer Service, 3251 Riverport Lane, Maryland Heights, MO 63043. Tel: 1-800-654-2452 (U.S. and Canada); 314-447-8871 (outside U.S. and Canada). Fax: 314-447-8029. E-mail: journalscustomerservice-usa@elsevier.com (for print support); journalsonlinesupport-usa@elsevier.com (for online support).**

Reprints. For copies of 100 or more, of articles in this publication, please contact the Commercial Reprints Department, Elsevier Inc., 360 Park Avenue South, New York, New York 10010-1710; Tel.: 212-633-3874, Fax: 212-633-3820, E-mail: reprints@elsevier.com.

Hematology/Oncology Clinics of North America is covered in *MEDLINE/PubMed (Index Medicus), EMBASE/ Excerpta Medica, and BIOSIS.*

Contributors

CONSULTING EDITORS

GEORGE P. CANELLOS, MD
William Rosenberg Professor of Medicine, Department of Medical Oncology, Dana-Farber Cancer Institute, Boston, Massachusetts, USA

H. FRANKLIN BUNN, MD
Professor of Medicine, Division of Hematology, Brigham and Women's Hospital, Harvard Medical School, Boston, Massachusetts, USA

EDITOR

ALI T. TAHER, MD, PhD, FRCP
Professor of Medicine, Hematology and Oncology, Department of Internal Medicine, Director, Naef K. Basile Cancer Institute, American University of Beirut Medical Center, Beirut, Lebanon

AUTHORS

YESIM AYDINOK, MD
Professor, Department of Pediatric Hematology and Oncology, Ege University Children's Hospital, Bornova, Izmir, Turkey

RAYAN BOU-FAKHREDIN, BSc
Department of Internal Medicine, American University of Beirut Medical Center, Beirut, Lebanon

FARID BOULAD, MD
Center for Cell Engineering, Department of Pediatrics, Memorial Sloan Kettering Cancer Center, New York, New York, USA

ANNALISA CABRIOLU, PhD
Center for Cell Engineering, Memorial Sloan Kettering Cancer Center, New York, New York, USA

MARIA DOMENICA CAPPELLINI, MD
Professor, Department of Medicine, Cà Granda Foundation IRCCS, Department of Clinical Science and Community, The University of Milan, Milano, Italy

KATIE T. CARLBERG, MD
Associate Hematologist/Oncologist, Hematology Oncology, UCSF Benioff Children's Hospital Oakland, Oakland, California, USA

DANIEL CORIU, MD, PhD
Professor, Fundeni Clinical Institute, University of Medicine and Pharmacy "Carol Davila," Bucharest, Romania

SUPACHAI EKWATTANAKIT, MD, PhD
Consultant Hematologist, Division of Hematology, Department of Medicine, Faculty of Medicine Siriraj Hospital, Mahidol University, Bangkok, Thailand

JULIANO LARA FERNANDES, MD, PhD, MBA
Cardiovascular Imaging Coordinator, Jose Michel Kalaf Research Institute, Radiologia Clinica de Campinas, Campinas, São Paulo, Brazil

MACIEJ W. GARBOWSKI, MD, PhD
Clinical Research Fellow, Haematology Department, University College London, Cancer Institute, UCL Cancer Institute, London, United Kingdom

AMALIRIS GUERRA, PhD
Department of Pediatrics, Division of Hematology, Children's Hospital of Philadelphia, Philadelphia, Pennsylvania, USA

RITAMA GUPTA, PhD
Department of Pediatrics, Division of Hematology, Children's Hospital of Philadelphia, Philadelphia, Pennsylvania, USA

DOUGLAS R. HIGGS, FMedSci, FRS
Molecular Hematology Unit, Medical Research Council, Weatherall Institute of Molecular Medicine, University of Oxford, John Radcliffe Hospital, Headington, United Kingdom; National Institute for Health Research, Oxford Biomedical Research Centre, Blood Theme, Oxford University Hospitals, Oxford, United Kingdom

FRANCO LOCATELLI, MD, PhD
Department of Pediatric Hematology and Oncology, IRCCS Bambino Gesù Children's Hospital, Roma, Italy; University of Pavia, Pavia, Italy

JORGE MANSILLA-SOTO, PhD
Center for Cell Engineering, Memorial Sloan Kettering Cancer Center, New York, New York, USA

ALESSIA MARCON, MD
Department of Medicine, Cà Granda Foundation IRCCS, Department of Clinical Science and Community, University of Milan, Milano, Italy

SACHITH METTANANDA, MBBS, MD, DPhil
Molecular Hematology Unit, Medical Research Council, Weatherall Institute of Molecular Medicine, University of Oxford, John Radcliffe Hospital, Headington, Oxford, United Kingdom; Department of Paediatrics, Faculty of Medicine, University of Kelaniya, Ragama, Sri Lanka

IRENE MOTTA, MD
Department of Medicine, Cà Granda Foundation IRCCS, Milano, Italy

KHALED M. MUSALLAM, MD, PhD
President, International Network of Hematology, London, United Kingdom

JOHN B. PORTER, MA, MD, FRCP, FRCPath
Professor, Haematology Department, University College London, Consultant and Head of Joint Red Cell Disorders Unit, UCLH and Whittington Hospitals, UCL Cancer Institute, London, United Kingdom

STEFANO RIVELLA, PhD
Professor, Department of Pediatrics, Division of Hematology, Children's Hospital of Philadelphia, Kwame Ohene-Frempong Chair on Sickle Cell Anemia, Cell and Molecular Biology Graduate Group (CAMB), University of Pennsylvania, Abramson Research Center, Philadelphia, Pennsylvania, USA

ISABELLE RIVIÈRE, PhD
Center for Cell Engineering, Memorial Sloan Kettering Cancer Center, New York, New York, USA

MICHEL SADELAIN, MD, PhD
Center for Cell Engineering, Memorial Sloan Kettering Cancer Center, New York, New York, USA

SYLVIA T. SINGER, MD
Associate Hematologist/Oncologist, Hematology Oncology, UCSF Benioff Children's Hospital Oakland, Oakland, California, USA

LUISA STROCCHIO, MD
Department of Pediatric Hematology and Oncology, IRCCS Bambino Gesù Children's Hospital, Roma, Italy

ALI T. TAHER, MD, PhD, FRCP
Professor of Medicine, Hematology and Oncology, Department of Internal Medicine, Director, Naef K. Basile Cancer Institute, American University of Beirut Medical Center, Beirut, Lebanon

ELLIOTT P. VICHINSKY, MD
Professor of Pediatrics, University of California San Francisco, San Francisco, California, USA; Medical Director, Hematology Oncology, UCSF Benioff Children's Hospital Oakland, Oakland, California, USA

VIP VIPRAKASIT, MD, DPhil(Oxon)
Siriraj Integrated Center of Excellence for Thalassemia (SiiCOE-T), Division of Hematology/Oncology, Professor, Department of Pediatrics, Faculty of Medicine Siriraj Hospital, Mahidol University, Bangkok, Thailand

DAVID J. WEATHERALL, MD, FRCP, FRS
Regius Professor of Medicine Emeritus, University of Oxford, Weatherall Institute of Molecular Medicine, John Radcliffe Hospital, Headington, Oxford, United Kingdom

Contents

The Evolving Spectrum of the Epidemiology of Thalassemia   165

David J. Weatherall

The thalassemias and other inherited disorders of hemoglobin are likely to remain a serious global health problem for the foreseeable future. Currently, they are most frequent in the tropical belt; an assessment of their true frequency and the likely cost of management for the governments of these countries will require a form of micromapping. Over recent years, there has been major progress toward better prevention and management of the thalassemias in richer countries; it is likely that, using the tools of molecular genetics, they will eventually be completely curable, although this is probably a long time in the future.

Molecular Basis and Genetic Modifiers of Thalassemia   177

Sachith Mettananda and Douglas R. Higgs

Thalassemia is a disorder of hemoglobin characterized by reduced or absent production of one of the globin chains in human red blood cells with relative excess of the other. Impaired synthesis of β-globin results in β-thalassemia, whereas defective synthesis of α-globin leads to α-thalassemia. Despite being a monogenic disorder, thalassemia exhibits remarkable clinical heterogeneity that is directly related to the intracellular imbalance between α- and β-like globin chains. Novel insights into the genetic modifiers have contributed to the understanding of the correlation between genotype and phenotype and are being explored as therapeutic pathways to cure this life-limiting disease.

Clinical Classification, Screening, and Diagnosis for Thalassemia   193

Vip Viprakasit and Supachai Ekwattanakit

At present, thalassemia diseases are classified into transfusion-dependent thalassemia and non–transfusion-dependent thalassemia. This classification is based on the clinical severity of the disease, determining whether patients require regular blood transfusions to survive (transfusion-dependent thalassemia) or not (non–transfusion-dependent thalassemia). In addition to the previous terminology of "thalassemia major" or "thalassemia intermedia," this classification has embraced all other forms of thalassemia syndromes, such as α-thalassemia, hemoglobin E/β-thalassemia, and combined α- and β-thalassemias. Definitive diagnosis of thalassemia and hemoglobinopathies requires a comprehensive workup, including complete blood count, hemoglobin analysis, and molecular studies to identify mutations of globin genes.

Stress erythropoiesis (SE) is characterized by an imbalance in erythroid proliferation and differentiation under increased demands of erythrocyte generation and tissue oxygenation. β-Thalassemia represents a chronic state of SE, called ineffective erythropoiesis (IE), exhibiting an expansion of erythroid-progenitor pool and deposition of alpha chains on erythrocyte membranes, causing cell death and anemia. Concurrently, there is a decrease in hepcidin expression and a subsequent state of iron overload. There are substantial investigative efforts to target increased iron absorption under IE. There are also avenues for targeting cell contact and signaling within erythroblastic islands under SE, for therapeutic benefits.

The hallmarks of thalassemias are ineffective erythropoiesis and peripheral hemolysis leading to a cascade of events responsible for several clinical complications. This pathophysiologic mechanism can be partially controlled by blood transfusions or by correction of the severity of ineffective erythropoiesis. Thalassemias include a spectrum of phenotypes. Two main groups can be clinically distinguished: transfusion-dependent (TDT) and non–transfusion-dependent (NTDT) thalassemia. Both conditions are characterized by several clinical complications along life; some are shared, whereas some have a higher prevalence in one group than in the other. The authors present the most common clinical complications in TDT and NTDT and their management.

The presence of a high incidence of thrombotic events, mainly in non–transfusion-dependent β-thalassemia syndromes, has led to the identification of a hypercoagulable state in patients with thalassemia. This article highlights the mechanisms leading to hypercoagulability in thalassemia. It also discusses the clinical experience and available evidence on prevention and management approaches.

The relationship between blood transfusion intensity, chelatable iron pools, and extrahepatic iron distribution is described in thalassemia. Risk factors for cardiosiderosis are discussed with particular reference to the balance of transfusional iron loading rate and transferrin-iron utilization rate as marked by plasma levels of soluble transferrin receptors. Low transfusion regimens increase residual erythropoiesis, allowing for apotransferrin-dependent clearance of non–transferrin-bound iron species otherwise destined for the myocardium. The impact of transfusion rates on chelation dosing required for iron balance is also shown.

Introduction of MRI techniques for identifying and monitoring tissue iron overload and the current understanding of iron homeostasis in transfusion-dependent (TDT) and non–transfusion-dependent thalassemia have allowed for a more robust administration of iron chelation therapies. The development of safe and efficient oral iron chelators and the insights gained from large-scale prospective studies using these agents have improved iron overload management. A significant reduction in iron toxicity–induced morbidity and mortality and improvements in quality of life were observed in TDT. The appropriate management of tissue-specific iron loading in TDT has been portrayed using evidence-based data obtained from investigational studies.

MRI is a key tool in the current management of patients with thalassemia. Given its capability of assessing iron overload in different organs noninvasively and without contrast, it has significant advantages over other metrics, including serum ferritin. Liver iron concentration can be measured either with relaxometry methods T2*/T2 or signal intensity ratio techniques. Myocardial iron can be assessed in the same examination through T2* imaging. In this article, the authors focus on showing how MRI evaluates iron in both organs and the clinical applications, as well as practical approaches to using this tool by clinicians taking care of patients with thalassemia.

As more women with transfusion-dependent thalassemia are seeking pregnancy, ensuring the best outcomes for both the mother and baby requires concerted, collaborative efforts between practitioners and the family. Proactive counseling, early fertility evaluation, recent developments in reproductive technology, and optimal management of iron overload have resulted in more successful pregnancies and the birth of healthy newborns. With advances in technology for prenatal screening and increased awareness to perform screening for hemoglobinopathies, healthy pregnancy outcomes have become the expectation. Topics that require further study include management that allows fertility preservation, improved noninvasive prenatal diagnostics methods for affected fetuses, the use of chelation therapy during pregnancy, and indications for and duration of anticoagulation.

Although recent advances in gene therapy are expected to increase the chance of disease cure in thalassemia major, at present hematopoietic stem cell transplantation (HSCT) remains the only consolidated curative approach for this disorder. The widest experience has been obtained in

HEMATOLOGY/ONCOLOGY
CLINICS OF NORTH AMERICA

Erratum

An error was made in the article on "Identification and Targeting of Kinase Alterations in Histiocytic Neoplasms" appearing in the August 2017 issue of *Hematology/Oncology Clinics of North America* (Volume 31, Issue 4). Reference number 13 is incorrect. The correct reference is: Satoh T, Smith A, Sarde A, et al. B-RAF Mutant Alleles Associated with Langerhans Cell Histiocytosis, a Granulomatous Pediatric Disease. PLoS One 2012;7(4):e33891. This correction has been made in the online version.

Hematol Oncol Clin N Am 32 (2018) xiii
https://doi.org/10.1016/j.hoc.2017.12.001
0889-8588/18

Preface

Thalassemia

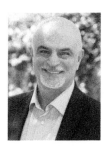

Ali T. Taher, MD, PhD, FRCP
Editor

Over the years, an increase in understanding of the underlying molecular and cellular mechanisms as well as the pathophysiology of thalassemia has caused a paradigm shift in diagnosis and treatment.

Several clinical forms of thalassemia exist and have been described. The disease hallmarks include an imbalance in the α/β-globin chain ratio, ineffective erythropoiesis, chronic hemolytic anemia, compensatory hemopoietic expansion, hypercoagulability, and increased intestinal iron absorption. Most patients with thalassemia are born in resource-poor countries, but modern migration patterns have altered the epidemiology of this disease, and patients with thalassemia are now found in areas such as Europe and North America. Despite the major advancements and the important improvements in safety of blood products and the management of iron overload through iron chelation therapy, several challenges remain.

This issue on thalassemia provides a comprehensive overview of major aspects of thalassemia starting with the molecular basis and genetic modifiers of the disease, its epidemiology, and clinical classification. We then move into the currently available screening and diagnostic modalities in addition to the main pathophysiologic mechanisms involved in this debilitating disease. These pathophysiologic mechanisms lead to an array of clinical manifestations involving numerous organ systems, which are thoroughly discussed. Conventional therapeutic modalities in thalassemia, which include transfusion and iron-chelation therapy, in addition to novel emerging therapies are also described. The issue concludes by focusing on the importance of improving the quality of life of all thalassemia patients through early diagnosis and good clinical management. We also highlight the importance of MRI use in clinical practice as a diagnostic modality that can allow better tailoring of iron-chelation therapy.

With the burden of transfusional iron overload affecting many organ systems with a wide spectrum of complications, it is necessary to acknowledge the importance of iron chelation therapy as a cornerstone in the optimal management of patients with

Hematol Oncol Clin N Am 32 (2018) xv–xvi
https://doi.org/10.1016/j.hoc.2017.12.003
0889-8588/18/© 2017 Published by Elsevier Inc.
hemonc.theclinics.com

thalassemia. An improved understanding of the pathophysiology and disease burden in patients with thalassemia has helped optimize management and construct the roadmap for the development of novel therapeutics. With the availability of several new treatment modalities, there is a need for comparative and combination clinical trials to design the best management approach. Nevertheless, the complexity of the disease itself may always imply the need for individualized therapy, and offering the right treatment approach to the right patient. Moreover, the focus of the future will always be on how to improve the quality of life of all thalassemia patients and pave the way for their integration into the rest of society and their future success.

Ali T. Taher, MD, PhD, FRCP
Department of Internal Medicine
American University of Beirut Medical Center
PO Box: 11-0236, Cairo Street, Hamra, Raid E Solh
Beirut 1107 2020, Lebanon

E-mail address:
ataher@aub.edu.lb

The Evolving Spectrum of the Epidemiology of Thalassemia

David J. Weatherall, MD, FRCP, FRS

KEYWORDS

- Thalassemia • Global frequency • Malaria • Future frequency
- North/South partnerships • Future control

KEY POINTS

- The current frequency and global load of the thalassemias are discussed.
- An estimation of the frequency for the foreseeable future is discussed.
- The reasons for the high frequency of thalassemia are discussed.
- The development of partnerships between the poor and richer countries for the better control and management of thalassemia is discussed.

INTRODUCTION

The inherited disorders of hemoglobin (Hb), which include sickle cell anemia and its variants and the thalassemias, are the most common monogenic diseases.[1,2] There are 2 main forms of thalassemia, α and β thalassemia. The α globin genes, which are duplicated, are on chromosome 16. A deletion of one of them is termed α^+ thalassemia, whereas if both of the pair are deleted it is termed α^0 thalassemia. Point mutations of the α genes are much less common; only one, Hb Constant Spring, occurs at a very high frequency in some populations. The single β globin genes are on chromosome 11. The β thalassemias result from more than 200 different mutations, and deletions are much less common. There is a very common structural Hb variant, Hb E, which is synthesized at a reduced rate and behaves like a very mild form of β thalassemia. When inherited together with β thalassemia, the result is Hb E β thalassemia, which is one of the most common forms of severe thalassemia in many parts of Asia.

Disclosure Statement: The author has nothing to disclose. Work from the author, which is described in this article, was funded by the Medical Research Council, The Wellcome Trust, and the Anthony Cerami and Ann Dunne Foundation for World Health.
University of Oxford, Weatherall Institute of Molecular Medicine, John Radcliffe Hospital, Headington, Oxford OX3 9DS, UK
E-mail address: liz.rose@imm.ox.ac.uk

The α^+ thalassemias alone are not associated with any severe hematologic changes; their major importance is that when they are inherited together with different forms of β thalassemia, they tend to reduce the severity of the disease. Coinheritance of α^+ and α^0 thalassemia results in a condition of variable severity called Hb H disease, whereas homozygosity for α^0 thalassemia results in hydrops fetalis and death in utero or early after birth. The β thalassemias are divided into β thalassemia major or intermedia depending on the severity of the particular mutations or the inheritance of phenotypic modifiers. Hb E β thalassemia is associated with remarkable variability of the phenotype, ranging from severe β thalassemia major through various levels of β thalassemia intermedia.

Although much progress has been made toward the prevention and management of the thalassemias in the richer countries, this is not the case for many of the poorer countries of the tropical belt. In this article, current knowledge about the world distribution and frequency is discussed together with the reasons for the very high frequency of the different forms of thalassemia. Particular emphasis is placed on likely changes in the frequency of thalassemia in the future and the effects of changes in the environment and of population movement on the global health load caused by this disease. The danger of its continued neglect by international health agencies is also discussed.

WORLD DISTRIBUTION

An approximate distribution of the α and β thalassemias is shown in **Figs. 1** and **2**, respectively, and summarized in references.[1,2] The α^+ thalassemias, which spread at high frequency right across the tropical belt from sub-Saharan Africa through the Middle East, South Asia, and Southeast Asia, are undoubtedly the most common of all single

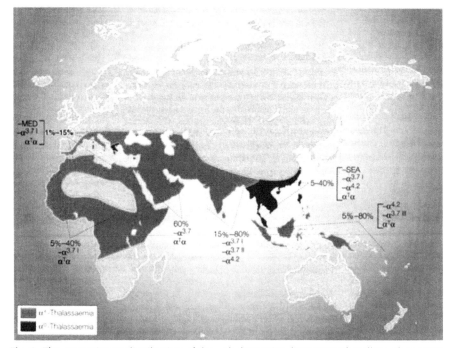

Fig. 1. The approximate distribution of the α thalassemias. (*From* Weatherall DJ. Phenotype-genotype relationships in monogenic disease: lessons from the thalassaemias. Nat Rev Genet 2001;2(4):245–55; with permission.)

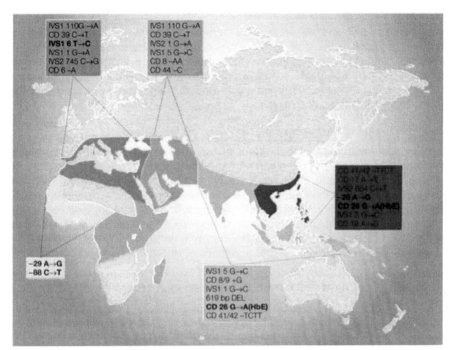

Fig. 2. The approximate distribution of the β thalassemias. (*From* Weatherall DJ. Phenotype-genotype relationships in monogenic disease: lessons from the thalassaemias. Nat Rev Genet 2001;2(4):245–55; with permission.)

gene disorders. Indeed, their heterozygote frequency in an area of North India and in parts of Southeast Asia seems to be going to fixation with frequency values of more than 75% of the population. The more severe form of α thalassemia, $α^0$ thalassemia, is less common and occurs at a high frequency in parts of the Mediterranean region and particularly in Southeast Asia. The β thalassemias are less common in sub-Saharan Africa and spread across the rest of the tropical belt at varying frequencies. Each of the high-frequency regions have their own particular β thalassemia mutations, a finding that suggests that in evolutionary terms they are fairly recent and have not had time to disperse equally across the tropical belt. Hb E is an extremely common structural Hb variant, occurring in South and Southeast Asia and reaching very high frequencies in parts of Southeast Asia, with 70% heterozygote rates in the Hb E triangle of North Thailand and Cambodia. Hence, Hb E β thalassemia is extremely common in this region.

The presence of thalassemia is not shown in the richer countries of Europe and the United States in **Figs. 1** and **2**. The disease occurs at various frequencies in all of these regions because of the increasing presence of immigrants from the tropical belt and will almost certainly increase in Europe as a reflection of the major increase of emigration from the Middle East at the current time.

DETERMINING THE ACCURATE FREQUENCY OF THE THALASSEMIAS IN DIFFERENT POPULATIONS
Standard Methods of Assessment

Particularly in the case of the poorer developing countries, it is extremely important for their governments to have reasonable knowledge regarding the cost of the prevention and management of thalassemia in their country. The usual method of determining its frequency in many countries has been to carry out the assessment in 1 or 2 centers and then extrapolate the data to the entire country. However, some years ago it was found that in Vanuatu and Vietnam there is remarkable variation in the frequency of the various forms of thalassemia over short geographic distances.[3,4] This finding was also observed later in Northwest India.[5] Until recently, there have been no other reports of micromapping of this type.

The Clinical Value of Micromapping

Recently, a study to determine the frequency of heterozygous carriers for common inherited Hb disorders has been carried out in more than 7500 adolescent children in 25 districts in Sri Lanka.[6] The results have disclosed a highly significant variation in frequency over very short geographic distances. As well as its evolutionary significance, this study had practical clinical implications. If this frequency calculation had been carried out by the usual approach of assessing it at 1 or 2 centers and then extrapolating the results to the entire population, it would have underestimated the births of β thalassemia major by 50% and those of HbE β thalassemia by 30%.

REASONS FOR THE HIGH FREQUENCY OF THE DIFFERENT FORMS OF THALASSEMIA
Malaria Resistance

Although many years of uncertainty have passed since J.B.S. Haldane[7] proposed that thalassemia was common in the Mediterranean region because of the heterozygote resistance against malaria, there is now extremely strong evidence that this is the case. This idea is particularly well described in the case of α thalassemia. For example, it has been shown in the northern coast of Papua New Guinea where the frequency of $α^+$ thalassemia is in excess of 70% of the population, there is strong resistance to malaria both by heterozygotes and homozygotes for this condition.[8] Similar findings have been described in the populations of Kenya.[9]

Early studies of the history of the distribution of malaria in the Mediterranean region showed that the highest frequencies were similar to those of β thalassemia,[2] and more recent studies have confirmed the relationship between this form of thalassemia and *Plasmodium falciparum* malaria.[1] Similarly, HbE has only reached high frequencies in populations with a high level of malaria.

These observations explain why the $α^+$ thalassemias are the most common single gene disorders in the world and why the β thalassemias have not reached such high frequencies. In the case of the $α^+$ thalassemias, there is malaria resistance to both heterozygotes and homozygotes; neither of these conditions have any clinical implications. In the case of the β thalassemias, there is heterozygote resistance; but homozygosity is associated with a severe clinical disorder. In this case, an equilibrium has been reached in which heterozygote resistance is counterbalanced by the clinical severity of homozygotes; hence, frequencies as high as the α thalassemias have not been attained.

The Mechanisms of Malaria Resistance

The increasing information about the mechanisms of resistance on the part of the thalassemias to malaria suggests that at least more than one mechanism is active in every form of the condition. In the case of the α thalassemias, it has been found that their red cells are deficient in complement receptor 1 (CR1). CR1 is a ligand for rosetting in which unaffected red cells adhere to parasite-infected cells, a phenomenon that is associated with severe forms of malaria due to vascular complications.[10] α thalassemia may also be involved in immunologic priming. Young children in parts of Asia have been found to be infected with the milder parasite *P vivax* in early life; because of cross immunity between *P vivax* and *P falciparum*, they may become more resistant to the latter and increase in number in later life.[11]

In the case of heterozygous β thalassemia, there is evidence of reduced invasion and growth of *P falciparum*; reduced adherence and rosetting, similar to that found in α thalassemia, has also been demonstrated. There are limited data on the relationship between Hb E and malaria. It only occurs at a high frequency in districts with a high frequency of malaria, and there have been reports of a reduced frequency in patients who are being admitted to the hospital with severe malaria.

It has been found that patients with Hb E β thalassemia are more prone to infection with *P vivax* malaria.[12] This finding is not surprising because this parasite is more prone to infect young red cell populations. This observation requires further study because *P vivax* can still be a quite serious form of malaria, and those with Hb E β thalassemia require a suitable form of prophylaxis.

Epistatic Interactions of Thalassemia and Hemoglobin Variants

Recent studies in Africa have shown that although individuals with α^+ thalassemia or sickle cell trait have significant protection against *P falciparum* malaria in those that inherit the genes for both variants, this protection is completely lost and they are as liable to have severe malaria as those who carry neither of these mutations.[13] These observations have recently explained the different frequencies of the sickle cell trait and different forms of thalassemia in the Mediterranean population and will undoubtedly be of great value for studying the population genetics of the thalassemias in the future.[14]

Malaria and the Different Frequencies of the Thalassemias Over Short Geographic Distances

As described earlier, a recent study[6] in Sri Lanka has demonstrated that there is a remarkable difference in frequency of the different forms of thalassemia over very short geographic distances. Because there are such excellent records of malaria frequency over the island over many years, first using spleen rates and later blood analysis, it has been possible to relate it to the frequency of thalassemia in different areas. The spleen is not palpable in thalassemia heterozygotes.[2]

It was found that there were significant differences in the frequency of malaria in different parts of the island. The frequency was closely related to the level of rainfall. It was significantly less in the southern parts of the island where rainfall is very heavy and where the lakes are being constantly refilled. The frequency of malaria in this environment compares with the much higher frequencies in the center and north of the island where the rainfall is limited and, hence, where sluggish pools of water provide a much more effective breeding ground for the mosquitoes. It was found that different frequencies of malaria in the island were significantly related to the varying frequency of different levels of thalassemia over short distances (**Fig. 3**). Although there are limited data for the dispersal and flight range of vectors, such data as there are suggest that the most common vector for *P falciparum*, *Anopheles culicifacies*, can probably travel only 1 to 2 km. This limited dispersal distance could also be a factor in the different frequency of the Hb variants over short distances. The latter may also relate to altitude; malarial transmission is gradually reduced to zero with increasing altitude. In the north coast of Papua New Guinea, the heterozygote frequency of α thalassemia exceeds 70% of the population, yet careful studies of the closely related mountains reveal no cases of α thalassemia at all.[15]

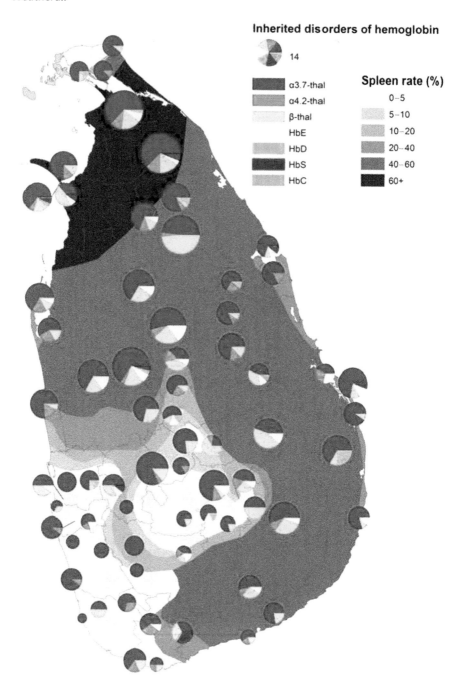

Fig. 3. The distribution of inherited disorders of Hb among more than 7000 adolescent children studied in 69 schools across Sri Lanka. Pie charts are proportional to the number of individuals with an inherited disorder of Hb. The boundaries of the 25 districts and the spleen rates from the 1921 to 1922 nationwide malaria survey (digitized from[26]) are shown in the background. thal, thalassemia. (*Adapted from* Premawardhena A, Allen A, Piel F, et al. The evolutionary and clinical implications of the uneven distribution of the frequency of the inherited hemoglobin variants over short geographic distances. Br J Haematol 2017;176(3):480; with permission.)

It seems, therefore, that the remarkable difference in frequency of the different forms of thalassemia over short geographic distances is very much related to the present or past frequency of malaria. Because the latter depends on different breeding requirements for the mosquito vectors, it seems likely that the same situation exists in many parts of the tropical belt.

Other Factors Involved in the Frequency of the Thalassemias

Given the extreme frequency of the thalassemias, it seems very likely that other factors must be involved as well as malaria. As mentioned earlier, there is some evidence that immune response plays a role, although more work is required in this area. Another important question relates to the frequency of consanguinity, particularly in the tropical belt. Unfortunately, there is very limited work being carried out to assess its frequency. Although consanguineous marriages are known to be an important factor for the frequency of all recessive genetic disorders and are thought to be common in many Asian countries very few studies of their frequency have been reported. In a recent family study in Sri Lanka,[6] marriage registrars asked a group of newly married couples to fill in a questionnaire regarding information about their relationship to their families and patterns of partner selection. Overall, the consanguinity rate was approximately 7% for the total island. Further studies of this type of families across the tropical belt is required.

Clinical Implications of the Studies of the Relative Distribution of the Thalassemias

It seems, therefore, that the remarkable difference in frequency of the different forms of thalassaemia over short geographic distances is largely, although not completely, related to the present or past frequency of malaria. Because the latter is strongly related to different environments and breeding requirements for the mosquito vectors, it seems likely that the same situation will exist in many parts of the tropical belt. These findings offer further evidence toward the importance of at least a limited form of micromapping as part of the management of thalassemia in the countries of the tropical belt. As discussed earlier, it provides a very much more accurate way of defining the genuine birth rate of the thalassemias, information that is essential for the governments of affected countries for assessing the financial aspects required for the prevention and management of the different forms of thalassemia. A more accurate assessment of the birth rate of babies with different forms of thalassemia, particularly in the poorer countries of the world, might also be helpful in persuading the international health agencies about their global importance.

THALASSEMIA FOR THE FORESEEABLE FUTURE

Major progress continues to be made toward the prevention and management of the thalassemias in the richer countries of the world. The application of genomics to the field looks very promising. Particularly because it is likely that progress in the latter work will still be some years before it reaches the clinic, especially in the poorer countries of the world, it is important that we try to assess the likely pattern of frequency of the thalassemias for the foreseeable future. Without this information, it will be difficult to persuade the international health agencies about the increasing finance required for the better control and management of these diseases in the poor countries of the world.

The Frequency of Thalassemia in the Foreseeable Future

Although some progress has been made toward the control of malaria, there is still widespread drug resistance; with the exception of protective bed nets, prophylactic approaches are still having limited success.[16,17] Even if malaria transmission is eradicated, it may take many generations, possibly up to 250 years, to have a significant effect on the frequency of the thalassemias.[18] Meanwhile, many of the poorer countries of the world may be going through an epidemiologic transition reflecting slow improvements in hygiene, nutrition, public health care, and other factors that are combining to reduce both neonatal and childhood mortality rates. It follows, therefore, that babies with severe forms of thalassemia who previously would have died undiagnosed early in life may be surviving to present for diagnosis and treatment. Hence, the global burden of disease caused by the thalassemias is likely to increase. Of course, much depends on how long it takes for the poorer countries to develop programs for the prevention and management of the different forms of thalassemia.

The Effects of Emigration

Most of the richer countries now have varying numbers of patients with thalassemia resulting from emigration from high-frequency tropical countries over many years. However, it seems that this phenomenon is increasing. A particularly good example is the United States.[19,20]

Once rare in North America, the thalassemias have become a major public health problem in some parts of the country. It is estimated that there is a 2000% increase in Asian and other at-risk populations emigrating to the United States in the last 3 decades. A screening program for the thalassemias in Californian newborn babies over 8 years demonstrated more than 500 with different forms of α thalassemia and 79 with different β thalassemias.

Given the many emigrants from the Middle East and related regions over the last few years, it seems likely that there will be a major increase in different forms of thalassemia throughout the richer countries of Europe.

Risks of Different Forms of Malaria for Some Types of Thalassemia

As mentioned earlier, not all forms of malaria offer resistance to carriers for different forms of thalassemia. It has been shown fairly recently that patients with Hb E β thalassemia are significantly more prone to infection with *P vivax* malaria.[11] Because this severe form of thalassemia is extremely common in many parts of Asia, its management in the future will depend on the prevention and treatment of this variety of malaria. Because the observations on the interaction between *P vivax* malaria and thalassemia have only been reported once from Sri Lanka,[12] further work is required to confirm the frequency of this interaction in countries like North India where HbE β thalassemia and *P vivax* malaria are both so common.

REQUIREMENTS FOR THE FUTURE

Considerable progress has been made toward the prevention and management of the different forms of thalassemia by centers in the richer countries; we are moving forward toward the successful applications of gene therapy toward a cure for many forms of thalassemia, although this will probably still take a long time. Regarding the very high frequencies of thalassemia over the tropical belt, some progress has been made; but, overall, the situation is still very unsatisfactory. In 2002, the World Health Organization (WHO) published a report entitled *Genomics and World Health*[21] that recommended the formation of what were called North/South and South/South partnerships as an approach to the control and management of common genetic diseases, such as the Hb disorders. These recommendations were later confirmed by the WHO Executive Board and at the 59th World Health Assembly. North/South indicates partnerships between centers in the rich countries with those in the poorer countries of the tropical belt, whereas South/South partnerships relate to those poorer countries in the tropical belt who have improved their management of thalassemia and other common genetic diseases sufficiently to help other countries in their vicinity where very little or no progress has been made. More recently, the inherited Hb disorders have been included in the current edition of the *Global Burden of Disease Study* and have been clearly defined as significant factors in the global burden of anemia.[22]

There seem to still be relatively small numbers of North/South partnerships even though they were encouraged by the WHO. An example of a partnership of this kind is that between the University of Oxford in the United Kingdom and the University of Toronto in Canada with Sri Lanka. This 20-year program has combined research into the many different forms of thalassemia in Sri Lanka together with capacity building, that is, training medical staff in the prevention and management of the severe forms of thalassemia in their country together with raising funds to build a new national thalassemia treatment center and various research laboratories for the study of these diseases.[23,24] This program has required sending some of the medical staff from Sri Lanka to Oxford for training purposes and journeys to Sri Lanka for the teaching staff from Oxford and Toronto at least four times per year. The program has developed quite well over the years and has had the approval of the Sri Lankan government.

There has been some progress toward the concept of the South/South partnerships. Several meetings have been arranged, mainly in Thailand, which are attended by representatives from many of the countries in South and Southeast Asia. Major attention has been focused on the current state of progress and available facilities for the management of the thalassemias. Also, particularly the teams in Thailand have been able to develop thalassemia programs with nearby countries where no such programs had previously existed.

Although it is still early days, it does seem as though programs of this type can be extremely valuable for the future management of the thalassemias, particularly in countries where little progress has hitherto been made.

One of the main problems with this approach is lack of financial support. The major international funding bodies, with a few exceptions, and the WHO and related international agencies do not seem to think that the thalassemias are worth supporting in comparison with infectious disease, cancer, or other common noninfectious disorders. It is vital, therefore, that they appreciate the global importance of the thalassemias. It is also important to modify the activities of some of the hematology societies of the richer countries. Over recent years, they have tended to have increasingly neglected the red cell in general and the Hb disorders in particular. This observation is mirrored by the relative lack of published work in their journals in this field with its major focus on other aspects of hematology.

It is also quite likely that some of the current problems of the thalassemia field relate to the quality of teaching of some aspects of hematology and tropical medicine, particularly in the richer countries of the world.[25] The further development of the North/South concept will certainly require improvement in the teaching of these subjects and of encouraging medical students and young trainees in hematology throughout the richer world to spend at least short periods of their training in the tropics to gain some experience of global diseases like the thalassemias.

SUMMARY

The thalassemias and other inherited disorders of Hb are likely to remain a serious global health problem for the foreseeable future. Currently, they are most frequent in the tropical belt; an assessment of their true frequency and the likely cost of management for the governments of these countries will require a form of micromapping. Over recent years, there has been major progress toward better prevention and management of the thalassemias in richer countries; it is likely that, using the tools of molecular genetics, they will eventually be completely curable, although this is probably a long time in the future. To facilitate the global management of these diseases, it will require North/South partnerships between rich and poor countries and related activities so that they can be better controlled over the tropical belt in the future. Unfortunately, the thalassemias are going through a phase of neglected diseases by the WHO, related international health bodies, and also by the hematology societies in the richer countries and, hence, the hematologic literature. With a few exceptions, they are also neglected by the fundraising bodies of the richer countries. It is vital that the current status of the thalassemias as increasingly common and severe global disorders is brought to the attention of the medical world as a whole.

ACKNOWLEDGMENTS

The author acknowledges the editors of *Nature Genetics* for allowing him to publish **Figs. 1** and **2**, which had been previously published in that journal and the editors of the *British Journal of Haematology* for allowing him to republish **Fig. 3**, which he had previously published in that journal. The article could not have been produced without the help of Liz Rose of the University of Oxford.

REFERENCES

1. Williams TN, Weatherall DJ. World distribution, population genetics, and health burden of the hemoglobinopathies. In: Weatherall DJ, Schechter AN, Nathan DG, editors. Cold spring harbor perspectives in medicine, vol. 2. New York: Cold Spring Harbor; 2012. p. a011692.
2. Weatherall DJ, Clegg JB. The thalassaemia syndromes. 4th edition. Oxford, United Kingdom: Blackwell Science; 2001.
3. Bowden DK, Hill AV, Higgs DR, et al. The relative roles of genetic factors, dietary deficiency and infection in anaemia in Vanuatu, Southwest Pacific. Lancet 1985; 2(8463):1025–8.
4. O'Riordan S, Hien TT, Miles K, et al. Large scale screening for haemoglobin disorders in southern Vietnam: implications for avoidance and management. Br J Haemat 2010;150(3):359–64.
5. Colah R, Gorakshakar A, Phanasgaonkar S, et al. Epidemiology of beta-thalassaemia in Western India: mapping the frequencies and mutations in sub-regions of Maharashtra and Gujarat. Br J Haemat 2010;149(5):739–47.
6. Premawardhena A, Allen A, Piel F, et al. The evolutionary and clinical implications of the uneven distribution of the frequency of the inherited haemoglobin variants over short geographical distances. Br J Haematol 2017;176(3):475–84.
7. Haldane JBS. The rate of mutation of human genes. Proc VIII Int Cong Genet Hereditas 1949;35:267–73.
8. Allen SJ, O'Donnell A, Alexander NDE, et al. a^+-thalassemia protects children against disease due to malaria and other infections. Proc Natl Acad Sci U S A 1997;94:14736–41.
9. Williams TN, Wambua S, Uyoga S, et al. Both heterozygous and homozygous alpha+ thalassemias protect against severe and fatal Plasmodium falciparum malaria on the coast of Kenya. Blood 2005;106(1):368–71.

10. Cockburn IA, Mackinnon MJ, O'Donnell A, et al. A human complement receptor 1 polymorphism that reduces Plasmodium falciparum rosetting confers protection against severe malaria. Proc Natl Acad Sci U S A 2004;101(1):272–7.
11. Williams TN, Maitland K, Bennett S, et al. High incidence of malaria in a-thalassaemic children. Nature 1996;383:522–5.
12. O'Donnell A, Premawardhena A, Arambepola M, et al. Interaction of malaria with a common form of severe thalassemia in an Asian population. Proc Natl Acad Sci U S A 2009;106:18716–21.
13. Williams TN, Mwangi TW, Wambua S, et al. Negative epistasis between the malaria-protective effects of alpha+-thalassemia and the sickle cell trait. Nat Genet 2005;37(11):1253–7.
14. Penman BS, Pybus OG, Weatherall DJ, et al. Epistatic interactions between genetic disorders of hemoglobin can explain why the sickle-cell gene is uncommon in the Mediterranean. Proc Natl Acad Sci U S A 2009;106(50):21242–6.
15. Flint J, Hill AVS, Bowden DK, et al. High frequencies of a thalassaemia are the result of natural selection by malaria. Nature 1986;321:744–9.
16. Greenwood BM, Bojang K, Whitty CJ, et al. Malaria. Lancet 2005;365(9469): 1487–98.
17. Greenwood B. New tools for malaria control - using them wisely. J Infect 2017; 74(Suppl 1):S23–6.
18. Cavalli-Sforza LL, Bodmer WF. The genetics of human populations. San Francisco (CA): USA: W.H. Freeman and Company; 1979. p. 776–7.
19. Vichinsky EP. Changing patterns of thalassemia worldwide. Ann N Y Acad Sci 2005;1054:18–24.
20. Vichinsky EP, MacKlin EA, Waye JS, et al. Changes in the epidemiology of thalassemia in North America: a new minority disease. Pediatr 2005;116(6):e818–25.
21. Weatherall DJ, Brock D, Chee HL. Genomics and world health. Geneva, Switzerland: World Health Organization; 2002.
22. GBD 2015 DALYs and HALE Collaborators. Global, regional, and national disability-adjusted life-years (DALYs) for 315 diseases and injuries and healthy life expectancy (HALE), 1990-2015: a systematic analysis for the global burden of disease study 2015. Lancet 2016;388(10053):1603–58.
23. de Silva S, Fisher CA, Premawardhena A, et al. Thalassaemia in Sri Lanka: implications for the future health burden of Asian populations. Sri Lanka thalassaemia study group. Lancet 2000;355(9206):786–91.
24. Olivieri NF, Thayalsuthan V, O'Donnell A, et al. Emerging insights in the management of hemoglobin E beta thalassemia. Ann N Y Acad Sci 2010;1202:155–7.
25. Hay D, Hatton CS, Weatherall DJ. The future of academic haematology. Br J Haematol 2017;176(5):721–7.
26. Gill CA. Some points in the epidemiology of malaria arising out of the study of the malaria epidemic in Ceylon in 1934-5. Trans Roy Soc Trop Med Hyg 1936;29(5): 427–80.

Molecular Basis and Genetic Modifiers of Thalassemia

Sachith Mettananda, MBBS, MD, DPhil[a,b], Douglas R. Higgs, FMedSci, FRS[a,c],*

KEYWORDS

- Thalassemia • Globin genes • Hemoglobin • Gene regulation • Phenotype-genotype
- Genetic modifiers • α-Globin

KEY POINTS

- Defective synthesis of α-globin caused by more than 120 deletional and nondeletional mutations in the α-globin genes and their regulatory elements are known to cause α-thalassemia.
- More than 250 mutations in and around the β-globin gene that affect multiple stages of gene expression cause β-thalassemia.
- In β-thalassemia, because of the absence of β-globin, unpaired α-globin chains precipitate in red blood cells and their precursors to cause hemolysis and ineffective erythropoiesis, leading to anemia.
- The clinical severity of β-thalassemia may be ameliorated via polymorphisms in the *Xmn1-HBG2* region, the *HBS1L-MYB* intergenic region, the *BCL11A* enhancer, and mutations in *KLF1*, all of which upregulate γ-globin.
- The clinical severity of β-thalassemia may also be ameliorated by coinheritance of α-thalassemia, which reduces the excess α-globin chains.

INTRODUCTION

Thalassemia is one of the most common monogenic disorders in the world.[1] It is estimated that nearly 70,000 children with various forms of thalassemia are born each year.[2] Thalassemia is particularly common in the traditional thalassemia belt, which extends from the Mediterranean region through sub-Saharan Africa and the Middle East to South and Southeast Asia.[3] The high prevalence of thalassemia

Conflicts of interest: Authors declare no conflicts of interest.
Disclosure statement: None of the authors have conflicting financial interests.
[a] Molecular Hematology Unit, Medical Research Council (MRC), Weatherall Institute of Molecular Medicine, University of Oxford, John Radcliffe Hospital, Headington, Oxford OX3 9DS, UK; [b] Department of Paediatrics, Faculty of Medicine, University of Kelaniya, Thalagolla Road, Ragama 11010, Sri Lanka; [c] National Institute for Health Research, Oxford Biomedical Research Centre, Blood Theme, Oxford University Hospitals, Headington, Oxford OX3 9DU, UK
* Corresponding author.
E-mail address: doug.higgs@imm.ox.ac.uk

Hematol Oncol Clin N Am 32 (2018) 177–191
https://doi.org/10.1016/j.hoc.2017.11.003
0889-8588/18/© 2017 Elsevier Inc. All rights reserved.

hemonc.theclinics.com

in these regions has been attributed to the selective advantage of carriers of thalassemia mutations against *Plasmodium falciparum* malaria, because prevalence of both conditions shows considerable overlap.[4] However, because of population migration, thalassemia has become an important health problem in most developed countries including the United Kingdom, Canada, and the United States.[5]

Most commonly the molecular defects that cause thalassemia lie within the human globin genes, which encode for α- and β-globin polypeptide chains of hemoglobin. Two α- and two β-globin chains, each conjugated with a heme moiety that is an iron-containing porphyrin derivative, form adult hemoglobin (hemoglobin A [HbA]), the specialized oxygen carrier molecule in human red blood cells (RBC).[6] Molecular defects in thalassemia lead to reduced or absent production of one of the globin chains with relative excess of the other; reduced or absent production of β-globin chains results in β-thalassemia, whereas defective synthesis of α-globin leads to α-thalassemia.

HUMAN α- AND β-GLOBIN GENE LOCI

The globin genes are possibly the most extensively studied and characterized gene loci in the human genome. The α- and β-globin gene loci are located in two different chromosomes. The human α-globin gene cluster is located on the short arm of chromosome 16 (16p13.3) close ($\sim$150 kilobase [kb]) to the telomere. In this 135-kb segment, globin genes are arranged in the order in which they are expressed during development: telomere-ζ-μ-α_2-α_1-centromere (**Fig. 1**).[7] Similarly, several β-like globin genes are located in the order of their expression during development

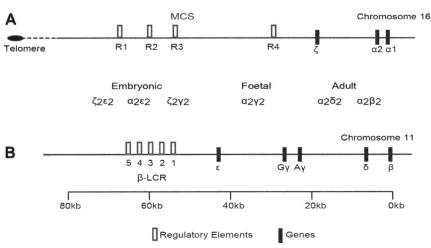

Fig. 1. Schematic diagram of α- and β-globin gene clusters and the types of hemoglobin produced at each developmental stage. Genes are arranged along the chromosome in the order in which they are expressed during development: (*A*) in the α-cluster ζ (embryonic) and α (embryonic, fetal, and adult); (*B*) in the β-cluster ϵ (embryonic), γ (fetal), and δ and β (adult). The four upstream regulatory elements of the α-locus are known as multispecies conserved sequences (MCS-) R1 to R4, whereas the five regulatory elements of the β-locus are collectively referred to as β-locus control region (β-LCR). (*Modified from* Mettananda S, Gibbons RJ, Higgs DR. alpha-Globin as a molecular target in the treatment of beta-thalassemia. Blood 2015;125(24):3695; with permission.)

in the human β-globin gene locus in chromosome 11 (11p). The arrangement of genes in this locus is, telomere-ε-^{G}γ-^{A}γ-δ-β-centromere.[8]

GLOBIN GENE EXPRESSION AND HEMOGLOBIN PRODUCTION DURING DEVELOPMENT

Throughout embryonic and fetal development, the site of erythropoiesis and hemoglobin production changes. During the early embryonic period, a transient cohort of embryonic RBCs originates in the blood islands of the yolk sac. Definitive hematopoietic stem cells (HSCs) then emerge from the ventral wall of the dorsal aorta, which migrate to the fetal liver midway in the first trimester. Around the time of birth, HSCs migrate to the bone marrow, which is the principal site of erythropoiesis for the rest of the life. Changes in the site of erythropoiesis are also associated with variations in the types of hemoglobin produced. Hemoglobin Gower-I ($\zeta_2\varepsilon_2$), hemoglobin Gower-II ($\alpha_2\varepsilon_2$), and hemoglobin Portland ($\zeta_2\gamma_2$) are produced during the embryonic stages, which are then switched, first, to hemoglobin F (HbF, $\alpha_2\gamma_2$) during the fetal stage and subsequently to HbA ($\alpha_2\beta_2$) and A₂ (HbA₂, $\alpha_2\delta_2$) after birth[9] (see **Fig. 1**).

These changes are the result of well-coordinated developmental-stage-specific expression of globin genes in α- and β-globin loci. At the α-globin locus, ζ- and α-globin are expressed during the embryonic period. However, the ζ-globin genes are silenced during fetal and postnatal stages. In the β-globin locus, ε- and γ-globin are expressed during embryonic and fetal periods, respectively, and then γ-globin is switched to β-globin (and to lesser extent δ-globin) after birth (**Fig. 2**).[1]

SYNTHESIS OF HEMOGLOBIN DURING ERYTHROPOIESIS

In humans, after birth, the bone marrow remains the predominant site of erythropoiesis throughout life. During erythropoiesis, multipotent HSCs that reside in the bone marrow differentiate through various progenitor stages to the earliest morphologically identifiable erythroid precursors: proerythroblasts. Thereafter, during terminal

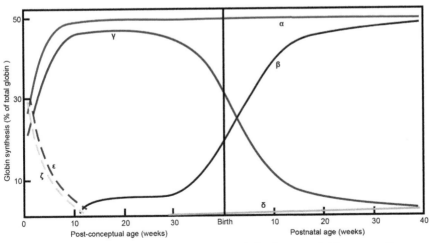

Fig. 2. Developmental-stage-specific expression of the human globin genes. ζ-, α- and ε-globin are the first globin genes to be expressed during embryonic erythropoiesis. During definitive erythropoiesis the ζ-globin genes are silenced and the γ-globin genes are switched on in the fetal stage. A second switch from γ-to β-globin occurs during the first few months after birth.

differentiation, proerythroblasts become progressively smaller and undergo nuclear condensation to differentiate into basophilic, polychromatophilic, and orthochromatic erythroblasts, which then enucleate to form reticulocytes and mature RBC.[10] Hemoglobin is first observed in pro- or basophilic erythroblasts, which is then produced exponentially during terminal differentiation to constitute 97% of the dry weight of mature RBC.[11] The synthesis of globin RNA is controlled through a complex interplay between transcriptional and epigenetic programs. Subsequently, there are many additional levels of post-transcriptional regulation involving RNA processing; translational control; and mechanisms to stabilize, chaperone, and degrade proteins.

REGULATION OF GLOBIN GENE EXPRESSION AND SWITCHING

Understanding the cellular mechanisms that govern expression of the α- and β-globin genes is essential to understand the molecular basis of thalassemia. Recent work by many research groups uncovering the mechanisms that regulate the expression of globin genes has provided useful insights into how α- and β-globin genes are switched on and off during erythropoiesis.

Expression of α-globin is controlled by four distant cis-acting regulatory elements (enhancers) situated 10 kb to 48 kb upstream of the genes (see Fig. 1).[7] These enhancers with conserved sequences underlying sites of DNase I hypersensitivity are collectively referred to as multispecies conserved sequences (MCS)-R1-4. Of these, through a variety of experiments including transient transfections, transgenic experiments, and naturally occurring human mutations, it has been shown that MCS-R2 (previously known as HS-40) is the strongest regulatory element enhancing the expression of α-globin.[12] During erythroid differentiation, expression of the human α-globin genes is initiated by demethylation of repressive chromatin signatures (H3K27me3) associated with the gene promoters.[13] As erythroid differentiation proceeds, erythroid transcription factors that include GATA-binding factor 1 (GATA1), nuclear factor-erythroid 2 (NF-E2), stem cell leukemia pentameric complex, and Kruppel-like factor 1 (KLF1) are recruited to the enhancers.[14] During this process, which initiates transcription of α-globin, physical interactions between enhancers and promoters are believed to occur through long-range, intrachromosomal interactions.[15]

As with α-globin, a cluster of distant cis-acting regulatory elements has also been identified at the β-globin locus. Five such enhancers that similarly underlie sites of DNase I hypersensitivity have been characterized and are collectively referred to as the locus control region (LCR).[16] In erythroid cells, the β-globin locus also establishes three-dimensional chromosomal interaction conformations to bring the LCR into proximity with gene promoters to initiate transcription.[17] This is associated with an active chromatin signature (H3K4me3 and H3K27me3) and recruitment of key erythroid transcription factors, which include LIM domain-binding protein 1 (LDB1), GATA1, Friend of GATA 1 (FOG1), KLF1, NF-E2, and stem cell leukemia (SCL) factor at the β-globin promoter.[18]

Another important consideration that has clinical and therapeutic implications is the understanding of factors that control the switch from γ- to β-globin expression and repression of γ-globin in adult human erythroid cells. Although the exact mechanisms are unclear, several transcription factors and proteins that suppress γ-globin have been identified. The B-cell lymphoma/leukemia 11A (BCL11A) protein is one of the best characterized transcriptional repressors of γ-globin, which is believed to coordinate the hemoglobin switch via multiprotein complexes recruited to the β-globin gene cluster. These complexes include erythroid transcription factors, GATA1 and FOG1; the Sex Determining Region Y-Box (SOX6); and Nucleosome remodeling deacetylase

(NuRD) complex.[19,20] The Direct repeat erythroid-definitive (DRED) complex, which is a tetrameric complex composed of Testosterone receptor (TR) 2 and TR4, DNA methyltransferase 1 (DNMT1), and lysine-specific histone demethylase 1 (LSD1) are also thought to repress γ-globin by binding to the direct repeat elements of the γ-globin promoter.[21] This complex also associates with additional corepressors that include NuRD and CoREST complexes that contain histone deacetylase 1 and 2.[22]

The erythroid transcription factor KLF1 is believed to mediate globin switching by directly activating β-globin and promoting expression of the γ-globin silencer BCL11A.[23,24] Moreover, hematopoietic transcription factor MYB is believed to repress γ-globin transcription indirectly by activating TR2/TR4 and KLF1.[21] More recently, another potent silencer known as leukemia/lymphoma-related factor (LRF) was identified.[25] BCL11A and LRF proteins interact with components of the NuRD complex, which serves a critical role in globin gene repression and may represent a common pathway through which silencers of γ-globin expression act.[8]

MOLECULAR DEFECTS DOWN-REGULATING α-GLOBIN EXPRESSION CAUSING α-THALASSEMIA

Defective synthesis of α-globin caused by mutations involving α-globin genes causes α-thalassemia. More than 120 such mutations have been reported (**Table 1**; for a comprehensive catalog see http://globin.cse.psu.edu/). Most of the mutations that give rise to α-thalassemia are deletions involving variable lengths of the α-globin locus. Normal individuals have four copies of the α-globin gene, two on each chromosome (denoted as 'αα/αα'), and a deletion can either remove one or both genes from a chromosome. Deletions that involve both α-globin genes (denoted as '--') and completely abolish the expression from a single chromosome are known as α^0-thalassemia, whereas deletions that remove one gene (denoted as '-α' or 'α-') and partially downregulate expression from a chromosome are known as α^+-thalassemia.[26] Rarely, deletions of the upstream enhancer elements (denoted as $[\alpha\alpha]^T$) cause α-thalassemia despite having normal α-globin genes. These deletions vary in length and remove variable combinations of enhancer elements; however, all such deletions reported to date remove the critical enhancer, MCS-R2.[27] Furthermore, very short deletions confined to the MCS-R2 enhancer leaving all other enhancers and genes intact are also known to cause α-thalassemia.[28–31]

Nondeletional mutations causing α-thalassemia are rare and include point mutations and oligonucleotide insertions or deletions. Although these mutations are confined to a single α-globin gene in a particular chromosome, the degree of α-globin reduction seen in nondeletional α^+-thalassemia is usually greater than α^+-thalassemia

Table 1
α-Thalassemia mutations

Type of Mutation	Genotype	Examples
Deletions		
Deletions that remove a single α-globin gene in a chromosome	-α or α-	$\alpha^{-3.7}$, $-\alpha^{4.2}$
Deletions that remove both α-globin genes in a single chromosome	--	$--^{MED\ I}$, $--^{SEA}$, $--^{THAI}$, $--^{FIL}$
Deletions that remove upstream regulatory elements	$(\alpha\alpha)^T$	$(\alpha\alpha)^{RA}$, $(\alpha\alpha)^{ALT}$, $(\alpha\alpha)^{JX}$
Nondeletional mutations	$\alpha^T\alpha$ or $\alpha\alpha^T$	$\alpha^{IVSI(-5nt)}\alpha$, $\alpha^{Constant\ Spring}\alpha$

caused by deletions and they often severely downregulate α-globin expression. This may be explained, at least partly, by the lack of any compensatory increase in expression of the remaining functional gene when the other is inactivated by a point mutation. Some severe forms of nondeletional α^+-thalassemia are caused by highly unstable α-globin variants produced by point mutations. Nondeletional α-thalassemia mutations may also effect various stages of gene expression including mRNA processing, mRNA translation, and protein stability.[32] An extremely rare *trans* acting mutation in the *ATRX* gene located in the X chromosome is also known to cause α-thalassemia associated with developmental delay, facial dysmorphism, and genital abnormalities in males (ATRX syndrome).[33] Although the exact mechanisms are yet unclear ATRX is believed to act as a chromatin remodeling protein facilitating expression of the α-globin.[34]

GENOTYPE-PHENOTYPE CORRELATION OF α-THALASSEMIA

The clinical severity of α-thalassemia depends on the number of functional α-globin genes (**Table 2**). Two (either caused by heterozygous α^0-thalassemia, --/$\alpha\alpha$, or homozygous α^+-thalassemia, -α/-α) or three (heterozygous α^+-thalassemia, -α/$\alpha\alpha$) functional α-globin genes (out of four, $\alpha\alpha$/$\alpha\alpha$) result in asymptomatic microcytic anemia and is referred to as α-thalassemia trait: the presence of three functional α-globin genes produces very mild hematologic changes (silent α-thalassemia). The inheritance of a single functional α-globin gene leads to hemoglobin H disease (--/-α), which usually produces the phenotype of nontransfusion-dependent thalassemia, whereas complete absence of functional α-globin genes (caused by homozygous α^0-thalassemia deleting all four genes, --/--) leads to lethal form of perinatal anemia called the hemoglobin Bart hydrops fetalis syndrome.[35]

The clinical outcome of nondeletional mutations of the α-globin gene and deletions removing the α-globin enhancers are complex. Nondeletional mutations, although confined to a single α-globin gene, result in greater reduction in α-globin expression than α^+-thalassemia caused by deletions.[32] Deletions of enhancers (MCS-R2, in particular) profoundly reduce expression of both α-globin genes in *cis*, but does not completely abolish it. This was evident from two patients: one who harbors a rare homozygous deletion of MCS-R2[28]; and another who is a compound heterozygote for a deletion of MCS-R2 and α^0-thalassemia,[36] presenting with clinical phenotype of hemoglobin H disease rather than hemoglobin Bart hydrops fetalis syndrome. However, removal of both MCS-R1 and MCS-R2 seems to severely reduce (>90%) α-globin expression.

Table 2
Genotype-phenotype correlation of α-thalassemia

Number of Functional α-Globin Genes	Clinical Phenotype	α-Globin Genotypes
4	Normal	$\alpha\alpha$/$\alpha\alpha$
3	α-Thalassemia trait (silent α-thalassemia)	- α/$\alpha\alpha$
2	α-Thalassemia trait	- α/- α, --/$\alpha\alpha$, $(\alpha\alpha)^T$/$\alpha\alpha$, $\alpha^T\alpha$/$\alpha\alpha$
1	Hemoglobin H disease	--/-α, $(\alpha\alpha)^T$/- α, $\alpha^T\alpha$/- α, $\alpha^T\alpha$/ $\alpha^T\alpha$, $(\alpha\alpha)^T$/$(\alpha\alpha)^T$
0	Hemoglobin Bart hydrops fetalis	--/--, α^T-/--

MOLECULAR DEFECTS CAUSING β-THALASSEMIA

β-Thalassemia is one of the most clinically significant forms of hemoglobinopathy in the world. More than 250 recessive mutations causing β-thalassemia have been identified to date (a complete updated list is available at http://globin.cse.psu. edu/hbvar/). In contrast to α-thalassemia, most of the mutations causing β-thalassemia are point mutations rather than large deletions. These include single-nucleotide substitutions and deletions and insertions of single nucleotides or oligonucleotides either in the gene or flanking regions. These mutations decrease the output of β-globin gene by affecting various stages of gene expression from gene transcription, through mRNA processing, to mRNA translation and protein stability **(Table 3)**.[37]

β-Thalassemia mutations are categorized into β^0-, β^+-, and β^{++}-thalassemia depending on the level of expression from the mutated globin gene and the extent to which β-chain output is reduced. Mutations that completely abolish the production of β-globin are known as β^0-thalassemia (severe), which include mutations of the initiation codon, nonsense mutations, frameshifts, and mutations involving RNA splicing and processing. In contrast, β^+-thalassemia alleles are characterized by mild to moderate reduction in β-chains caused by mutations in the promoter area (either the CACCC or TATA box), the polyadenylation signal, and the 5′ or 3′ untranslated region or splicing abnormalities. Furthermore, β^{++}-thalassemia alleles are caused by mutations in the promoter or 5′untranslated region of mRNA and they have only subtle effects on the production of β-globin chains.[38]

Table 3 β-Thalassemia mutations		
Type of Mutation	**Severity Type**	**Examples**
Point mutations		
Transcriptional mutations		
Promoter regulatory elements	β^+ or β^{++}	– 101 (C > T)
5′ UTR	β^+ or β^{++}	CAP +1 (A > C)
Mutations involving RNA processing		
Splice junction	β^0	IVS1-1 (G > T)
Consensus splice sites	β^0 or β^+	IVS1-5 (G > C)
Cryptic splice sites	β^0 or β^+	IVS1–110 (G > A), CD26 (GAG > AAG)
RNA cleavage - Poly A signal	β^+ or β^{++}	AATAAA > AATGAA
Others in 3′ UTR	β^{++}	Term CD +6, C > G
Mutations involving RNA translation		
Initiation codon	β^0	ATG > ATA
Nonsense codons	β^0	CD39 (CAG > TAG), CD17 (AAG > TAG)
Frameshift	β^0	CD41/42 (–TTCT)
Deletions		
Deletions confined to β-globin gene	β^0	– 619 bp deletion
Deletions extending to other genes	β^0	$(\epsilon\gamma\delta\beta)^0$-thalassemia, $(\delta\beta)^0$-thalassemia
Deletions of the LCR	β^0	

Abbreviation: UTR, untranslated region.

Adapted from Thein SL. Molecular basis of beta thalassemia and potential therapeutic targets. Blood Cells Mol Dis 2017:[pii:S1079-9796(17)30210-3]; with permission.

The worldwide distribution of different mutations correlates with regional and ethnic distributions. In the Mediterranean and Middle East, IVS1–110 (G > A) and CD39 (CAG > TAG) are reported as common mutations. IVS1-5 (G > C) is commonly found in South Asia, whereas CD41/42 (–TTCT) mutation is the commonest in Southeast Asia.[39] Of all β-thalassemia mutations, CD26 (GAG > AAG), which is particularly common in South and Southeast Asia, requires a special mention. This mutation is caused by the substitution of guanine by adenine at codon 26, which results in structurally abnormal hemoglobin E consisting of $\alpha_2\beta^E_2$ globin chains.[40] However, the abnormal DNA sequence also activates a cryptic splice site, which leads to a 16-nucleotide deletion of the 3′ end of exon-1, creating a stop codon to causes aberrant splicing (represents 5%–8% of total mRNA) and decreased rate of splicing (3- to 5-fold reduction)[41] to reduce the amount of correctly spliced β^E-globin mRNA, thus giving rise to underproduction of this mRNA and the phenotype of β-thalassemia.[41]

Some other β-globin chain variants, although synthesized in normal amounts, are extremely unstable and are not capable of forming stable hemoglobin tetramers. These mutations cause functional deficiency of β-globin and result in the phenotype of β-thalassemia even when present in a single copy. Such mutations are referred to as dominantly inherited β-thalassemia.[42]

Less commonly, deletions involving the β-globin gene may cause β-thalassemia. The most common form is a 619-bp deletion that removes only the β-globin gene; however, several other deletions extend beyond β-globin and involve the δ-, γ-, and ε-globin genes.[43] Vary rarely, similar to the α-locus, deletions of the upstream LCR results in β-thalassemia, despite the linked β-globin genes being normal. These deletions have only been found in the heterozygous state; none has been reported in the homozygous state, presumably because those embryos do not survive beyond early gestation due to the absence of expression of the embryonic (ε-globin) and fetal (γ-globin) β-like globin chains.[38]

In rare instances, β-thalassemia defects do not lie in the β-globin locus but in different chromosomes. One of these is linked to a mutation in the gene encoding the general transcription factor TFIIH resulting in β-thalassemia associated with xeroderma pigmentosum and tricothiodystrophy.[44] Some mutations in the erythroid-specific transcription factor GATA-1 on the X chromosome have also been reported to cause β-thalassemia in association with thrombocytopenia.[45] Furthermore, class 2 or 3 mutations in *KLF1* result in dysregulation of globin gene synthesis and increased levels of HbF (hereditary persistence of HbF) and HbA_2 mimicking β-thalassemia.[46]

MOLECULAR AND CELLULAR PATHOLOGY OF β-THALASSEMIA

During every stage of normal erythropoiesis, production of α-like and β-like globin chains is closely balanced to prevent an accumulation of free globin chains, which damage RBCs. In patients with β-thalassemia, there is absent or reduced production of β-globin; however, the production of α-globin continues normally leading to an excess of α-globin within RBCs. This unbalanced production of α-globin chains is the main pathophysiologic mechanism causing anemia in β-thalassemia.[47]

In normal RBCs, the damaging effects of small amounts of free α-globin chains are counteracted by the erythroid-specific molecular chaperone, α-hemoglobin stabilizing protein, which binds to and stabilizes free α-chains by promoting protein folding and resistance to protease digestion.[48] Excess α-globin chains are destroyed by proteolysis. In patients with β-thalassemia, the levels of free α-globin chains are far in excess of the capacity of α-hemoglobin stabilizing protein to chaperone and the proteolytic system to remove unpaired α-globin and the resulting unstable, free α-chains undergo auto-oxidation. This process leads to formation of α-globin monomers, which contain oxidized ferric iron (α-hemichromes) and reactive oxygen species (ROS), which trigger a cascade of events leading to hemolysis and ineffective erythropoiesis (**Fig. 3**).[49]

The α-globin monomers are degraded via several pathways including a ubiquitin-dependent proteolytic pathway, an autophagy pathway, and a nonenzymatic pathway triggered by ROS that results in release of hemin (heme containing oxidized ferric iron) and free iron, which then lodges in the cell membrane.[47,50] In this unstable conformation, both the heme group and iron may participate in redox reactions leading to further generation of ROS, which damage cellular proteins, lipids, and nucleic acids. ROS-induced alterations in membrane deformability and stability through partial oxidation of protein band 4.1 and defective assembly of spectrin-actin-band 4.1 membrane skeleton complex are the main mechanisms of hemolysis in β-thalassemia.[51] In addition, oxidant injury leads to clustering of band 3, which in turn produces a neoantigen that binds to IgG and complement, thereby facilitating removal by macrophages.[52]

Ineffective erythropoiesis, however, is not explained by membrane damage and seems to be caused by enhanced apoptosis.[53] Apoptosis in β-thalassemia RBC is probably mediated through Fas cell surface death receptor (FAS) and FAS-ligand pathway, which is triggered by high levels of ROS. In addition, overexpression of

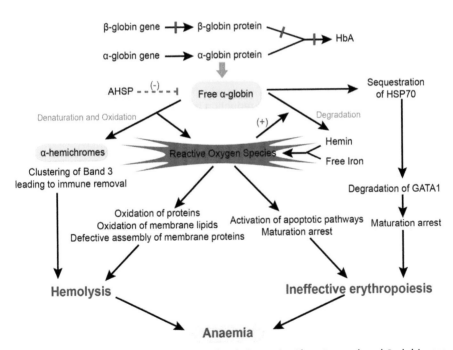

Fig. 3. Molecular and cellular pathology of β-thalassemia. Absent or reduced β-globin production leads to an unbalanced excess of α-globin chains, which then triggers a cascade of events through the generation of reactive oxygen species resulting in hemolysis of mature red blood cells and destruction of immature erythroid precursors in the bone marrow (ineffective erythropoiesis). AHSP, α-hemoglobin stabilizing protein; HSP70, heat shock protein 70. (*Modified from* Mettananda S, Gibbons RJ, Higgs DR. alpha-Globin as a molecular target in the treatment of beta-thalassemia. Blood 2015;125(24):3696; with permission.)

growth differentiation factor (GDF) 11 in response to high ROS results in terminal erythroid maturation arrest, contributing to ineffective erythropoiesis. The action of GDF11 is believed to be mediated via Activin receptor (ActR) IIA, which is a surface receptor found on the erythroid cell membrane.[54] Additionally, heat shock protein 70 (HSP70) interacts directly with free α-globin chains and thereby becomes sequestered in the cytoplasm. This prevents HSP70 from performing its normal physiologic role of protecting GATA1 from proteolytic cleavage and the resultant premature degradation of GATA1 causes maturation arrest and apoptosis of polychromatic erythroblasts.[55] In summary, the existing evidence clearly suggests that the excess free α-globin chains are directly responsible for hemolysis and ineffective erythropoiesis, which are the two primary pathophysiologic mechanisms that cause anemia in patients with β-thalassemia.

GENOTYPE-PHENOTYPE CORRELATION AND GENETIC MODIFIERS OF β-THALASSEMIA

Despite being a typical monogenic disorder, β-thalassemia exhibits a remarkable clinical heterogeneity with a broad spectrum of disease severity (**Fig. 4**).[56] Individuals with β-thalassemia trait are asymptomatic, have minor hematologic abnormalities, and do not require RBC transfusions. Individuals at the most severe end of the spectrum have transfusion-dependent anemia and require regular life-long RBC transfusions: these patients are homozygotes or compound heterozygotes for thalassemia mutations (β-thalassemia major). Another substantial proportion of patients with β-thalassemia have a less severe form of thalassemia. They require only occasional RBC transfusions and are thus said to have nontransfusion-dependent anemia: a situation that has previously been referred to as β-thalassemia intermedia.

    This clinical heterogeneity is partly explained by the nature of mutations. β^0-thalassemia mutations, which cause complete abolition of β-globin gene expression, give rise to severe forms of the disease. Conversely, β^{+}- and β^{++}-thalassemia mutations, which result in only moderate to mild reduction in β-globin synthesis, are often associated with less severe phenotypes.[57] However, there are remarkable variations in severity even in patients who inherit identical β-thalassemia mutations. This is explained through the pathophysiology and cellular pathology of β-thalassemia and several genetic modifiers have been well characterized and studied. Because the pathophysiology of β-thalassemia results from the accumulation of unpaired α-globin chains in erythroid cells and their precursors, the clinical severity is directly related to the degree of imbalance between α- and β-like globin chains. Conditions that increase

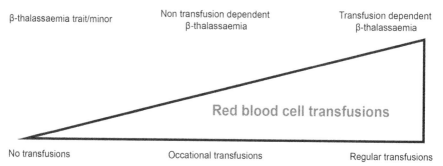

Fig. 4. Spectrum of clinical severity of β-thalassemia. Severity of β-thalassemia varies from asymptomatic anemia, which does not require transfusion (β-thalassemia trait), to severe transfusion-dependent β-thalassemia.

this imbalance exacerbate the severity, whereas conditions that reduce the globin chain imbalance ameliorate the severity of β-thalassemia (**Box 1**).

GENETIC MODIFIERS THAT WORSEN THE SEVERITY OF β-THALASSEMIA

Individuals with heterozygous β-thalassemia mutations who are generally asymptomatic sometimes manifest clinical features of β-thalassemia intermedia. This occurs for two main reasons. First, some β-thalassemia mutations encode highly unstable β-globin chain variants, which are not capable of forming stable hemoglobin tetramers. These dominantly inherited β-thalassemia mutations cause clinical features even in the heterozygous state.[42] Second, some individuals inherit more than four copies of the α-globin gene. When more than the usual number of α-globin genes (ααα/αα, ααα/ααα, αααα/αα) are coinherited with heterozygous β-thalassemia, it worsens the excess of α-globin and tips the globin chain imbalance still further, converting a clinically asymptomatic state to thalassemia intermedia.[58]

GENETIC MODIFIERS THAT AMELIORATE SEVERITY OF β-THALASSEMIA

By contrast, conditions that improve the α- to β-globin balance by either increasing the β-like globin output or by decreasing α-globin production improve the clinical severity of β-thalassemia. Again, this occurs for two main reasons: in natural conditions that increase the production of γ-globin, and in α-thalassemia.

Several genetic modifiers that upregulate γ-globin expression have now been established. Certain deletions involving the β-globin locus (eg, δβ⁰-thalassemia) are associated with higher than normal levels of γ-globin, sufficient to partially compensate for the absence of β-globin.[38] Next, several molecular, genetic linkage and genome-wide association studies have identified three quantitative trait loci that are associated with increased production of γ-globin and HbF. The *Xmn1-HBG2* polymorphism in the β-globin cluster and polymorphisms in the *HBS1L-MYB* intergenic region on chromosome 6q23 and the *BCL11A* enhancer on chromosome 2p16 have all been shown to increase γ-globin expression.[19,59,60] Recently, it was also shown that certain mutations of the *KLF1* gene increase the production of HbF, which in turn ameliorates the clinical severity of β-thalassemia.[61,62]

Similarly, several family, cohort, and case-control studies have reported that the coinheritance of α-thalassemia ameliorates the severity of β-thalassemia.[47] These

---

Box 1
Genetic modifiers of β-thalassemia

- Factors that worsen clinical phenotype of heterozygous β-thalassemia
  - ○ Dominantly inherited β-thalassemia mutations
  - ○ Coinheritance of excess α-globin genes (ααα/αα, ααα/ααα, αααα/αα)

- Factors that ameliorate clinical phenotype of homozygous or compound heterozygous β-thalassemia
  - ○ Inheritance of mild (β⁺ or β⁺⁺) mutations
  - ○ Increased synthesis of γ-globin and hemoglobin F
    - ■ δβ⁰-thalassemia
    - ■ *Xmn1-HBG2* polymorphism at $^{G}\gamma$ (−158 C > T)
    - ■ Polymorphisms at *BCL11A* on chromosome 2p16
    - ■ Polymorphisms at *HBS1L-MYB* intergenic region or *MYB* on chromosome 6q23
    - ■ *KLF1* mutations
  - ○ Coinheritance of α-thalassemia

studies have shown that deletion of one or two α-globin genes (-α/αα, --/αα, or -α/-α) is associated with a milder disease in most patients with β-thalassemia and in some circumstances transforms the phenotype from transfusion-dependent thalassemia to thalassemia intermedia.

SUMMARY

More than 250 mutations in and around the β-globin gene and cis-acting enhancers that affect multiple stages of gene expression are known to cause β-thalassemia. These mutations lead to absent or reduced synthesis of β-globin, which then result in an excess of free α-globin chains that precipitate in RBCs and their precursors to cause hemolysis and ineffective erythropoiesis leading to anemia. Despite being an archetypal monogenic disorder, β-thalassemia exhibits a remarkable clinical heterogeneity that is explained by its pathophysiology and molecular basis and is directly related to the intracellular imbalance between α- and β-like globin chains. β-Globin mutations, which cause milder reductions in the synthesis of β-globin, genetic polymorphisms, which cause up-regulation of γ-globin, and coinheritance of α-thalassemia ameliorate severity of β-thalassemia. With the advent of novel molecular-based therapies, these genetic modifiers have created great enthusiasm within the field to investigate the associated therapeutic pathways to find a cure for this life-limiting disease.[23,63,64]

ACKNOWLEDGMENTS

The authors thank Anuja Premawardhena of University of Kelaniya, Sri Lanka and Mohsin Badat of Weatherall Institute of Molecular Medicine, University of Oxford, UK for suggestions and critically reading the article.

REFERENCES

1. Higgs DR, Engel JD, Stamatoyannopoulos G. Thalassaemia. Lancet 2012; 379(9813):373–83.
2. Weatherall DJ. The inherited diseases of hemoglobin are an emerging global health burden. Blood 2010;115(22):4331–6.
3. Weatherall DJ. The challenge of haemoglobinopathies in resource-poor countries. Br J Haematol 2011;154(6):736–44.
4. Weatherall DJ. Genetic variation and susceptibility to infection: the red cell and malaria. Br J Haematol 2008;141(3):276–86.
5. Fucharoen S, Weatherall DJ. Progress toward the control and management of the thalassemias. Hematol Oncol Clin North Am 2016;30(2):359–71.
6. Weatherall DJ, Clegg JB. The thalassaemia syndromes. 4th edition. Oxford, United Kingdom: Blackwell Science; 2001.
7. Hughes JR, Cheng JF, Ventress N, et al. Annotation of cis-regulatory elements by identification, subclassification, and functional assessment of multispecies conserved sequences. Proc Natl Acad Sci U S A 2005;102(28):9830–5.
8. Smith EC, Orkin SH. Hemoglobin genetics: recent contributions of GWAS and gene editing. Hum Mol Genet 2016;25(R2):R99–105.
9. Stamatoyannopoulos G. Control of globin gene expression during development and erythroid differentiation. Exp Hematol 2005;33(3):259–71.
10. Nandakumar SK, Ulirsch JC, Sankaran VG. Advances in understanding erythropoiesis: evolving perspectives. Br J Haematol 2016;173(2):206–18.

11. Weed RI, Reed CF, Berg G. Is hemoglobin an essential structural component of human erythrocyte membranes? J Clin Invest 1963;42:581–8.
12. Mettananda S, Gibbons RJ, Higgs DR. Understanding alpha-globin gene regulation and implications for the treatment of beta-thalassemia. Ann N Y Acad Sci 2016;1368(1):16–24.
13. Vernimmen D, Lynch MD, De Gobbi M, et al. Polycomb eviction as a new distant enhancer function. Genes Development 2011;25(15):1583–8.
14. De Gobbi M, Anguita E, Hughes J, et al. Tissue-specific histone modification and transcription factor binding in alpha globin gene expression. Blood 2007;110(13): 4503–10.
15. Vernimmen D, Marques-Kranc F, Sharpe JA, et al. Chromosome looping at the human alpha-globin locus is mediated via the major upstream regulatory element (HS -40). Blood 2009;114(19):4253–60.
16. Tuan D, London IM. Mapping of DNase I-hypersensitive sites in the upstream DNA of human embryonic epsilon-globin gene in K562 leukemia cells. Proc Natl Acad Sci U S A 1984;81(9):2718–22.
17. Deng W, Rupon JW, Krivega I, et al. Reactivation of developmentally silenced globin genes by forced chromatin looping. Cell 2014;158(4):849–60.
18. Lee WS, McColl B, Maksimovic J, et al. Epigenetic interplay at the beta-globin locus. Biochim Biophys Acta 2017;1860(4):393–404.
19. Sankaran VG, Menne TF, Xu J, et al. Human fetal hemoglobin expression is regulated by the developmental stage-specific repressor BCL11A. Science 2008; 322(5909):1839–42.
20. Xu J, Sankaran VG, Ni M, et al. Transcriptional silencing of {gamma}-globin by BCL11A involves long-range interactions and cooperation with SOX6. Genes Development 2010;24(8):783–98.
21. Suzuki M, Yamamoto M, Engel JD. Fetal globin gene repressors as drug targets for molecular therapies to treat the beta-globinopathies. Mol Cell Biol 2014; 34(19):3560–9.
22. Cui S, Kolodziej KE, Obara N, et al. Nuclear receptors TR2 and TR4 recruit multiple epigenetic transcriptional corepressors that associate specifically with the embryonic beta-type globin promoters in differentiated adult erythroid cells. Mol Cell Biol 2011;31(16):3298–311.
23. Bauer DE, Kamran SC, Orkin SH. Reawakening fetal hemoglobin: prospects for new therapies for the beta-globin disorders. Blood 2012;120(15):2945–53.
24. Zhou D, Liu K, Sun CW, et al. KLF1 regulates BCL11A expression and gamma- to beta-globin gene switching. Nat Genet 2010;42(9):742–4.
25. Masuda T, Wang X, Maeda M, et al. Transcription factors LRF and BCL11A independently repress expression of fetal hemoglobin. Science 2016;351(6270): 285–9.
26. Higgs DR. The molecular basis of alpha-thalassemia. Cold Spring Harb Perspect Med 2013;3(1):a011718.
27. Higgs DR, Wood WG. Long-range regulation of alpha globin gene expression during erythropoiesis. Curr Opin Hematol 2008;15(3):176–83.
28. Coelho A, Picanco I, Seuanes F, et al. Novel large deletions in the human alpha-globin gene cluster: clarifying the HS-40 long-range regulatory role in the native chromosome environment. Blood Cell Mol Dis 2010;45(2):147–53.
29. Wu MY, He Y, Yan JM, et al. A novel selective deletion of the major alpha-globin regulatory element (MCS-R2) causing alpha-thalassaemia. Br J Haematol 2017; 176(6):984–6.

30. Sollaino MC, Paglietti ME, Loi D, et al. Homozygous deletion of the major alpha-globin regulatory element (MCS-R2) responsible for a severe case of hemoglobin H disease. Blood 2010;116(12):2193–4.
31. Phylipsen M, Prior JF, Lim E, et al. Thalassemia in Western Australia: 11 novel deletions characterized by multiplex ligation-dependent probe amplification. Blood Cell Mol Dis 2010;44(3):146–51.
32. Harteveld CL, Higgs DR. Alpha-thalassaemia. Orphanet J Rare Dis 2010;5:13.
33. Gibbons R. Alpha thalassaemia-mental retardation, X linked. Orphanet J Rare Dis 2006;1:15.
34. Clynes D, Higgs DR, Gibbons RJ. The chromatin remodeller ATRX: a repeat offender in human disease. Trends Biochem Sci 2013;38(9):461–6.
35. Piel FB, Weatherall DJ. The alpha-thalassemias. N Engl J Med 2014;371(20):1908–16.
36. Huang LY, Yan JM, Zhou JY, et al. A severe case of hemoglobin H disease due to compound heterozygosity for deletion of the major alpha-globin regulatory element (MCS-R2) and alpha0-thalassemia. Acta Haematol 2017;138(1):61–4.
37. Thein SL. Molecular basis of beta thalassemia and potential therapeutic targets. Blood Cell Mol Dis 2017 [pii:S1079–9796(17)30210-3].
38. Thein SL. The molecular basis of beta-thalassemia. Cold Spring Harbor Perspect Med 2013;3(5):a011700.
39. Weatherall DJ. Phenotype-genotype relationships in monogenic disease: lessons from the thalassaemias. Nat Rev Genet 2001;2(4):245–55.
40. Fucharoen S, Weatherall DJ. The hemoglobin E thalassemias. Cold Spring Harbor Perspect Med 2012;2(8) [pii:a011734].
41. Orkin SH, Kazazian HH Jr, Antonarakis SE, et al. Abnormal RNA processing due to the exon mutation of beta E-globin gene. Nature 1982;300(5894):768–9.
42. Thein SL. Is it dominantly inherited beta thalassaemia or just a beta-chain variant that is highly unstable? Br J Haematol 1999;107(1):12–21.
43. Shang X, Xu X. Update in the genetics of thalassemia: what clinicians need to know. Best Pract Res Clin Obstet Gynaecol 2017;39:3–15.
44. Viprakasit V, Gibbons RJ, Broughton BC, et al. Mutations in the general transcription factor TFIIH result in beta-thalassaemia in individuals with trichothiodystrophy. Hum Mol Genet 2001;10(24):2797–802.
45. Origa R. beta-Thalassemia. Genet Med 2017;19(6):609–19.
46. Perkins A, Xu X, Higgs DR, et al. Kruppeling erythropoiesis: an unexpected broad spectrum of human red blood cell disorders due to KLF1 variants. Blood 2016;127(15):1856–62.
47. Mettananda S, Gibbons RJ, Higgs DR. alpha-Globin as a molecular target in the treatment of beta-thalassemia. Blood 2015;125(24):3694–701.
48. Voon HP, Vadolas J. Controlling alpha-globin: a review of alpha-globin expression and its impact on beta-thalassemia. Haematologica 2008;93(12):1868–76.
49. Shinar E, Rachmilewitz EA. Haemoglobinopathies and red cell membrane function. Baillieres Clin Haematol 1993;6(2):357–69.
50. Khandros E, Thom CS, D'Souza J, et al. Integrated protein quality-control pathways regulate free alpha-globin in murine beta-thalassemia. Blood 2012;119(22):5265–75.
51. Schrier SL. Pathophysiology of thalassemia. Curr Opin Hematol 2002;9(2):123–6.
52. Yuan J, Kannan R, Shinar E, et al. Isolation, characterization, and immunoprecipitation studies of immune complexes from membranes of beta-thalassemic erythrocytes. Blood 1992;79(11):3007–13.

53. Ribeil JA, Arlet JB, Dussiot M, et al. Ineffective erythropoiesis in beta -thalassemia. ScientificWorldJournal 2013;2013:394295.
54. Dussiot M, Maciel TT, Fricot A, et al. An activin receptor IIA ligand trap corrects ineffective erythropoiesis in beta-thalassemia. Nat Med 2014;20(4):398–407.
55. Arlet JB, Ribeil JA, Guillem F, et al. HSP70 sequestration by free alpha-globin promotes ineffective erythropoiesis in beta-thalassaemia. Nature 2014;514(7521): 242–6.
56. Musallam KM, Rivella S, Vichinsky E, et al. Non-transfusion-dependent thalassemias. Haematologica 2013;98(6):833–44.
57. Danjou F, Anni F, Galanello R. Beta-thalassemia: from genotype to phenotype. Haematologica 2011;96(11):1573–5.
58. Thein SL. Genetic association studies in beta-hemoglobinopathies. Hematology Am Soc Hematol Educ Program 2013;2013:354–61.
59. Menzel S, Garner C, Gut I, et al. A QTL influencing F cell production maps to a gene encoding a zinc-finger protein on chromosome 2p15. Nat Genet 2007; 39(10):1197–9.
60. Thein SL, Menzel S, Peng X, et al. Intergenic variants of HBS1L-MYB are responsible for a major quantitative trait locus on chromosome 6q23 influencing fetal hemoglobin levels in adults. Proc Natl Acad Sci U S A 2007;104(27):11346–51.
61. Borg J, Papadopoulos P, Georgitsi M, et al. Haploinsufficiency for the erythroid transcription factor KLF1 causes hereditary persistence of fetal hemoglobin. Nat Genet 2010;42(9):801–5.
62. Liu D, Zhang X, Yu L, et al. KLF1 mutations are relatively more common in a thalassemia endemic region and ameliorate the severity of beta-thalassemia. Blood 2014;124(5):803–11.
63. Mettananda S, Fisher CA, Sloane-Stanley JA, et al. Selective silencing of alpha-globin by the histone demethylase inhibitor IOX1: a potentially new pathway for treatment of beta-thalassemia. Haematologica 2017;102(3):e80–4.
64. Makis A, Hatzimichael E, Papassotiriou I, et al. 2017 Clinical trials update in new treatments of beta-thalassemia. Am J Hematol 2016;91(11):1135–45.

Clinical Classification, Screening and Diagnosis for Thalassemia

Vip Viprakasit, MD, DPhil(Oxon)[a],*, Supachai Ekwattanakit, MD, PhD[b]

KEYWORDS

- Transfusion-dependent thalassemia (TDT)
- Non–transfusion-dependent thalassemia (NTDT) • Diagnosis • Screening

KEY POINTS

- Diagnosis of thalassemia and hemoglobinopathies requires a comprehensive evaluation combining red blood cell phenotypes, hemoglobin profiles, and DNA analysis.
- A recent classification of thalassemia syndrome is based on the patients' clinical severity that is their transfusion requirement, not genotypes.
- Hemoglobin analysis can be performed at any age; however, interpretation requires age-specific reference ranges.
- Genetic analysis for globin mutations are required to confirm the clinical diagnosis and are indispensable for genetic counseling, genetic risk calculation, prenatal, and preimplantation genetic testing.

INTRODUCTION

Over the past decade, our knowledge of the clinical diagnosis and management of thalassemia has progressed extensively. In recent years, the most critical change in clinical diagnosis is a new classification that has been simplified and help guiding clinical management from thalassemia intermedia (TI) into non–transfusion-dependent thalassemia (NTDT) and thalassemia major (TM) into transfusion-dependent thalassemia (TDT) based on their requirement of regular blood transfusions to survive. This new classification has included several other forms of thalassemia syndromes beside β-thalassemia diseases (β-TI and β-TM) that have been a prototype of

Disclosure Statement: All authors have nothing to declare.
[a] Siriraj Integrated Center of Excellence for Thalassemia (SiiCOE-T) and Division of Hematology/Oncology, Department of Pediatrics, Faculty of Medicine Siriraj Hospital, Mahidol University, 2 Wanglang Road, Siriraj, Bangkoknoi, Bangkok 10700, Thailand; [b] Division of Hematology, Department of Medicine, Faculty of Medicine Siriraj Hospital, Mahidol University, 2 Wanglang Road, Siriraj, Bangkoknoi, Bangkok 10700, Thailand
* Corresponding author.
E-mail address: vip.vip@mahidol.ac.th

Hematol Oncol Clin N Am 32 (2018) 193–211
https://doi.org/10.1016/j.hoc.2017.11.006
hemonc.theclinics.com

thalassemia syndromes for many years. In addition, the medical technology for screening and definitively diagnosing thalassemia traits and diseases has also been improved and are the subjects of our review in this article. However, the classification of thalassemia continues to rely on clinical presentation and severity. Diagnostic tests, including molecular analyses, can only guide but not yet replace clinical evaluation and judgment.

CLINICAL CLASSIFICATION OF THALASSEMIA

Disorders of hemoglobin (Hb) are characterized according to pathologic defects on globin chain production; a quantitative defect or "thalassemia," mainly α-thalassemia and β-thalassemia, and a qualitative defect, namely hemoglobinopathy (or structural Hb variants), and, last, hereditary persistence of fetal Hb. Interactions of these 3 types of globin defects result in a wide array of thalassemia syndromes and related diseases.[1]

Thalassemia has a wide spectrum of clinical severity, which was previously used for a clinical classification of thalassemia into TM, TI, and thalassemia minor. The term TM describes patients who have severe anemia presenting early in life and requiring lifelong blood transfusions and iron chelation, whereas thalassemia minor, at the other end of clinical spectrum, are persons with asymptomatic, mild anemia and a heterozygous condition (trait) of thalassemia. The latter group requires no transfusion, but genetic counseling. TI are highly diverse group of patients with various clinical severities from mild, moderate, to moderately severe anemia, requiring no blood transfusions to occasional and frequent blood transfusions. Moreover, these clinical entities are dynamic; patients with TI particularly might require more frequent or even regular transfusions if they develop several complications owing to thalassemia, such as pulmonary hypertension, extramedullary hematopoietic masses, or chronic ulceration. In addition, early published articles and guidelines addressed mainly the clinical management and complications of TM (mostly homozygous β-thalassemia or β-TM).[2] This classification has left out several clinical thalassemia syndromes, especially α-thalassemia and the hemoglobinopathies, such as Hb E/β-thalassemia.

Recently, a concept of clinical diagnosis of thalassemia syndromes has changed dramatically owing to several clinical research and observational findings focusing on the clinical management and complications of TI showing that, even they were called a milder group according to the degree of anemia and transfusion requirement, patients with TI could develop serious complications later in their lives. Better monitoring and treatment with better outcomes are increasingly important.[3] In 2012, the new terminology for a clinical classification of thalassemia (TDT and NTDT) was proposed and then adopted by the Thalassemia International Federation in their recent guidelines and publications.[4,5] Differentiation of a new thalassemia patient as either TDT or NTDT requires a careful clinical evaluation using several clinical and hematological parameters, particularly baseline Hb levels (**Fig. 1**). Most patients with β-TM and those who have survived Hb Bart's hydrops have a very severe phenotype and could be easily classified as TDT. However, in patients with other thalassemia syndromes, particularly Hb E/β-thalassemia, usually present during an intercurrent infection that is causing an acute hemolytic crisis that can make their presentation to be more serious, with an enlarged spleen and a low Hb level with symptomatic anemia.[6] It is recommended to follow such patients for at least 3 to 6 months to observe their clinical severity at their true baseline before a diagnosis of TDT or NTDT is made.

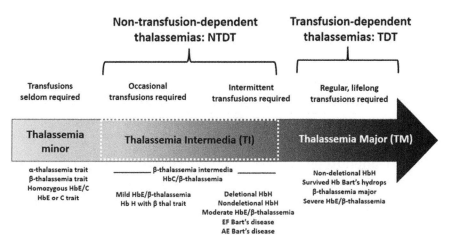

Fig. 1. The clinical spectrum of thalassemia syndromes based on their requirement of regular blood transfusions into non–transfusion dependent thalassemia (NTDT) and transfusion-dependent thalassemia (TDT). The *arrow* shows a spectrum of clinical heterogeneity from asymptomatic (or with mild anemia) in thalassemia carriers (or thalassemia minor) to mild, moderate and severe thalassemia diseases, NTDT and TDT. The previous terminology of thalassemia intermedia (TI) and thalassemia major (TM) are shown inside the *arrow* and refers to the similar concept of clinical severity in thalassemia syndromes. (*Modified from* Taher A, Vichinsky E, Musallam K, et al. Introduction [Chapter 1]. In: Weatherall D, editor. Guidelines for the management of non transfusion dependent thalassaemia (NTDT). Nicosia (Cyprus): Thalassaemia International Federation; 2013. p. 1; with permission.)

Transfusion-Dependent Thalassemia

Patients with TDT are those who require regular transfusions for survival, which consist of β-TM (homozygous $β^0$-thalassemia or Cooley's anemia), severe Hb E/β-thalassemia, severe nondeletional Hb H disease, and those who survived Hb Bart's hydrops fetalis.[4]

Clinical presentation, history, and physical examination

Clinical onset of the first presentation for severe α- and β-thalassemia are different as a result of a physiologic Hb switching during fetal and infant development. In Hb Bart's hydrops fetalis, the most severe form of α-thalassemia with deletions of all 4 α-globin genes (−/−), severe anemia occurs in utero, resulting in fetal hydrops. Without intrauterine blood transfusion and regular transfusions after birth, these patients could not survive.[7] In severe nondeletional Hb H disease, the affected neonate has severe anemia from birth and usually has neonatal jaundice, requiring regular transfusions.[8] Also, there are several case reports of hydrops fetalis resulting from nondeletional Hb H disease, so-called Hb H hydrops fetalis.[9–17] For homozygous β-thalassemia or β-TM, the first clinical presentation usually occurs between the first 6 months and 2 years of life, as the γ-globin genes (producing Hb F) physiologically is switched off. These patients can present with symptoms of severe anemia (Hb <7 g/dL), pallor, jaundice, irritability, feeding problems, failure to thrive, skeletal deformities, abdominal enlargement owing to progressive splenomegaly and hepatomegaly, or recurrent episodes of infection (see **Fig. 1**; and **Fig. 2, Table 1**). Subsequently, they require regular blood transfusions to survive.

Physical examination at first presentation in patients with TDT reveals inactive infants with inappropriate growth and development, marked anemia, moderate to marked jaundice, and huge hepatosplenomegaly; some patients exhibit

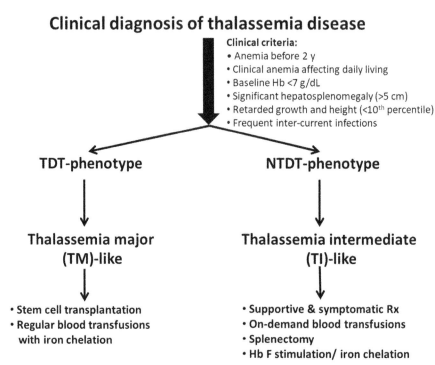

Clinical diagnosis of thalassemia disease

Clinical criteria:
• Anemia before 2 y
• Clinical anemia affecting daily living
• Baseline Hb <7 g/dL
• Significant hepatosplenomegaly (>5 cm)
• Retarded growth and height (<10th percentile)
• Frequent inter-current infections

TDT-phenotype

NTDT-phenotype

Thalassemia major
(TM)-like

Thalassemia intermediate
(TI)-like

• Stem cell transplantation
• Regular blood transfusions
  with iron chelation

• Supportive & symptomatic Rx
• On-demand blood transfusions
• Splenectomy
• Hb F stimulation/ iron chelation

Fig. 2. Differential characteristics for diagnosis of transfusion-dependent thalassemia (TDT) versus and non–transfusion-dependent thalassemia (NTDT) to guide further clinical management. Hb, hemoglobin.

thalassemic facie. For TDT who have been inadequately treated or untreated, a degree of growth retardation, bony changes, and organomegaly becomes more apparent. These skeletal changes include deformities of the long bones (legs) and craniofacial changes (frontal bossing, malar prominence, depressed nasal bridge, and hypertrophy of the maxillae, which tends to expose the upper teeth), and osteoporosis.[18] Whereas in properly treated children with TDT, minimal or no abnormal findings on physical examination are expected. However, in severe cases, even if they have been treated with adequate transfusion, progressive splenomegaly may still occur.[19]

Non–Transfusion-Dependent Thalassemia

The term NTDT is used for a group of thalassemia patients who do not require regular blood transfusions for survival; however, they may require occasional transfusions during periods of physiologic stress, such as infection or pregnancy.[20,21] Also patient with NTDT may require more regular transfusions later in life owing to complications of the disease, including the development of splenomegaly.[21] NTDT includes a wide spectrum of clinical severity with mild to moderately severe chronic anemia that can hamper physiologic processes such as growth and development, and result in diverse clinical complications later in life.[3,22,23] Generally, NTDT can be categorized into 3 main groups according to molecular defect, β-TI, Hb E/β-thalassemia, and Hb H disease.[20] A clinical diagnosis of NTDT requires both clinical and laboratory information as discussed elsewhere in this article (see **Figs. 1** and **2, Table 1**).

Table 1
Diagnosis of 4 common thalassemia diseases

	β-TM	β-TI	Hb E/β-Thalassemia	Hb H
Steady-state Hb levels	<5 g/dL	~7–10 g/dL	Mild 9–11 g/dL Moderately severe 6–7 g/dL Severe 4–5 g/dL	2.6–13.3 g/dL
Blood smear	Red cell microcytosis and hypochromia Nucleated RBC, target cells, irregularly crenated RBC, evidence of hemolysis such as increased reticulocytes (5%–10%) and nucleated RBCs			
Other RBC findings	Positive acid elution test		Numerous target cells Positive acid elution test	Inclusion bodies Numerous basophilic stippling in Hb H/Hb CS
HPLC Electrophoresis	Hb F up to 100% Hb A$_2$↑	Hb F 10%–50% (up to 100%) Hb A$_2$ >4%	Hb E (40%–60%) Hb F (60%–40%) ±Hb A (with β$^+$-thal) Hb A$_2$ increased	Variable Hb H (0.8%–40%) Hb A$_2$ decreased Possible presence of Hb CS, Hb PS, etc
DNA analysis	• Common known mutations of both β^0 and β$^+$-thal mutations in population specific set can be done by PCR-based methods. • For rare or unusual mutations, a direct sequencing or array analysis is required. • Other analysis for β-TI included α- and β-globin mutations, *Xmn I* polymorphism, and other QTLs			• GAP-PCR developed for common α-thalassemia deletions and RDB for nondeletional mutations • For unknown mutations, Southern blotting, MLPA analysis and gene sequencing required

Abbreviations: Hb, hemoglobin; Hb CS, Hb Constant Spring; MLPA, multiplex ligation-dependent probe amplification; PCR, polymerase chain reaction; QTL, quantitative trait loci; RBC, red blood cells; RDB, reverse dot blot; TI, thalassemia intermedia; TM, thalassemia major.

Adapted from Viprakasit V, Origa R. Genetic basis, pathophysiology and diagnosis. In: Cappellini MD, Cohen A, Porter J, et al, editors. Guidelines for the Management of Transfusion Dependent Thalassaemia (TDT). 3rd edition. Nicosia (Cyprus): Thalassaemia International Federation; 2014; with permission.

Clinical presentation, history, and physical examination

In patients with NTDT, the first clinical presentation often is symptomatic anemia with a concurrent episode of infection occurring early in life, usually when they are older than 2 years of age. Consequently, blood transfusion may be required in patients who have moderate to severe anemia.[21] On the other end of NTDT spectrum, many patients do well and are diagnosed as having NTDT later in life during screening for blood donation, a routine health checkup, family planning consultation, or when seeking medical attention owing to unrelated condition. Also, in several cases, the diagnosis of NTDT is made when a thalassemia-related complication, such as symptomatic gallstones or chronic leg ulcer, occurs. To determine the clinical severity of thalassemia, especially in the former group, it is critical to carefully follow these babies or young children presenting with hemolytic crisis, whether they are truly NTDT or TDT by determining the steady-state Hb levels after the acute illness has resolved. However, some patients with NTDT may require frequent or even regular transfusion therapy owing to delayed growth and development during childhood. Adult patients with NTDT may require more regular transfusions owing to late complications, especially progressive anemia secondary to increased splenomegaly.[21]

Physical examination in patients with NTDT can be vastly differed owing to several factors, including age, baseline Hb levels, degree of hemolysis and extramedullary hematopoiesis, and the frequency of previous transfusions.[3,24] Patients with a more severe form of NTDT without adequate treatment during childhood may have a short stature, moderate to marked pallor with moderate jaundice, and moderate to severe hepatosplenomegaly. These abnormal findings could be improved if they were treated with regular blood transfusions.[24] For those with a milder form of NTDT, physical examination may reveal mild anemia and otherwise unremarkable findings, or mild splenomegaly.[24] In those with a modest degree of anemia, a low-grade systolic ejection murmur (hemic murmur) at the left upper sternal border may be evident. It is also important to look for signs of thalassemia-related complications, for example, delayed pubic hair, breast, and testis development (delayed puberty), abnormal skeletal changes (thalassemic facie), and abnormal heart sound (loud P2 for pulmonary hypertension).

SCREENING AND DIAGNOSIS OF THALASSEMIA

In general, the screening and diagnostic algorithm for thalassemia can be divided into 2 levels—population and individual—in which different approaches have been implemented owing to different objectives of screening. The screening methods used in a population approach that focused on identification of thalassemia and Hb variant traits are described. Last, comprehensive diagnostic tests for thalassemia confirmation are discussed. All currently available laboratory tests for screening and confirmation of thalassemia traits and diseases with-related characteristics such as accuracy, validity, and availability are summarized in **Table 2**.

Screening Tests for Thalassemia Carriers in a Population Approach

Several large-scale screening programs to identify thalassemia carriers have been proposed.[25–30] The main purpose of screening for thalassemia carrier status is to identify couples at risk of having offspring with severe thalassemia diseases, such as β-TM, Hb E/β-thalassemia, and Hb Bart's hydrops fetalis as the first part of a prevention and control program for thalassemia syndromes in several parts of the world.[30] All these programs are based on heterozygote (carrier) detection, couple at-risk identification, genetic counseling, and fetal diagnosis. Screening programs can vary in details owing

Table 2
Summary of available screening and diagnostic methods for thalassemia diagnosis

	Affordability	Accuracy	Sensitivity	Reproducibility	Simplicity	Validation
Screening tools						
Osmotic fragility	++++	+++	+++	+++	++++	++++
Mean corpuscular volume	+++	++++	++++	++++	++++	++++
DCIP	++++	+++	+++	+++	++++	++++
Carrier diagnosis						
HPLC/LPLC	++	++++	++++	++++	+++	++++
Capillary electrophoresis	+++	?	++++	++++	++++	?
Isoelectric focusing	+++	++	++++	++++	++	++++
Mutation specific detection-α-thalassemia						
GAP-PCR for α^0-thalassemia	++++	++++	+++	++++	++++	++++
ARMS-α-thalassemia	++++	++++	+++	+++	++++	++++
RDB-α-thalassemia	+++	++++	++++	++++	++	++++
Mismatched-PCR RFLP for HbCS/PS	+++	++++	+++++	++++	++	++++
HRM for α-thalassemia	+	+++	??	??	+	+++
Real-time GAP-PCR	+	++++	+++++	+++	+	++++
Genomic scanning for α-thalassemia						
Direct $\alpha2$ and $\alpha1$ globin sequencing	++	+++++	+++++	++++	++++	++++
MLPA for α-globin cluster	+	++++	++++	++++	++	++++
CGH array	+	++++	+++++	++++	++	++++
Mutation specific detection-β-thalassemia						
ARMS-β-thalassemia	++++	++++	+++	+++	++++	++++
RDB-β-thalassemia	+++	++++	++++	++++	++	++++
PCR-RFLP/sizing	+++	++++	+++++	++++	++	++++
HRM for β-thalassemia	+	+++	??	??	+	+++
GAP-PCR for β-globin deletions	++++	++++	+++	++++	++++	++++

(continued on next page)

Table 2
(*continued*)

	Affordability	Accuracy	Sensitivity	Reproducibility	Simplicity	Validation
Genomic scanning for β-thalassemia						
dHPLC	?	++++	+++++	?	?	++++
DGGE/SSCP	++	++++	++++	++++	+	++++
Direct β-globin sequencing	++	+++++	+++++	++++	++++	++++
MLPA for α-globin cluster	+	++++	++++	++++	++	++++
CGH array	+	++++	+++++	++++	++	++++

Abbreviations: ARMS, allele-related mutations specific; CGH, comparative genomic hybridization; DCIP, dichlorophenol indophenol precipitation test; DGGE, denaturing gradient gel electrophoresis; dHPLC, denaturing HPLC; Hb, hemoglobin; HPLC, high-performance liquid chromatography; HRM, high-resolution melting analysis; LPLC, low-performance liquid chromatography; MLPA, multiple ligation probe assay; PCR, polymerase chain reaction; RDB, reverse dot blot; RFLP, restriction fragment length polymorphism; SSCP, single strand conformation polymorphism.

to different prevalences of thalassemia types in any given country—α-thalassemia, β-thalassemia, and Hb variant and available technology and resources. The target population for screening includes teenagers or school children, preconception, and early pregnancy. Alternatively, a thalassemia screening can be done in the neonatal period through a newborn screening program,[27,31,32] but this measure is beyond the scope of this review. In this part of article, selected and widely used methods in thalassemia screening are described, in terms of principles, advantages, and disadvantages.

One-tube osmotic fragility test
The one-tube osmotic fragility test (OTOFT), originally described by Parpart and colleagues in 1947,[33] is used to measure erythrocyte resistance to hemolysis while being exposed to varying concentrations of a saline solution. In a hypotonic solution, water enters the red blood cell (RBC), resulting in swelling and eventually RBC lysis. The susceptibility of this osmotic hemolysis is a function of surface area to volume ratio. In thalassemia, RBCs have a low cellular Hb, resulting in an increase in osmotic resistance compared with a normal RBC. Generally, a small drop of fresh whole blood (20 μL) is used and pipetted into buffered NaCl solution (typically 0.36% NaCl) or glycerine-saline in a test tube.[34] The tube is mixed and left at room temperature for 15 to 30 minutes (according to each protocol) and the degree of hemolysis is assessed by visual inspection or photometrical measurement. A clear solution is interpreted as a negative result and a cloudy appearance as a positive result.

Advantages The OTOFT is a simple, fast, and inexpensive method requiring no sophisticated equipment. It has been validated for use as a preliminary screening method for thalassemia carrier status and provides good sensitivity (87.0%-100%) and specificity (59%-100% for thalassemias and Hb E carrier screening; 34.1%-83.7% for β-thalassemia carrier screening).[35–39] In a complex interaction such as combined α-thalassemia and β-thalassemia trait, this test can result in borderline mean corpuscular volume (MCV) value (discussed elsewhere in this article) and a normal Hb A_2 level. However, OTOFT can be positive in this situation.[36]

Disadvantages There are several factors that could affect the sensitivity of OTOFT. In β-thalassemia carrier screening, coinheritance of α-thalassemia, Hb E trait, Hb S trait, some Hb variants, glucose-6-phosphate dehydrogenase deficiency, or Southeast Asian ovalocytosis can lead to a false-positive OTOFT.[34,39,40] Iron deficiency anemia (IDA) also affects OTOFT, causing a false-positive rate of up to 63.9% in a study from Egypt, where the population has a high prevalence rate of IDA.[35] Moreover, nearly 10% of normal subjects have a false-positive OTOFT result.[34] To improve the efficacy of OTOFT, several studies compared its sensitivity and specificity using different buffered solutions.[34,41–43] So far, there is no consensus on a standard recommendation about the most suitable protocol for OTOFT.

Red blood cell indices: Mean corpuscular volume and mean corpuscular hemoglobin
An automated blood cell analyzer is one of the most important instruments in the modern hematology laboratory. In general, a blood sample is aspirated and separated into different fluidic streams, which contain different buffer solutions to achieve specific purposes of analysis, for an example, measuring Hbs in RBC using specific reagents such as Drapkin's solution. Briefly, measurements of each parameter occur under a principle of flow cytometry, as a single cell in fluidic stream passing through a laser beam and signals are collected from a series of detectors. For RBC indices, MCV, RBC count, Hb concentration, and RBC distribution width are measured directly, whereas hematocrit, mean cell Hb (MCH), and MCH concentration are calculated from these primary measurements. For thalassemia screening, an MCV of less than 80 fL and/or an MCH of less than 27 pg are generally used as cutoff levels for a positive screening result.[18] These cutoff levels are derived from –2 standard deviations of the normal distribution of MCV and MCH from normal population.

Advantages MCV and MCH are provided from an automated machine, which provides a rapid, cost effective, reproducible, and accurate analysis.

Disadvantages Several conditions such as IDA and anemia of inflammation can affect RBC indices, especially MCV, and these values could be as low as those found for thalassemia traits. Normal ranges of MCV vary by age in infants and young children.[44] In addition, there is variation in the MCV from different automated blood cell counters, although MCH cutoff levels seem to be more consistent among all analyzers.[45] Therefore, it is suggested to validate the cutoff levels for each analyzer used in a screening program.[45] It is well-noted that a low MCV is not suitable for screening Hb E carriers and individuals with single α-globin gene deletion ($-\alpha^{3.7}$ and $-\alpha^{4.2}$) or nondeletional α-globin gene mutations (ie, Hb Constant Spring [Hb CS] and Hb Quong Sze).[46] Moreover, the interaction of heterozygous β-thalassemia with α-thalassemia trait alone or with glucose-6-phosphate dehydrogenase deficiency may lead to normal MCV and a false-negative result for thalassemia screening.[30,47] Therefore, screening of thalassemia carriers by using RBC indices alone in a population with a high prevalence of α-thalassemia, β-thalassemia, and Hb E is not sufficient.[48]

Dichlorophenol indophenol precipitation test
As mentioned, RBC indices have a limitation on detecting Hb E traits. Screening of Hb E with the dichlorophenol indophenol (DCIP) test has been described since 1976.[49] Unstable Hb E results from the mutation on the β-globin gene at codon 26 (GAG > AAG), leading to a substitution of amino acid from glutamine to lysine, which can be oxidized by DCIP dye at a neutral pH. Apart from Hb E, other unstable Hbs such as Hb H can also be precipitated by this test. Technically, 20 μL of fresh whole blood is added to 2 mL of DCIP reagent. After gently mixing and incubation at 37°C for 15 minutes, 20 μL of stopping reagent is added to eliminate and decolorize excess DCIP dye.[25] Tests were interpreted by visualization by the naked eye. A clear solution

is interpreted as a negative result and a cloudy appearance or the presence of precipitation of Hb as a positive result.

Advantages The DCIP precipitation test for Hb E has been validated extensively and has a sensitivity of 98.1% to 100% and a specificity of 65.4% to 100%.[25,36–38] Also, it is a simple, fast, and economical technique.

Disadvantages Interpretation of a positive DCIP test could be difficult sometimes; equivocal or false-positive results were found in several compound heterozygotes of Hb variants, such as Hb S with Hb C and Hb S with Hb F.[50] Owing to the high false-positive rate, a new screening test for Hb E has been developed and showed satisfactory result with high sensitivity (100%) and specificity (99.1%-100%).[43,51] However, this test is not widely available and still needs to be validated further.

A combination of thalassemia screening techniques
A combination of one-tube osmotic fragility test and dichlorophenol indophenol tests To improve the sensitivity and specificity of screening methods, several authors have suggested using a combination of the previously mentioned techniques. A combination of OTOFT and DCIP has been extensively validated and the sensitivity and specificity of these methods were 99.2% to 100% and 79.3% to 97.1%, respectively.[37,52,53]

Although both methods are easy to perform, an appropriate interpretation of results requires a well-trained staff. False-positive rates were reported at between 15.5% and 36.1%.[25,37,54,55] A study in Thailand showed that this high false-positive rate led to a high economic burden for a confirmatory diagnosis by Hb analysis; however, a trend of false-positive rates during the first 10-year period decreased owing to training program and staff experience.[54] Another explanation for the high false-positive rate is a high prevalence of other milder forms of thalassemia and/or IDA.[25,54,55]

A combination of mean corpuscular volume and dichlorophenol indophenol testing The sensitivity and specificity of these combined tests were 99.4% to 100% and 76.2% to 98.93%, respectively,[52,55] and they have been proved to be cost effective in a thalassemia prevention program.[56] This combination is currently recommended to be used widely in Thailand[30] (**Fig. 3**). This model for a thalassemia screening program could be applied in resource-limited countries.

In summary, in countries with limited health resources, the use of MCV plus DCIP screening tests would help in selecting individuals requiring for a referral to a central laboratory for further definitive diagnosis for thalassemia.

Diagnostic Tests for Thalassemia
Interpretation of the peripheral blood smear
An important diagnostic tool for thalassemia is the interpretation of the peripheral blood smear (**Fig. 4**). Typical RBC morphology in thalassemia disease demonstrates microcytosis, hypochromia, apparent anisocytosis (variation in cell size), and poikilocytosis (variation in shape). Normally, microcytes can be evaluated by comparing the size of RBC with those of nucleus of small lymphocytes (see **Fig. 4**A, C, E, F). Hypochromic RBCs are those with increased diameter of central pallor of RBCs, more than one-third of their diameter. Anisopoikilocytosis results from various abnormal RBC morphology including schistocytes, microspherocytes, target cells, polychromasia, and nucleated RBCs (erythroblasts). The number of erythroblasts is related to the degree of anemia and is markedly increased after splenectomy (see **Fig. 4**D).[1]

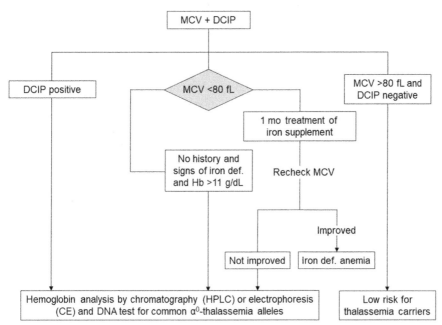

Fig. 3. Summary of a simple screening for thalassemia control program using mean corpuscular volume (MCV) and dichlorophenol indophenol precipitation (DCIP) tests. CE, capillary electrophoresis; def., deficiency; HPLC, high-performance liquid chromatography. (*Modified from* Viprakasit V, Limwongse C, Sukpanichnant S, et al. Problems in determining thalassemia carrier status in a program for prevention and control of severe thalassemia syndromes: a lesson from Thailand. Clin Chem Lab Med 2013;51(8):1612; with permission.)

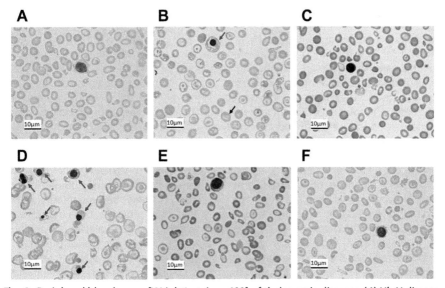

Fig. 4. Peripheral blood smear [Wright's stain, ×400] of thalassemia diseases. (*A*) Hb H disease. (*B*) Hb H/Hb CS disease. (*C*) β-Thalassemia intermedia. (*D*) Homozygous β-thalassemia (after splenectomy). (*E*) Hb E/β⁰-thalassemia. (*F*) AE Bart's disease (Hb H disease with Hb E trait). Basophilic stippling and nucleated red blood cells are shown by *black arrows* and *red arrows*, respectively.

In α-thalassemia, Hb H (see **Fig. 4**A), and Hb H/Hb CS disease (see **Fig. 4**B), the degree of anisopoikilocytosis varies according to the degree of hemolysis, with a higher hemolysis causing higher anisopoikilocytosis. Basophilic stippling of RBCs, small basophilic granules in RBCs representing ribosomes, are markedly present in the peripheral blood smear of those with Hb H/Hb CS disease or homozygous Hb CS. However, it can be apparently detected in those with acute anemia caused by any causes, even from normal individuals. In β-thalassemia diseases (see **Fig. 4**C, D) and Hb E/β-thalassemia (see **Fig. 4**E), anisopoikilocytosis is more prominent than those in a steady state of α-thalassemia (Hb H disease), reflecting greater ongoing active hemolysis and ineffective hematopoiesis in β-thalassemia syndromes.

For thalassemia carriers, RBC morphologic changes are less severe than in affected individuals.[1] Only hypochromic and microcytic red cells are evident, although numerous target cells can be found in Hb E homozygotes.[57] Erythroblasts are normally undetectable. Of note, it is recommended that an interpretation of the peripheral blood smear can only suggest those with thalassemia diseases from other causes of anemia, such as IDA or anemia of inflammation; however, it is not possible to define a specific type of thalassemia diseases based solely on RBC morphology.

Hemoglobin analysis

Hb analysis is an important laboratory evaluation to provide a presumptive identification and diagnosis of thalassemia and/or Hb variants diagnosis. However, to provide an accurate diagnosis, clinical information is needed, which includes age, ethnicity, history and onset of anemia, pregnancy status, history of blood transfusion (and the most recent date of transfusion), and family history. All this information is crucial for the interpretation of an Hb analysis. With an age-matched reference range, an Hb analysis could be performed at any age, even in the neonatal period.[32] Also, RBC indices and peripheral blood smears are helpful for obtaining a better interpretation of Hb analysis. There are several platforms of Hb analyzers, including Hb electrophoresis using cellulose acetate membrane (at pH 8.6), acid agarose (at pH 6.0) or citrate agar gel, isoelectric focusing, low-performance liquid chromatography, high-performance liquid chromatography (HPLC), and capillary electrophoresis (see **Table 2**).[58,59] Each method uses different principles to separate different species of Hb molecules, but some are tedious and obsolete.[59] At present there are 3 main platforms of Hb analyses commonly used. First, isoelectric focusing is a sensitive method, giving a good separation of Hb variants. However, isoelectric focusing requires considerably greater expertise for interpretation than acid agarose or citrate agar electrophoresis, because adducted Hb fractions could also be separated and might hamper interpretation.[59] HPLC provides an automated system with a good resolution to discriminate different Hb species.[60,61] HPLC has been widely adopted worldwide and the manufacturer has provided a standard library of Hb variants to help guiding presumptive diagnosis of thalassemia and Hb variants (https://hemoglobins.bio-rad.com). However, HPLC has a limitation to detect and quantify the percentages of Hb Bart's and Hb H based on their widely used β-thal short program; both substances are important in the diagnosis of α-thalassemia syndromes. Moreover, this technique has a low sensitivity to detect α-globin variants in particular Hb CS (a termination codon mutation of the α2 gene). In addition, it could not separate Hb A_2 from Hb E; therefore, these 2 Hb species are eluted into the same retention time, and the interpretation of Hb E traits and homozygous Hb E are based on the summation of both Hb E and Hb A_2 percentages.[57,62] Recently, a new capillary electrophoresis platform has become increasingly adopted in many laboratories, especially in the regions where Hb E and α-thalassemias are highly prevalent, such as Thailand. This new platform can provide an improving detection and quantification for Hb Bart's, Hb H, Hb CS, and Hb Q-Thailand (combined deletion and point mutation on the same allele) for both disease conditions and heterozygotes (**Fig. 5**). In addition, it can also separate Hb E from Hb A$_2$, this property can be useful when it comes to distinguishing between homozygous Hb E and Hb E/β-thalassemia.[62] Examples of different individuals with normal and various α- and β-thalassemia syndromes are shown in **Figs. 5** and **6**.

DNA or molecular analysis

Because thalassemia and hemoglobinopathy are mainly caused by mutations in globin genes, the molecular analysis of DNA sequences is the most definitive diagnosis modality for such conditions. At present, there are several measures to study the molecular basis of globin disorders. In principle, molecular studies of thalassemia could be divided into 2 main categories: mutation-specific detection and genome scanning (see **Table 2**). Mutation-specific detection makes use the information from any given population on their common profiles of both α-globin and β-globin mutations (deletions, point mutations, or gene rearrangements) to generate a panel of mutation

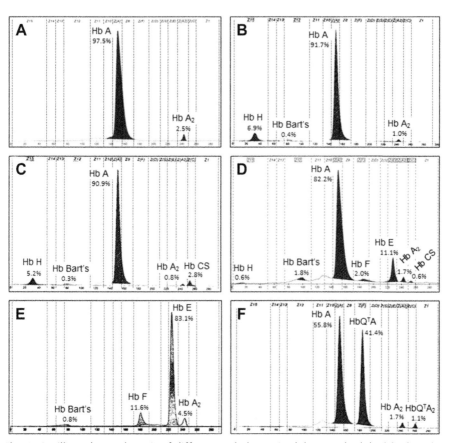

Fig. 5. Capillary electrophoresis of different α-thalassemia. (*A*) Normal adult. (*B*) Hb H disease. (*C*) Hb H/Hb CS disease. (*D*) AE Bart's CS disease (Hb H/Hb CS disease with Hb E heterozygote). (*E*) EF Bart's disease (Hb H disease with Hb E homozygote). (*F*) Hb Q-Thailand trait (an α globin variant). Hb, hemoglobin. ([*C, E*] *Courtesy of* N. Siritanaratkul, MD, Bangkok, Thailand.)

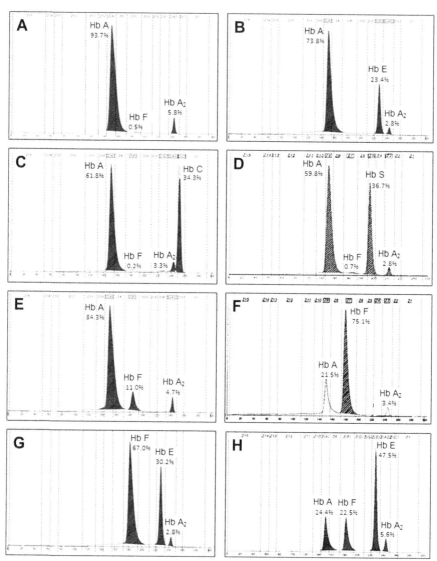

Fig. 6. Capillary electrophoresis of different β-thalassemia. (*A*) β-Thalassemia heterozygote. (*B*) Hb E heterozygote. (*C*) Hb C heterozygote. (*D*) Hb S heterozygote. (*E*) β-thalassemia intermedia. (*F*) Homozygous β-thalassemia (after transfusion). (*G*) Hb E/β⁰-thalassemia. (*H*) Hb E/β⁺-thalassemia. Hb, hemoglobin. ([*D, F*] *Courtesy of* N. Siritanaratkul, MD, Bangkok, Thailand.)

detection, and uses different polymerase chain reaction (PCR)-based methods to identify these known mutations. There are several molecular techniques used to detect known mutations, including GAP-PCR using conventional[63] or real-time detection (for gene deletions or insertions),[64] allele-related mutations specific PCR,[65-67] reverse dot blot hybridization[68] or array-based detection,[69] mismatched-PCR restriction fragment length polymorphism,[70] and analyses of a high-resolution melting curve (for point or small nucleotide changes).[71,72] Although this approach can provide a robust, cost-effective, and more rapid measure to identify causative mutations, it has also a limitation in that it cannot detect unknown or rare variations, which might not be included into the panels. Therefore, genome scanning (by denaturing gradient gel electrophoresis,[73] denaturing HPLC,[74] or single strand conformation polymorphism,[75] etc) and direct sequencing of the whole globin genes would be useful in such situations.[70] In addition, for genome deletions or rearrangement, a multiple ligation probe amplification assay has increasingly been adopted, because it can be used to scan the globin clusters first to determine the possibility of gene deletions, duplications, or rearrangement.[76] However, there would be a need for further confirmation by breakpoint identification using a CGH array.[77] Although this approach can detect almost all possible globin mutations causing thalassemia, it is costly, requires a high level of expertise, is not widely validated, and is available only in limited laboratories in the world (see **Table 2**).

In general, these mutation analyses would be critical for the confirmation of thalassemia diagnoses in only a few selected cases for whom the basic hematology and Hb analysis described could not provide a conclusive diagnosis. However, these molecular analyses would be indispensable in a program for the prevention and control of thalassemia syndromes because the mutation data would be required for genetic counseling, genetic risk calculation in the offspring, and prenatal and preimplantation genetic diagnosis. In addition, DNA analysis could help in predicting the clinical severity and guiding clinical management; milder β-globin mutations (β^+-thal) usually are associated with milder phenotypes, as been shown in Hb E/β-thalassemia.[78]

SUMMARY

Thalassemia diseases are classified into TDT and NTDT, based on patients' clinical severity whether they require regular blood transfusions to survive (TDT) or not (NTDT). Screening and definitive diagnoses of thalassemia and hemoglobinopathies require a comprehensive evaluation, from clinical history, physical examination, and laboratory results, including a complete blood count, Hb profiles, and molecular studies. There are several screening tools used in population screening. Clinicians need to understand the advantages and disadvantages of each laboratory method to select an appropriate diagnostic test and accurately interpret the results. An Hb analysis could be performed at any age; however, interpretation requires age-specific reference ranges. Genetic analysis for globin mutations are required to confirm clinical diagnosis in some but not all cases. Nevertheless, DNA testing would be indispensable for genetic counseling, risk calculation, and prenatal genetic diagnosis.

REFERENCES

1. Weatherall DJ, Clegg JB. The thalassaemia syndromes. 4th edition. Oxford: Blackwell Science; 2001.
2. Cappellini MD, Cohen A, Eleftheriou A, et al. Guidelines for the clinical management of thalassaemia. 2nd Revised edition. Nicosia (CY): Thalassaemia International Federation; 2008.
3. Taher AT, Musallam KM, Karimi M, et al. Overview on practices in thalassemia intermedia management aiming for lowering complication rates across a region of endemicity: the OPTIMAL CARE study. Blood 2010;115(10):1886–92.
4. Cappellini MD, Cohen A, Porter J, et al, editors. Guidelines for the management of transfusion dependent thalassaemia (TDT). 3rd edition. Nicosia (Cyprus): Thalassaemia International Federation; 2014.

5. Taher A, Vichinsky E, Musallam K, et al, editors. Guidelines for the management of non transfusion dependent thalassaemia (NTDT). Nicosia (Cyprus): Thalassaemia International Federation; 2013.

6. Taher AT, Cappellini MD, Musallam KM. Recent advances and treatment challenges in patients with non-transfusion-dependent thalassemia. Blood Rev 2012;26(Suppl 1):S1–2.

7. Songdej D, Babbs C, Higgs DR. An international registry of survivors with Hb Bart's hydrops fetalis syndrome. Blood 2017;129(10):1251–9.

8. Viprakasit V. Alpha thalassemia syndromes: from clinical and molecular diagnosis to bedside management. EHA Hematol Educ Program 2013;7:329–38.

9. Chan V, Chan TK, Liang ST, et al. Hydrops fetalis due to an unusual form of Hb H disease. Blood 1985;66(1):224–8.

10. Chan V, Chan VW, Tang M, et al. Molecular defects in Hb H hydrops fetalis. Br J Haematol 1997;96(2):224–8.

11. He S, Zheng C, Meng D, et al. Hb H Hydrops Fetalis Syndrome Caused by Association of the - -(SEA) Deletion and Hb Constant Spring (HBA2: c.427T > C) Mutation in a Chinese Family. Hemoglobin 2015;39(3):216–9.

12. Li DZ, Liao C, Li J, et al. Hemoglobin H hydrops fetalis syndrome resulting from the association of the - -SEA deletion and the alphaQuong Szealpha mutation in a Chinese woman. Eur J Haematol 2005;75(3):259–61.

13. Li J, Liao C, Zhou JY, et al. Phenotypic variability in a Chinese family with nondeletional Hb H-Hb Quong Sze disease. Hemoglobin 2011;35(4):430–3.

14. Lorey F, Charoenkwan P, Witkowska HE, et al. Hb H hydrops foetalis syndrome: a case report and review of literature. Br J Haematol 2001;115(1):72–8.

15. McBride KL, Snow K, Kubik KS, et al. Hb Dartmouth [alpha66(E15)Leu–>Pro (alpha2) (CTG–>CCG)]: a novel alpha2-globin gene mutation associated with severe neonatal anemia when inherited in trans with Southeast Asian alpha-thalassemia-1. Hemoglobin 2001;25(4):375–82.

16. Viprakasit V, Green S, Height S, et al. Hb H hydrops fetalis syndrome associated with the interaction of two common determinants of alpha thalassaemia (–MED/(alpha)TSaudi(alpha)). Br J Haematol 2002;117(3):759–62.

17. Zainal NZ, Alauddin H, Ahmad S, et al. alpha-Thalassemia with Haemoglobin Adana mutation: prenatal diagnosis. Malays J Pathol 2014;36(3):207–11.

18. Viprakasit V, Origa R. Genetic basis, pathophysiology and diagnosis [Chapter 1]. In: Cappellini MD, Cohen A, Porter J, et al, editors. Guidelines for the management of transfusion dependent thalassaemia (TDT). 3rd edition. Nicosia (CY): Thalassaemia International Federation; 2014. p. 14–26.

19. de Montalembert M, Girot R, Revillon Y, et al. Partial splenectomy in homozygous beta thalassaemia. Arch Dis Child 1990;65(3):304–7.

20. Weatherall DJ. The definition and epidemiology of non-transfusion-dependent thalassemia. Blood Rev 2012;26(Suppl 1):S3–6.

21. Taher AT, Radwan A, Viprakasit V. When to consider transfusion therapy for patients with non-transfusion-dependent thalassaemia. Vox Sang 2015;108(1):1–10.

22. Taher AT, Musallam KM, Cappellini MD, et al. Optimal management of beta thalassaemia intermedia. Br J Haematol 2011;152(5):512–23.

23. Taher AT, Musallam KM, Karimi M, et al. Splenectomy and thrombosis: the case of thalassemia intermedia. J Thromb Haemost 2010;8(10):2152–8.

24. Viprakasit V, Tyan P, Rodmai S, et al. Identification and key management of non-transfusion-dependent thalassaemia patients: not a rare but potentially underrecognised condition. Orphanet J Rare Dis 2014;9:131.

25. Fucharoen G, Sanchaisuriya K, Sae-ung N, et al. A simplified screening strategy for thalassaemia and haemoglobin E in rural communities in south-east Asia. Bull World Health Organ 2004;82(5):364–72.
26. Silvestroni E, Bianco I. Screening for microcytemia in Italy: analysis of data collected in the past 30 years. Am J Hum Genet 1975;27(2):198–212.
27. Bain BJ. Haemoglobinopathy diagnosis: algorithms, lessons and pitfalls. Blood Rev 2011;25(5):205–13.
28. Harteveld CL. State of the art and new developments in molecular diagnostics for hemoglobinopathies in multiethnic societies. Int J Lab Hematol 2014;36(1):1–12.
29. Cao A, Congiu R, Sollaino MC, et al. Thalassaemia and glucose-6-phosphate dehydrogenase screening in 13- to 14-year-old students of the Sardinian population: preliminary findings. Community Genet 2008;11(3):121–8.
30. Viprakasit V, Limwongse C, Sukpanichnant S, et al. Problems in determining thalassemia carrier status in a program for prevention and control of severe thalassemia syndromes: a lesson from Thailand. Clin Chem Lab Med 2013;51(8):1605–14.
31. Streetly A, Latinovic R, Hall K, et al. Implementation of universal newborn bloodspot screening for sickle cell disease and other clinically significant haemoglobinopathies in England: screening results for 2005-7. J Clin Pathol 2009;62(1):26–30.
32. Jindatanmanusan P, Riolueang S, Glomglao W, et al. Diagnostic applications of newborn screening for alpha-thalassaemias, haemoglobins E and H disorders using isoelectric focusing on dry blood spots. Ann Clin Biochem 2014;51(Pt 2):237–47.
33. Parpart AK, Lorenz PB, Parpart ER, et al. The osmotic resistance (fragility) of human red cells. J Clin Invest 1947;26(4):636–40.
34. Kattamis C, Efremov G, Pootrakul S. Effectiveness of one tube osmotic fragility screening in detecting beta-thalassaemia trait. J Med Genet 1981;18(4):266–70.
35. El-Beshlawy A, Kaddah N, Moustafa A, et al. Screening for beta-thalassaemia carriers in Egypt: significance of the osmotic fragility test. East Mediterr Health J 2007;13(4):780–6.
36. Fucharoen S, Fucharoen G, Sanchaisuriya K, et al. Molecular analysis of a Thai beta-thalassaemia heterozygote with normal haemoglobin A2 level: implication for population screening. Ann Clin Biochem 2002;39(Pt 1):44–9.
37. Sangkitporn S, Sangnoi A, Supangwiput O, et al. Validation of osmotic fragility test and dichlorophenol indophenol precipitation test for screening of thalassemia and Hb E. Southeast Asian J Trop Med Public Health 2005;36(6):1538–42.
38. Winichagoon P, Thitivichianlert A, Lebnak T, et al. Screening for the carriers of thalassemias and abnormal hemoglobins at the community level. Southeast Asian J Trop Med Public Health 2002;33(Suppl 2):145–50.
39. Penman BS, Gupta S, Weatherall DJ. Epistasis and the sensitivity of phenotypic screens for beta thalassaemia. Br J Haematol 2015;169(1):117–28.
40. Fucharoen G, Fucharoen S, Singsanan S, et al. Coexistence of Southeast Asian ovalocytosis and beta-thalassemia: a molecular and hematological analysis. Am J Hematol 2007;82(5):381–5.
41. Chow J, Phelan L, Bain BJ. Evaluation of single-tube osmotic fragility as a screening test for thalassemia. Am J Hematol 2005;79(3):198–201.
42. Panyasai S, Sringam P, Fucharoen G, et al. A simplified screening for alpha-thalassemia 1 (SEA type) using a combination of a modified osmotic fragility test and a direct PCR on whole blood cell lysates. Acta Haematol 2002;108(2):74–8.
43. Wanapirak C, Sirichotiyakul S, Luewan S, et al. Comparison of the accuracy of dichlorophenolindophenol (DCIP), modified DCIP, and hemoglobin E tests to screen for the HbE trait in pregnant women. Int J Gynaecol Obstet 2009;107(1):59–60.

44. Gajjar R, Jalazo E. Hematology [Chapter 14]. In: Flerlage J, Engorn B, editors. The Harriet Lane handbook: a manual for pediatric house officers. 20th edition. Philadelphia: Saunders/Elsevier; 2015. p. 305–33.
45. Chaitraiphop C, Sanchaisuriya K, Inthavong S, et al. Thalassemia screening using different automated blood cell counters: consideration of appropriate cutoff values. Clin Lab 2016;62(4):545–52.
46. Chan LC, Ma SK, Chan AY, et al. Should we screen for globin gene mutations in blood samples with mean corpuscular volume (MCV) greater than 80 fL in areas with a high prevalence of thalassaemia? J Clin Pathol 2001;54(4):317–20.
47. Melis MA, Pirastu M, Galanello R, et al. Phenotypic effect of heterozygous alpha and beta 0-thalassemia interaction. Blood 1983;62(1):226–9.
48. Maccioni L, Cao A. Osmotic fragility test in heterozygotes for alpha and beta thalassaemia. J Med Genet 1985;22(5):374–6.
49. Kulapongs P, Sangunasermsri T, Mertz G, et al. Dichlorophenol indophenol (DCIP) precipitation test: a new screening test of Hb E and H. J Paediatr Soc Thai 1976;15:1–7.
50. Chapple L, Harris A, Phelan L, et al. Reassessment of a simple chemical method using DCIP for screening for haemoglobin E. J Clin Pathol 2006;59(1):74–6.
51. Sirichotiyakul S, Tongprasert F, Tongsong T. Screening for hemoglobin E trait in pregnant women. Int J Gynaecol Obstet 2004;86(3):390–1.
52. Prayongratana K, Polprasert C, Raungrongmorakot K, et al. Low cost combination of DCIP and MCV was better than that of DCIP and OF in the screening for hemoglobin E. J Med Assoc Thai 2008;91(10):1499–504.
53. Savongsy O, Fucharoen S, Fucharoen G, et al. Thalassemia and hemoglobinopathies in pregnant Lao women: carrier screening, prevalence and molecular basis. Ann Hematol 2008;87(8):647–54.
54. Jopang Y, Thinkhamrop B, Puangpruk R, et al. False positive rates of thalassemia screening in rural clinical setting: 10-year experience in Thailand. Southeast Asian J Trop Med Public Health 2009;40(3):576–80.
55. Sanchaisuriya K, Fucharoen S, Fucharoen G, et al. A reliable screening protocol for thalassemia and hemoglobinopathies in pregnancy: an alternative approach to electronic blood cell counting. Am J Clin Pathol 2005;123(1):113–8.
56. Ratanasiri T, Charoenthong C, Komwilaisak R, et al. Prenatal prevention for severe thalassemia disease at Srinagarind Hospital. J Med Assoc Thai 2006; 89(Suppl 4):S87–93.
57. Tachavanich K, Viprakasit V, Chinchang W, et al. Clinical and hematological phenotype of homozygous hemoglobin E: revisit of a benign condition with hidden reproductive risk. Southeast Asian J Trop Med Public Health 2009;40(2): 306–16.
58. Barrett AN, Saminathan R, Choolani M. Thalassaemia screening and confirmation of carriers in parents. Best Pract Res Clin Obstet Gynaecol 2017;39:27–40.
59. Bain BJ. Laboratory techniques for the identification of abnormalities of globin chain synthesis. Haemoglobinopathy diagnosis. 2nd edition. Malden (MA): Blackwell; 2006. p. 26–62.
60. Joutovsky A, Hadzi-Nesic J, Nardi MA. HPLC retention time as a diagnostic tool for hemoglobin variants and hemoglobinopathies: a study of 60000 samples in a clinical diagnostic laboratory. Clin Chem 2004;50(10):1736–47.
61. Szuberski J, Oliveira JL, Hoyer JD. A comprehensive analysis of hemoglobin variants by high-performance liquid chromatography (HPLC). Int J Lab Hematol 2012;34(6):594–604.

62. Sae-ung N, Srivorakun H, Fucharoen G, et al. Phenotypic expression of hemoglobins A(2), E and F in various hemoglobin E related disorders. Blood Cells Mol Dis 2012;48(1):11–6.
63. Tan AS, Quah TC, Low PS, et al. A rapid and reliable 7-deletion multiplex polymerase chain reaction assay for alpha-thalassemia. Blood 2001;98(1):250–1.
64. Kho SL, Chua KH, George E, et al. A novel gap-PCR with high resolution melting analysis for the detection of alpha-thalassaemia Southeast Asian and Filipino beta degrees -thalassaemia deletion. Sci Rep 2015;5:13937.
65. Eng B, Patterson M, Walker L, et al. Detection of severe nondeletional alpha-thalassemia mutations using a single-tube multiplex ARMS assay. Genet Test 2001;5(4):327–9.
66. Viprakasit V, Tachavanich K, Suwantol L, et al. Allele related mutation specific-polymerase chain reaction for rapid diagnosis of Hb New York (beta 113 (G15) Val->Glu, beta(CD113 GTG->GAG)). J Med Assoc Thai 2002;85(Suppl 2): S558–63.
67. Viprakasit V, Chinchang W, Pung-Amritt P, et al. Identification of Hb Q-India (alpha64 Asp->His) in Thailand. Hematology 2004;9(2):151–5.
68. Sutcharitchan P, Saiki R, Huisman TH, et al. Reverse dot-blot detection of the African-American beta-thalassemia mutations. Blood 1995;86(4):1580–5.
69. Chan K, Wong MS, Chan TK, et al. A thalassaemia array for Southeast Asia. Br J Haematol 2004;124(2):232–9.
70. Viprakasit V, Tanphaichitr VS, Pung-Amritt P, et al. Clinical phenotypes and molecular characterization of Hb H-Pakse disease. Haematologica 2002;87(2):117–25.
71. Sirichotiyakul S, Wanapirak C, Saetung R, et al. High resolution DNA melting analysis: an application for prenatal control of alpha-thalassemia. Prenat Diagn 2010; 30(4):348–51.
72. Pornprasert S, Sukunthamala K, Kunyanone N, et al. Analysis of real-time PCR cycle threshold of alpha-thalassemia-1 Southeast Asian type deletion using fetal cell-free DNA in maternal plasma for noninvasive prenatal diagnosis of Bart's hydrops fetalis. J Med Assoc Thai 2010;93(11):1243–8.
73. Harteveld KL, Heister AJ, Giordano PC, et al. Rapid detection of point mutations and polymorphisms of the alpha-globin genes by DGGE and SSCA. Hum Mutat 1996;7(2):114–22.
74. Hung CC, Lee CN, Chen CP, et al. Molecular assay of -alpha(3.7) and -alpha(4.2) deletions causing alpha-thalassemia by denaturing high-performance liquid chromatography. Clin Biochem 2007;40(11):817–21.
75. Chinchang W, Viprakasit V, Pung-Amritt P, et al. Molecular analysis of unknown beta-globin gene mutations using polymerase chain reaction-single strand conformation polymorphism (PCR-SSCP) technique and its application in Thai families with beta-thalassemias and beta-globin variants. Clin Biochem 2005; 38(11):987–96.
76. Harteveld CL, Voskamp A, Phylipsen M, et al. Nine unknown rearrangements in 16p13.3 and 11p15.4 causing alpha- and beta-thalassaemia characterised by high resolution multiplex ligation-dependent probe amplification. J Med Genet 2005;42(12):922–31.
77. Blattner A, Brunner-Agten S, Ludin K, et al. Detection of germline rearrangements in patients with alpha- and beta-thalassemia using high resolution array CGH. Blood Cells Mol Dis 2013;51(1):39–47.
78. Viprakasit V, Tanphaichitr VS, Chinchang W, et al. Evaluation of alpha hemoglobin stabilizing protein (AHSP) as a genetic modifier in patients with beta thalassemia. Blood 2004;103(9):3296–9.

Ineffective Erythropoiesis: Anemia and Iron Overload

Ritama Gupta, PhD[a], Khaled M. Musallam, MD, PhD[b],
Ali T. Taher, MD, PhD, FRCP[c], Stefano Rivella, PhD[a,d,*]

KEYWORDS

- Erythroblastic island • Hepcidin and iron homeostasis
- Stress and ineffective erythropoiesis • Iron overload

KEY POINTS

- Stress erythropoiesis (SE) is characterized by an imbalance in erythroid proliferation and differentiation under increased demands of erythrocyte generation and tissue oxygenation.
- β-thalassemia represents a chronic state of SE, called ineffective erythropoiesis (IE), exhibiting an expansion of erythroid-progenitor pool and deposition of alpha chains on erythrocyte membranes, causing cell death and anemia. Concurrently, there is a decrease in hepcidin expression and a subsequent state of iron overload.
- There are substantial investigative efforts to target increased iron absorption under IE, by genetic and pharmacologic agents. There are also avenues for targeting cell-contact and signaling within erythroblastic islands under SE for therapeutic benefits.

Erythrocytes are the primary carrier of oxygen in vertebrate systems. The oxygen-carrying capacity of erythrocytes stems from their key constituent heme, capable of binding to iron and delivering oxygen to tissue through circulating red blood cells (RBCs). As a result, erythropoiesis and iron levels are tightly linked in mammalian

Conflict of Interest Statement: K.M. Musallam received honoraria from Novartis, Celgene, and CRISPR Therapeutics. A.T. Taher received research support and honoraria from Novartis and research support from Celgene and Roche. S. Rivella is a member of scientific advisory board of Ionis Pharmaceuticals. S. Rivella is sponsored by Ionis Pharmaceuticals. R. Gupta declares no conflict of interest. Work related to this article was funded by grants from the NIH-NIDDK: R01 DK095112 and R01 DK090554 (S. Rivella).

[a] Department of Pediatrics, Division of Hematology, Children's Hospital of Philadelphia (CHOP), 3401 Civic Center Boulevard, Philadelphia, PA 19104, USA; [b] International Network of Hematology, London WC1V 6AX, UK; [c] Department of Internal Medicine, American University of Beirut Medical Center, PO Box: 11-0236, Cairo Street, Hamra, Raid E Solh, Beirut 1107 2020, Lebanon; [d] Children's Hospital of Philadelphia (CHOP), Cell and Molecular Biology Graduate Group (CAMB), University of Pennsylvania, Abramson Research Center, 3615 Civic Center Boulevard, Room 316B, Philadelphia, PA 19104, USA
* Corresponding author. Children's Hospital of Philadelphia (CHoP), Cell and Molecular Biology Graduate Group (CAMB), University of Pennsylvania, Abramson Research Center, 3615 Civic Center Boulevard, Room 316B, Philadelphia, PA 19104.
E-mail address: rivellas@email.chop.edu

Hematol Oncol Clin N Am 32 (2018) 213–221
https://doi.org/10.1016/j.hoc.2017.11.009
0889-8588/18/© 2017 Elsevier Inc. All rights reserved.

hemonc.theclinics.com

systems in order to maintain a healthy balance of iron utilization for the generation of new erythroblasts and iron recycling from senescent erythrocytes.

Iron has unique properties that make it crucial to the functioning of the mammalian physiologic system. One such property is its interconversion from the ferric (Fe^{3+}) to the ferrous (Fe^{2+}) form.[1] Although this makes iron an essential component of oxygen-carrying proteins like hemoglobin and myoglobin, as well as many redox enzymes, it also allows iron to generate harmful oxidative radicals.[2] This dichotomous nature of iron functioning requires this element to be tightly regulated. Loss of this regulation is the underlying cause of many disorders, with symptoms ranging from anemia to hemochromatosis (iron overload). Although many of these disorders have been identified and some characterized, their underlying molecular mechanisms have only recently begun to be elucidated.

ERYTHROPOIESIS AND THE ERYTHROBLASTIC ISLAND

Erythropoiesis occurs in specialized niches within the bone marrow and the spleen consisting of a central nursing macrophage surrounded by erythroid cells in different stages of differentiation. Although the first erythroblastic island was observed by Bessis and colleagues[3] through electron micrographs, long-term liquid cultures of bone marrow cells have also been used to generate erythroblastic islands in vitro. Erythroblastic islands have also been isolated and cultured from the spleens of phlebotomized mice, whereby the central stromal macrophage extended cytoplasmic processes to surrounding erythroblasts with the erythrobalsts also exhibiting differentiation.[4] Moreover, cell-to-cell adhesion has been shown to be a key factor regulating erythroid differentiation in an erythroblastic island. Adhesion within an erythroblastic island is not only mediated by the erythroblast macrophage protein, as demonstrated extensively using knock-out mice of this protein that are embryonic lethal, but also by the intracellular adhesion molecule-4 (ICAM-4) such that mice lacking ICAM-4 shows significantly reduced erythroblastic islands.[5] Furthermore, blocking the interaction between ICAM-4 on erythroid cells and α-V integrin on macrophages results in a marked reduction of erythroblastic islands.[6] Interaction between vascular cell adhesion protein 1 (VCAM-1) and Beta-1 integrin has also been implicated in erythroid macrophage contact within the erythroblastic island[7] (**Fig. 1**).

Erythropoiesis within erythroblastic islands consists of multiple developmental stages. Erythroid progenitor proliferation begins as multipotent hematopoietic stem cells proliferate and differentiate into the burst-forming unit-erythroid stage, which in turn gives rise to the colony-forming unit-erythroid. Terminal erythroid differentiation begins at the proerythroblast stage. This stage undergoes 3 consecutive mitoses to generate basophilic erythroblast followed by polychromatic erythroblast and then orthochromatic erythroblasts. The orthochromatic cells expel their nuclei to generate reticulocytes, which undergo further changes to give rise to erythrocytes or RBCs.[8] The different stages of terminal erythroid differentiation have been elucidated both by sequencing of RNA and by morphology.[9]

Hepcidin and Iron Homeostasis

Hepcidin (HAMP) is considered a key regulatory molecule of systemic iron homeostasis, produced primarily by hepatocytes.[10,11] HAMP acts as a negative regulator of iron availability by preventing the export of iron from duodenal enterocytes, hepatocytes, macrophages, and placental trophoblasts. High levels of HAMP trigger hypoferremia, as evidenced by studies whereby a single dose of 50 ug of HAMP in mice caused a rapid decrease in serum iron in 1 hour. HAMP carries out this negative regulation of

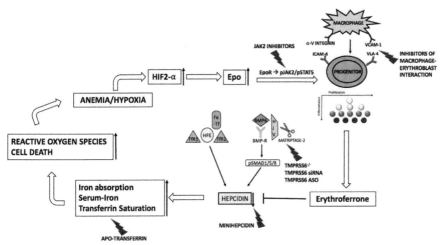

Fig. 1. Ineffective erythropoiesis and its therapeutic targeting. Epo, erythropoietin; EpoR, erythropoietin receptor.

iron availability by directly binding to and degrading the iron exporter ferroportin (FPN).[12,13] In a feedback loop, HAMP in itself is also regulated by the element it controls: iron. This regulation happens such that when iron levels are plentiful, HAMP expression is upregulated. Conversely, under conditions of iron deficiency, HAMP expression is downregulated, releasing iron into circulation, thereby increasing transferrin (TF) saturation and plasma iron levels.[14–17]

One pathway controlling HAMP expression involves iron availability and the presence of holo-TF. This pathway controlling HAMP expression is mediated by the membrane protein HFE. Under conditions of high serum iron levels and TF saturation or increased concentrations of holo-TF, the membrane protein HFE, generally sequestered away by binding to TF receptor 1 (TFR1), is displaced to TF receptor 2 (TFR2), thereby forming an Fe-TF, HFE, TFR2 complex. This complex has been implicated in upregulating the transcription of HAMP[18–20] (see **Fig. 1**). The key pathway in inducing expression of HAMP involves BMP6, binding to the bone morphogenic protein (BMP) receptor I and II complex, including the BMP coreceptor hemojuvelin (HJV), which confers sensitivity of binding. Activation of the BMP receptor leads to phosphorylation of SMAD1/5/8 in the cytosol, and the latter then goes on to interact and form a complex with SMAD 4, which translocates to the nucleus and induces the expression of HAMP.[21–24] A serine protease Matriptase-2 encoded by the TMPRSS6 gene is capable of cleaving the BMP coreceptor HJV (see **Fig. 1**). Thus, it negatively regulates the expression of HAMP such that TMPRSS6$^{-/-}$ mice have severe iron deficiency anemia.[25–29]

Stress and Ineffective Erythropoiesis

Erythropoiesis is driven by the kidney hormone erythropoietin (EPO) (see **Fig. 1**). EPO binding to the EPO-receptor triggers activation of Janus kinase 2 (JAK2) and phosphorylated JAK2 can bind to signal transducers and activators of transcription 5 (STAT5) wherein the JAK2-STAT5 complex translocates to the nucleus and induces expression of target genes,[30] including but not limited to iron responsive element binding protein 2 and antiapoptotic factors, such as BCL-XL.[31] Under conditions of acute blood loss or demands for increased oxygenation, the existing cellular hypoxia controls EPO expression through hypoxia inducible factor alpha 2. Upregulated EPO expression elicits an increased erythropoietic response, referred to as stress erythropoiesis. Stress erythropoiesis is characterized by an imbalance of erythroid proliferation and the differentiation axis, resulting in an expansion of the erythroid progenitor pool to meet the demands of increased RBC generation and oxygenation. Erythropoiesis extends to extramedullary sites, such as the liver and the spleen; indeed, splenomegaly is another hallmark of stress erythropoiesis. Under these conditions, increased iron absorption is facilitated by the erythroid factor erythroferrone (ERFE) produced by erythroid progenitors, which act on the liver by an as-yet-unknown mechanism to suppress HAMP expression.[30,32] This process, with a concurrent upregulation of EPO, works to increase the generation of RBCs, iron availability, and oxygenation of tissues under conditions of stress erythropoiesis.[30]

A chronic state of stress, erythropoiesis seen in certain disorders is referred to as ineffective erythropoiesis. Under ineffective erythropoiesis, the imbalance of erythroid proliferation and differentiation is characterized by an increase in erythroblast proliferation that fails to differentiate and give rise to enucleate RBCs, thereby resulting in anemia. The disease model of β-thalassemia has been used to study and characterize ineffective erythropoiesis. In the face of a lack of decreased generation of beta globin chains, there is an accumulation of alpha chains that get deposited on erythroid membranes, generating hemichromes, causing substantial oxidative stress and cell death. As result of this, despite an expansion of the erythroid progenitor pool, a continuous state of chronic stress erythropoiesis ensues and the expanded pool of erythroid precursors are unable to generate RBCs. The resulting anemia is also accompanied by a decrease in expression of HAMP, thereby increasing iron availability. Indeed, it has been shown that ERFE expression is upregulated in the mouse model of β-thalassemia intermedia ($Hbb^{th3/+}$).[33] Thus, despite the inability to generate RBCs due to apoptosis of erythroid precursors, the ineffective erythropoiesis in β-thalassemia is characterized by increased serum EPO levels and concurrent decrease in HAMP levels, leading to increased iron absorption and iron overload.

The pathophysiology of ineffective erythropoiesis has been attributed in part to macrophages, which are a key component of erythroblastic islands within the bone marrow and the spleen. Depletion of macrophages by clodronate-encapsulated liposomes or by using CD169 DTR mice substantially ameliorated anemia and splenomegaly seen in a mouse model of β-thalassemia intermedia.[34,35] The various proteins and pathways implicated in maintaining contact between the central nursing macrophage and surrounding erythroblasts, including focal adhesion kinase signaling downstream of alpha4beta1 integrin, potentially contributes to the macrophage-mediated pathophysiology seen in the ineffective erythropoiesis of β-thalassemia. The underlying mechanism of this remains unknown.

There are also other factors that have also been implicated in anemia associated with ineffective erythropoiesis seen in β-thalassemia, primarily associated with the imbalance of alpha-beta chains. One such factor is heat shock protein 70 (HSP 70), which translocates to the nucleus and protects the erythroid transcription factor GATA1 from cleavage by caspase 3. In in vitro studies of human BM erythroblasts from β-thalassemic patients have shown that HSP 70 is sequestered by alpha chains as a result of which GATA1 is cleaved and erythroid maturation is impaired. Another factor is growth differentiation factor 11 (GDF11), a member of the transforming growth factor beta super family that has been shown to be elevated in both β-thalassemia and another disorder exhibiting some hallmarks of ineffective erythropoiesis, myelodysplastic syndrome. There is also work to indicate that blocking GDF11 using trap ligands can reduce precipitation of alpha globin chains on erythroid membranes and subsequent oxidative stress, although the complete mechanism has not been completely elucidated.[36,37]

In the absence of transfusion therapy, ineffective erythropoiesis in β-thalassemia patients is associated with local bone defects due to marrow expansion and the appearance of extramedullary hematopoietic pseudotumors. It is also associated with several clinical sequelae because of the resulting anemia and iron overload. A hypercoagulable state due to premature red cell death has also been described in this patient population, leading to frequent thrombotic and other vascular events.[38–42]

Iron Overload and Its Therapeutic Targeting

Downregulated HAMP and its subsequent impact on iron homeostasis results in increased iron absorption and a state of iron overload and ensuing oxidative stress. Primary disorders of iron overload include hereditary hemochromatosis (HH), the most common cause of which is mutations in the gene HFE. β-thalassemia is also associated with iron overload due to HAMP downregulation by ineffective erythropoiesis, as stated earlier. Although iron loading from increased intestinal absorption in β-thalassemia is slower than that secondary to regular transfusion therapy, it can still reach clinically significant thresholds associated with serious morbidity. Other iron overloading anemias that exhibit some hallmarks of ineffective erythropoiesis are autosomal recessive disorders caused by mutations in Codenin-1 (CDA-1).[43] GDF15 has been found to downregulate HAMP in vitro and is upregulated in patients with both β-thalassemia and CDA-1, indicating that this factor might be an important biomarker of ineffective erythropoiesis and iron overload. The exact role of this factor in ineffective erythropoiesis, if at all, remains debatable.[44,45]

Several avenues have been explored to target the ineffective erythropoiesis and iron overload in mouse models of nontransfusion-dependent β-thalassemia (see Fig. 1). Given the significant role of TMPRSS6 in cleaving HAMP, genetic or pharmacologic depletion of TMPRSS6 has been the subject of much study. TMPRSS6−/− mice crossed with a mouse model of β-thalassemia intermedia ($Hbb^{th3/+}$) resulted in improved splenomegaly, anemia, and iron loading.[60] Moreover, targeting TMPRSS6 using small interfering RNA (siRNA) and antisense oligonucleotides (ASOs) significantly improved anemia and reduced hemichrome formation in $Hbb^{th3/+}$ mice.[46,47] TMPRSS6 ASOs were also able to decrease serum iron TF saturation and liver iron accumulation in HFE-/- mice exhibiting HH.[48] Additionally, minihepcidins, which are small molecule agonists mimetic of HAMP activity and are capable of binding to and degrading FPN, have also been used in preclinical studies of $Hbb^{th3/+}$ mice showing amelioration of anemia and symptoms of ineffective erythropoiesis.[49] The minihepcidins, TMPRSS6 ASO, and TMPRSS6 siRNA therapies have also been used in combination with the treatment of the iron chelator deferiprone to target organ iron content under conditions of ameliorating ineffective erythropoiesis.[49–51] Additional therapies that have also been in use involve the administration of Apo TF in $Hbb^{th3/+}$ as well as $Hbb^{th1/th1}$ animals showing a substantial decrease in iron overload, hemichrome formation, and improvement of anemia.[43,52] Other preclinical studies encompassing therapies to ameliorate ineffective erythropoiesis include the use of JAK2 inhibitors. Given the role of the JAK2-STAT5 pathway in EPO production under hypoxic conditions and stress erythropoiesis, these seem to be an ideal possibility for therapeutic targeting. Indeed, the use of JAK2 inhibitor in animals affected by β-thalassemia shows significant reduction of splenomegaly and improvement of anemia.[53] Additionally, ligand traps based on the extracellular domains of activing receptors, such as RAP011 and RAP536, which target GDF11, have been shown to improve the erythroid precursor to mature RBC ratio in both $Hbb^{th3/+}$ and $Hbb^{th1/th1}$ animals, with amelioration of splenomegaly, anemia, and iron-overloading conditions.[54]

CONCLUDING REMARKS

The current understanding of iron homeostasis and its dysregulation warrants a 2-pronged approach at combating iron overload under conditions of ineffective erythropoiesis. The first one involves a reduction of iron absorption. Both preclinical and preliminary clinical studies show promise in reducing the burden of iron excess, with or without the combination of iron chelators, the latter being in clinical use to treat iron overload. However, the second approach points toward the possible iron-independent role of macrophages within erythroblastic island under stress erythropoiesis. Macrophage-erythroblast interactions could trigger signaling that promotes erythroid proliferation, tipping the balance of erythroid proliferation versus differentiation, that is, characteristic of pathophysiologic stress erythropoiesis in β-thalassemia. Understanding the proteins and pathways involved in these interactions within the erythroblastic island might be key to identifying new therapeutic targets for ameliorating the symptoms of ineffective erythropoiesis. There is substantial investigative appreciation for both these approaches; it is hoped that this will help us better understand and treat iron overload and ineffective erythropoiesis in clinical settings.

ACKNOWLEDGMENTS

The authors extend special thanks to Ping La (Children's Hospital of Philadelphia) for helpful discussion and support.

REFERENCES

1. Lewis GK, Drickamer HG. High pressure Mossbauer resonance studies of the conversion of Fe(III) to Fe(II) in Ferric halides. Proc Natl Acad Sci U S A 1968;61(2):414–21.
2. Rice-Evans C, Baysal E. Iron-mediated oxidative stress in erythrocytes. Biochem J 1987;244(1):191–6.
3. Bessis M, Mize C, Prenant M. Erythropoiesis: comparison of in vivo and in vitro amplification. Blood cells 1978;4(102):155–74.
4. Sadahira Y, Mori M, Kimoto T. Isolation and short-term culture of mouse splenic erythroblastic islands. Cell Struct Func 1990;15(1):59–65.
5. Chasis JA. Erythroblastic islands: specialized microenvironmental niches for erythropoiesis. Curr Opin Hematol 2006;13(3):137–41.
6. Mohandas N, Chasis JA. The erythroid niche: molecular processes occurring within erythroblastic islands. Transfus Clin Biol 2010;17(3):110–1.
7. Sadahira Y, Yoshino T, Monobe Y. Very late activation antigen 4-vascular cell adhesion molecule 1 interaction is involved in the formation of erythroblastic islands. J Exp Med 1995;181(1):411–5.
8. Liu J, Zhang J, Ginzburg Y, et al. Qualitative analysis of murine terminal erythroid differentiation in vivo: novel method to study normal and disordered erythropoiesis. Blood 2013;121(8):e43–9.
9. Hu J, Liu J, Xue F, et al. Isolation and functional characterization of human erythroblasts at distinct stages: implications for understanding of normal and disordered erythropoiesis in vivo. Blood 2013;121(16):3246–53.
10. Park CH, Valore EV, Waring AJ, et al. Hepcidin, a urinary antimicrobial peptide synthesized in the liver. J Biol Chem 2001;276(11):7806–10.

11. Fleming RE, Sly WS. Hepcidin: a putative iron regulatory hormone relevant to hereditary hemochromatosis and the anemia of chronic disease. Proc Natl Acad Sci U S A 2001;98(15):8160–2.

12. Rivera S, Nemeth E, Gabayan V, et al. Synthetic hepcidin causes rapid dose dependent hypoferremia and is concentrated in ferroportin containing organs. Blood 2005;106(6):2196–9.

13. Fleming RE, Sly WS. Mechanisms of iron accumulation in hereditary hemochromatosis. Annu Rev Physiol 2002;64:663–80.

14. Nemeth E, Tuttle MS, Powelson J, et al. Hepcidin regulates cellular iron efflux by binding to ferroportin and inducing its internalization. Science 2004;306(5704): 2090–3.

15. Nicolas G, Chauvet C, Viatte L, et al. The gene encoding the iron regulatory peptide hepcidin is regulated by anemia hypoxia and inflammation. J Clin Invest 2002;110(7):1037–44.

16. Frazer DM, Wilkins SJ, Becker EM, et al. Hepcidin expression inversely correlates with the expression of duodenal iron transporters and iron absorption in rats. Gastroenterology 2002;123(3):835–44.

17. Nicolas G, Viatte L, Lou DQ, et al. Constitutive iron expression prevents iron overload in a mouse model of hemochromatosis. Nat Genet 2003;34(1):97–101.

18. Adamsky K, Weizer O, Amariglio N, et al. Decreased hepcidin mRNA expression in thalassemic mice. Br J Haematol 2004;124(1):123–4.

19. Papanikolaou G, Samuels ME, Ludwig EH, et al. Mutations in HFE2 cause iron overload in chromosome 1q-linked juvenile hemochoromatosis. Nat Genet 2004;36(1):77–82.

20. Feder JN, Penny DM, Irrinki A, et al. The hemochromatosis gene product complexes with the transferrin receptor and lowers its affinity for ligand binding. Proc Natl Acad Sci U S A 1998;95(4):1472–7.

21. West AP Jr, Bennett MJ, Sellers VM, et al. Comparison of the interactions of transferrin receptor and transferrin receptor 2 with transferrin and the hereditary hemochromatosis protein HFE. J Biol Chem 2000;275(49):38135–8.

22. Goswami T, Andrews NC. Hereditary hemochromatosis protein HFE interaction with transferrin receptor 2 suggests a molecular mechanism for mammalian iron sensing. J Biol Chem 2006;281(39):28494–8.

23. Andriopoulos B Jr, Corradini E, Xia Y, et al. BMP6 is a key endogenous regulator of hepcidin expression and iron metabolism. Nat Genet 2009;41(4):482–7.

24. Meynard D, Kautz L, Darnaud V, et al. Lack of bone morphogenic protein BMP6 induces mass iron overload. Nat Genet 2009;41(4):478–81.

25. Zhang AS, Gao J, Koeberl DD, et al. The role of hepatocyte hemojuvelin in the regulation of bone morphogenic protein-6 and hepcidin expression in vivo. J Biol Chem 2010;285(22):16416–23.

26. Nili M, Shinde U, Rotwein P. Soluble repulsive guidance molecule c/hemojuvelin is a broad spectrum bone morphogenetic protein (BMP) antagonist and inhibits both BMP2- and BMP6-mediated signaling and gene expression. J Biol Chem 2010;285(32):24783–92.

27. Silvestri L, Pagani A, Nai A, et al. The serine protease matriptase-2 (TMPRSS6) inhibits hepcidin activation by cleaving membrane hemojuvelin. Cell Metab 2008;8(6):502–11.

28. Du X, She E, Gelbart T, et al. The serine protease TMPRSS6 is required to sense iron deficiency. Science 2008;320(5879):1088–92.

29. Casu C, Rivella S. Iron age: novel targets for iron overload. Hematology Am Soc Hematol Educ Program 2014;2014(1):216–21.

30. Camaschella C, Nai A. Ineffective erythropoiesis and regulation of iron status in iron loading anaemias. Br J Haematol 2016;172(4):512–23.
31. Kautz L, Jung G, Valore EV, et al. Identification of erythroferrone as an erythroid regulator of iron metabolism. Nat Genet 2014;46(7):678–84.
32. Kautz L, Jung G, Du X, et al. Erythroferrone contributes to hepcidin suppression and iron overload in a mouse model of β-thalassemia. Blood 2015;126(17): 2031–7.
33. Chow A, Huggins M, Ahmed J, et al. CD169+ macrophages provide a niche promoting erythropoiesis under homeostasis and stress. Nat Med 2013;19(4): 429–36.
34. Ramos P, Casu C, Gardenghi S, et al. Macrophages support pathological erythropoiesis in polycythemia vera and β-thalassemia. Nat Med 2013;19(4):437–45.
35. Arlet JB, Ribeil JA, Guillem F, et al. HSP70 sequestration by free α-globin promotes ineffective erythropoiesis in β-thalassaemia. Nature 2014;514(7521): 242–6.
36. Dussiot M, Maciel TT, Fricot A, et al. An activin receptor IIA ligand trap corrects ineffective erythropoiesis in β-thalassemia. Nat Med 2014;20(4):398–407.
37. Rivella S. The role of ineffective erythropoiesis in non-transfusion-dependent thalassemia. Blood Rev 2012;26(Suppl 1):S12–5.
38. Taher A, Isma'eel H, Mehio G, et al. Prevalence of thromboembolic events among 8,860 patients with thalassaemia major and intermedia in the Mediterranean area and Iran. Thromb Haemost 2006;96:488–91.
39. Musallam KM, Taher AT, Karimi M, et al. Cerebral infarction in beta-thalassemia intermedia: breaking the silence. Thromb Res 2012;130:695–702.
40. Musallam KM, Cappellini MD, Wood JC, et al. Elevated liver iron concentration is a marker of increased morbidity in patients with beta thalassemia intermedia. Haematologica 2011;96:1605–12.
41. Musallam KM, Rivella S, Vichinsky E, et al. Non-transfusion-dependent thalassemias. Haematologica 2013;98:833–44.
42. Taher AT, Musallam KM, Saliba AN, et al. Hemoglobin level and morbidity in non-transfusion-dependent thalassemia. Blood Cells Mol Dis 2015;55:108–9.
43. Gelderman MP, Baek JH, Yalamanoglu A, et al. Reversal of hemochromatosis by apotransferrin in non-transfused and transfused Hbbth3/+ (heterozygous B1/B2 globin gene deletion) mice. Haematologica 2015;100(5):611–22.
44. Tamary H, Shalev H, Perez-Avraham G, et al. Elevated growth differentiation factor 15 expression in patients with congenital dyserythropoietic anemia type I. Blood 2008;112(13):5241–4.
45. Tanno T, Bhanu NV, Oneal PA, et al. High levels of GDF15 in thalassemia suppress expression of the iron regulatory protein hepcidin. Nat Med 2007;13(9): 1096–101.
46. Nai A, Pagani A, Mandelli G, et al. Deletion of TMPRSS6 attenuates the phenotype in a mouse model of β-thalassemia. Blood 2012;119(21):5021–9.
47. Schmidt PJ, Toudjarska I, Sendamarai AK, et al. An RNAi therapeutic targeting TMPRSS6 decreases iron overload in Hfe(-/-) mice and ameliorates anemia and iron overload in murine β-thalassemia intermedia. Blood 2013;121(7): 1200–8.
48. Guo S, Casu C, Gardenghi S, et al. Reducing TMPRSS6 ameliorates hemochromatosis and β-thalassemia in mice. J Clin Invest 2013;123(4):1531–41.
49. Casu C, Oikonomidou PR, Chen H, et al. Minihepcidin peptides as disease modifiers in mice affected by β-thalassemia and polycythemia vera. Blood 2016; 128(2):265–76.

50. Casu C, Aghajan M, Oikonomidou PR, et al. Combination of TMPRSS6- ASO and the iron chelator deferiprone improves erythropoiesis and reduces iron overload in a mouse model of beta-thalassemia intermedia. Haematologica 2016;101(1): e8–11.
51. Schmidt PJ, Racie T, Westerman M, et al. Combination therapy with a TMPRSS6 RNAi-therapeutic and the oral iron chelator deferiprone additively diminishes secondary iron overload in a mouse model of β-thalassemia intermedia. Am J Hematol 2015;90(4):310–3.
52. Li H, Choesang T, Bao W, et al. Decreasing TfR1 expression reverses anemia and hepcidin suppression in β-thalassemic mice. Blood 2017;129(11):1514–26.
53. Libani IV, Guy EC, Melchiori L, et al. Decreased differentiation of erythroid cells exacerbates ineffective erythropoiesis in beta-thalassemia. Blood 2008;112(3): 875–85.
54. Suragani RN, Cadena SM, Cawley SM, et al. Transforming growth factor-β superfamily ligand trap ACE-536 corrects anemia by promoting late-stage erythropoiesis. Nat Med 2014;20(4):408–14.

Clinical Complications and Their Management

Alessia Marcon, MD[a,b], Irene Motta, MD[a], Ali T. Taher, MD, PhD, FRCP[c],
Maria Domenica Cappellini, MD[a,b],*

KEYWORDS

- Thalassemia • Ineffective erythropoiesis • Iron overload • Heart failure
- Liver disease • Endocrinopathies

KEY POINTS

- Thalassemia syndromes, clinically speaking, include transfusion-dependent and non–transfusion dependent forms.
- Ineffective erythropoiesis, chronic hemolytic anemia, compensatory hemopoietic expansion, hypercoagulability, and increased intestinal iron absorption are the hallmarks of thalassemias due to the α/β globin chain imbalance and are responsible for several clinical complications.
- Iron overload, secondary to increased iron absorption and to blood transfusions, causes organ damage.
- Treatment of anemia and iron overload may prevent clinical complications.
- In patients with thalassemia standard management for specific morbidities, beyond transfusion and iron chelation, should be considered.

INTRODUCTION

Clinical complications in thalassemias are systemic, and they are the consequence of the underlying pathophysiologic mechanisms, namely, ineffective erythropoiesis, chronic hemolytic anemia, compensatory hemopoietic expansion, and increased intestinal iron absorption. In the severe forms clinical complications can be the consequence of the treatment with red blood cell transfusions, which lead to iron overload. Nevertheless some complications are present similarly in patients with transfusion-dependent thalassemia (TDT) and in patients with non-TDT (NTDT), while some others

Disclosure: M.D. Cappellini is a member of the scientific board for Celgene and Sanofi Genzyme; A.T. Taher is a member of the scientific board for Celgene and Novartis.
[a] Department of Medicine, Cà Granda Foundation IRCCS, Via Francesco Sforza 35, Milano 20122, Italy; [b] Department of Clinical Science and Community, University of Milan, Via Francesco Sforza 35, Milano 20122, Italy; [c] Department of Internal Medicine, American University of Beirut Medical Center, 2nd floor, Building 5, PO Box 11-0236, Riad-El-Solh Beirut, Beirut 1107 2020, Lebanon
* Corresponding author. Fondazione IRCCS Ca Granda Policlinico, Via Francesco Sforza 35, Milano 20122, Italy.
E-mail address: maria.cappellini@unimi.it

Hematol Oncol Clin N Am 32 (2018) 223–236
https://doi.org/10.1016/j.hoc.2017.11.005
0889-8588/18/© 2017 Elsevier Inc. All rights reserved.

hemonc.theclinics.com

can be more prevalent in one or the other form.[1] In this review we discuss the most clinically relevant complications, comparing the presentation and the characteristics in TDT and in NTDT (**Table 1** and **Fig. 1**).

CARDIAC COMPLICATIONS
Cardiac Dysfunction

Despite great improvement in the clinical management of thalassemia, cardiovascular involvement represents a well-known complication and remains the primary cause of mortality in TDT and less frequently contributes to morbidity in patients with NTDT.[2,3]

The two forms of the disease have common basic underlying pathophysiologic mechanisms that affect the heart in a different extent.

In TDT, cardiac iron overload is mainly due to blood transfusions, whereas, in NTDT, iron accumulates to a lesser extent in the heart because it is due to increased intestinal iron absorption and accumulates mainly in the liver. In TDT, the heart failure due to accumulation of iron within myocytes is a major risk of death. Cardiac iron deposition occurs mainly in the ventricle, with greater accumulation in the epicardium. Moreover, free labile iron interacts with calcium channels and leads to impaired myocardial contractility.[4–6]

Patients with considerable myocardial iron overload may remain free of symptoms for a long time; once myocardial dysfunction develops, symptoms are related to the degree of ventricular impairment. In more advanced stages, clinical presentations are equivalent to those seen with any severe heart failure and may include dyspnea, peripheral edema, hepatic congestion, and severe exercise limitation. It is important to underline that iron overload complications, even when severe, may be reversed by intensive chelation therapy.

In NTDT, the heart involvement may be due to other cardiovascular causes than iron overload, such as pulmonary hypertension (PH) and thrombosis (see Hypercoagulability and Vascular Disease).

A mechanism of heart dysfunction, which is common to TDT and NTDT, is represented by an increased workload on the heart; in NTDT, because of chronic anemia,

Table 1
The difference in complications between transfusion-dependent thalassemia and non–transfusion-dependent thalassemia

Complications	TDT	NTDT	Management
Cardiac dysfunction	+++	+	Iron chelation + standard care
Arrhythmias	+	++	Standard care
Viral hepatitis	+++	+	HBV vaccination, antiviral therapy
Hepatic fibrosis, cirrhosis, and cancer	++	+++	Standard care
Growth retardation Sexual development	++	+	Transfusion + chelation + hormones
Glucose intolerance/diabetes	++	+	Standard care
Bone disease	++	+++	Standard care + specific therapy
Extramedullary hematopoietic masses	+	+++	Hypertransfusion, HU, radiation
Thrombosis	+	+++	Anticoagulation, transfusion
Pulmonary hypertension	+	+++	Standard care, sildenafil, bosentan
Leg ulcers	+	++	Topic measures, HU

Abbreviations: HBV, hepatitis B virus; HU, hydroxyurea.

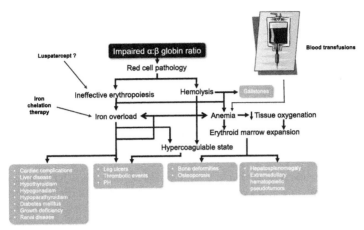

Fig. 1. Summary of the pathophysiologic mechanisms and the clinical complications in thalassemias. Ineffective erythropoiesis and compensatory mechanisms drive clinical complications. The outcome can be modified by blood transfusions and iron chelation or reducing ineffective erythropoiesis. PH, pulmonary hypertension.

the increased cardiac output represents one of the basic pathophysiologic mechanisms of cardiovascular involvement. Patients with TDT, even if well transfused, also present some degree of high cardiac output.[7]

Other factors contributing to the development of cardiovascular complications are represented by endocrinopathies, infections, hemolysis-induced tissue injury and vascular involvement, valvular involvement, and hypercoagulability.[8] The regular assessment of cardiac status in patients with thalassemia should include regular controls of electrocardiogram (ECG), ECG recording for 24 hours, echocardiography and, if available, cardiac MRI (MRI T2*).

Cardiac MRI represents the gold standard for monitoring patients with thalassemia because it can provide a precise estimation of cardiac iron burden as well as left and right ventricular volumes.[4,5] Echocardiography is a noninvasive tool to monitor the ejection fraction, cardiac volumes, and pulmonary arterial pressure (PAP).[9]

Prevention of iron loading with an appropriate and regular iron chelation therapy is mandatory to prevent or to control heart dysfunction, and intensive chelation (high doses in monotherapy or combined therapy) has to be implemented in case of heart failure.[10–12] Impaired myocardial function may also require specific cardiac treatment, including angiotensin-converting enzyme (ACE) inhibitors, beta-blockers, and diuretics (furosemide and/or aldosterone antagonists). In patients with thalassemia, the dose can be limited by hypotension. If ACE inhibitors are not tolerated, angiotensin II receptor antagonists can be used.

Arrhythmia

Cardiac iron overload may also affect the heart conduction system; for this reason, conduction delays and heart block can occur in patients with thalassemia.

Ectopic activity, usually supraventricular but occasionally ventricular, can produce symptoms requiring prophylactic drug treatment (often with beta-blockers); these events can trigger more sustained arrhythmias, particularly atrial fibrillation (AF). For most supraventricular arrhythmias, the reassurance of patients is generally appropriate. AF is the most commonly encountered arrhythmia[13] and is promoted by the combination of iron overload and dilatation of the left atrium. Atrial or multifocal atrial tachycardia can also develop.

Beta-blockers are a good first-line therapy. When AF occurs in presence of severe myocardial iron overload, the chelation regimen should be intensified. In uncontrolled or persistent AF, antiarrhythmic therapy and rhythm control with amiodarone may be attempted. Catheter ablation may also be considered.[14] Anticoagulation is generally recommended in the presence of AF, heart failure, or if the medical history is positive for stroke. Amiodarone is the drug of choice in the acute setting because of its broad spectrum of action and modest impairment of cardiac function; however, long-term therapy is associated with an increased risk of hypothyroidism; therapy can often be terminated after 6 to 12 months.[15]

Arrhythmias are life threatening in the presence of heart failure but can also be the first sign of cardiac decompensation in patients with normal cardiac function but with severe myocardial iron overload. MRI T2* is a good tool for arrhythmia prediction, although arrhythmic events may occur with normal T2* values. Careful tailoring of chelation therapy according to the T2* value may help diminish event rates.

Sudden death is relatively rare in thalassemia in the modern era of iron chelation, but historical data suggest an association with increased QT dispersion consistent with torsades de pointes as a possible mechanism.[16]

Acute pericarditis before the era of regular therapy occurred very often, but now the effective management of thalassemia has significantly limited the occurrence of this complication. As in the case of pericarditis, the better management of anemia and iron overload and the enhanced quality of the transfused blood have also reduced the rate of acute myocarditis in thalassemia.[6]

LIVER DISEASE

Liver disease is one of the major complications in patients with thalassemia.[17,18] Liver damage is multifactorial; it is due to iron overload (See Gupta R and colleagues', "Ineffective Erythropoiesis, Anemia, and Iron Overload," in this issue), which is the main causative factor in both TDT and NTDT, and to viral hepatitis, especially hepatitis C virus (HCV) and hepatitis B virus (HBV). Angelucci and colleagues[19] showed, in a series of liver biopsies from patients with thalassemia who underwent bone marrow transplant and who did not receive any treatment of iron overload or HCV, that iron overload and HCV infection are independent risk factors for hepatic fibrosis progression. Moreover, their concomitant presence results in an increased risk of developing liver fibrosis. Nowadays, liver fibrosis can be assessed by transient elastography (TE), a noninvasive method, whereas liver biopsy can be limited to selected cases. FerriScan (Resonance Health, Burswood, Australia) and MRI T2* are today the major noninvasive methods used to confirm and quantify organ iron excess.[17] Both improvement in chelation therapy and the availability of new drugs for hepatitis virus represent amelioration in the management of liver disease in patients with thalassemia. However, the aging of patients expose them to other hepatotoxic factors, such as dysmetabolism and alcohol. Chronic liver disease can progress to cirrhosis with its risk of hepatocellular carcinoma (HCC), an increasing complication due to longer survival.

Iron Overload

Free or nontransferrin-bound iron is the major mediator of hepatic and extrahepatic tissue damage.[20] It enters the hepatocytes and generates reactive-oxygen species, resulting in damage to lipids, proteins, DNA, and subcellular organelles, including lysosomes and mitochondria. This injury can result in cellular dysfunction, apoptosis, and necrosis. For iron overload treatment and evaluation see specific sections.

Viral Hepatitis

Patients affected by thalassemia are exposed to the blood transfusion–related risk of infection. In the prescreening era (1970s for HVB, 1992 for HCV), hepatitis viral infections, particularly HCV and HBV, were very common.

The prevalence of HBV and HCV varies according to the prevalence in the different regions of the world. The prevalence of patients with thalassemia with positive hepatitis B surface antigen ranges from 0.3% to 5.7%, with a higher prevalence of HBV chronic infection in Asia and Southeast Asia countries.[21] A safe and effective vaccine against HBV infection has been available since 1981, and its administration in infants has resulted in a significant decrease in prevalence in many parts of the world.[22]

Anti-HBV drugs include interferon and nucleos(t)ide analogues (lamivudine, adefovir, entecavir, telbivudine, and tenofovir); however, these drugs are expensive and may not be available in all regions of the world.[17]

Anti–hepatitis C antibodies are detected in 4.4% to 85.4% of patients with thalassemia, with a high prevalence in Italy.[23,24] The concomitant presence of iron overload and HCV infection in patients with thalassemia has been demonstrated to increase the risk of hepatic fibrosis progression.[19]

Originally, the treatment of hepatitis C was a combination of pegylated interferon and ribavirin that demonstrated a sustained viral response (SVR) in the 25% to 64% of patients with thalassemia.[25] However, ribavirin causes hemolysis, worsening anemia in these patients, with an increase in the transfusion requirement. During the last years, the treatment of HCV infection dramatically changed and several interferon-free regimens are now available. According to the recent European Association for the Study of the Liver's treatment recommendations on hepatitis C, patients with hemoglobinopathies should be treated with an interferon-free regimen, without ribavirin. However, patients with hemoglobinopathies have been excluded from the major clinical trials that led to the approval of direct-acting antivirals (DAAs).[26]

So far, few data are available about the use of DAAs in patients affected by thalassemia, some limited to case reports. Recently, Origa and colleagues[27] published an observational study in an Italian cohort of patients with hemoglobinopathies and HCV infection and advanced liver fibrosis treated with different DAA regimens. A total of 130 out of 139 (93.5%) achieved an SVR, data similar to patients without hemoglobinopathies. Moreover, successful treatment with DAAs was associated with significant reduction of liver enzymes and serum ferritin.[27]

A randomized, placebo-controlled, phase III C-EDGE IBLD (ClinicalTrials.gov: NCT02252016) study to assess the safety and efficacy of elbasvir/grazoprevir in patients with inherited bleeding disorders and HCV infection, including thalassemia, has been recently published. One hundred out of 107 patients (93.5%) achieved SVR 12 weeks after the end of the treatment (SVR12). Among the 41 patients with thalassemia, 40 (97.6%) showed an SVR12.[28]

Hepatocellular Carcinoma

The incidence of HCC has increased during the last decades. An Italian study showed that the number of HCCs significantly increased between 1993 and 1997 and 2008 and 2012 (8–31 diagnosis, respectively).[29]

The onset of HCC is anticipated in patients with thalassemia compared with the general population because of the presence of the aforementioned risk factors.[30] HCC at present is more common in patients with NTDT who are aged older than 40 years compared with patients with TDT, because of a severe liver iron overload that in some cases remains untreated.[1]

ENDOCRINE COMPLICATIONS

Endocrine complications were very common in patients with thalassemia in the pre-chelation era because they are mainly related to endogenous (hemolysis) and exogenous (transfusional) iron overload. Most of the alive patients with thalassemia who are aged older than 30 years have some endocrine complications due to poor iron chelation in their first decade of life.[31] The anterior pituitary gland is particularly sensitive to iron associated free radicals; for this reason, even a low amount of iron deposition in this gland during childhood can interfere with its function.[32]

As a matter of fact, the prevalence of endocrine disease as reported in the past years is significantly decreasing because of more optimal iron chelation and serum ferritin. Endocrinopathies are more prevalent in patients with TDT, whereas hypogonadism, hypothyroidism, and diabetes mellitus are quite rare in NTDT. Although patients with NTDT generally experience late puberty, they have normal sexual development and are usually fertile.

Hypogonadotropic Hypogonadism

Secondary hypogonadism, often referred to as hypogonadotropic hypogonadism (HH), is the most frequent endocrinopathy in patients with TDT. Nowadays, the incidence rate of hypogonadism, in both sexes, varies considerably according to the adherence to the conventional treatment ranging from less than 50% to 100%.[33] HH in thalassemia is caused by iron deposits in the pituitary gland and gonads in an early age, but it can also be related to anemia during the first months of life. Before puberty, pituitary dysfunction is difficult to detect because of the immaturity of the hypothalamic-pituitary-gonadal axis. In males clinical presentations of HH includes lack, delay, and/or block of pubertal sexual maturation and, in adult life, decreased libido, erectile dysfunction, worsened sense of well-being, and lower quality of life. Spermatogenesis is impaired, and the volume of ejaculate is decreased. Low serum concentrations of testosterone and gonadotropins confirm the diagnosis.[34] In females, hypogonadism is clinically diagnosed by the absence of pubertal development or discontinuation or regression of the maturation of secondary sex characteristics. Low serum concentrations of sexual hormones and gonadotropins confirm the diagnosis. Hormone replacement therapy must be introduced in the absence of clinical contraindications to alleviate symptoms of sexual hormone deficiency and also to prevent long-term complications, such as osteoporosis. Many adult patients with thalassemia are subfertile due to HH. Spermatogenesis and ovulation can be induced by the administration of human chorionic gonadotropin. Assisted reproductive techniques are usually needed.[35] The young population of patients with thalassemia is much less hypogonadic due to an adequate regular transfusion and chelation therapy. Although adult patients with NTDT have a normal puberty and are fertile, they may have early menopause and severe osteoporosis.

Growth Hormone Deficiency

The pathogenesis of growth failure in thalassemia syndromes is multifactorial,[36] including chronic anemia, iron overload, and chelation toxicity. Other contributing factors include others endocrinopathies, chronic liver disease, and, in patients living in poor countries, malnutrition. Growth hormone (GH) deficiency can be found in adult patients through a GH stimulation test in case of a strong clinical suspicion and in patients with at least one other pituitary hormone deficiency and low or low-normal insulinlike growth factor 1 level. Treatment of GH deficiency, when established, is substitutive therapy with subcutaneous recombinant GH.

Hypothyroidism

Hypothyroidism is an endocrine complication strongly correlated with anemia and iron overload.[37] It is relatively rare in well-treated patients with TDT. As for other endocrinopathies, hypothyroidism is not frequent in patients with NTDT but sometimes can be observed late in life or in the presence of antithyroid antibodies positivity.[38] In patients with subclinical hypothyroidism, a regular follow-up is recommended with an intensification of iron chelation therapy if required (inadequate iron overload control); a low dose of levothyroxine can be evaluated for specific cases. For patients with clinical hypothyroidism, a therapy with levothyroxine is indicated in order to maintain normal thyrotropin levels.

Diabetes

Diabetes mellitus is a complication found in 20% to 30% of adult patients with β-thalassemia worldwide. It is strongly associated with iron overload. Presumably, diabetes is preceded by insulin resistance and hyperinsulinemia. The risk of developing diabetes/impaired glucose tolerance depends on the efficacy of iron chelation, and the risk factors include poor compliance and late initiation of chelation therapy and family predisposition. Hemoglobin (Hb) A_{1c}, the gold standard test to assess glycemic control in diabetic patients, cannot be used in hemoglobinopathies because of alterations in Hb balance in those patients. Usually fructosamine, which can provide an evaluation of glucose metabolism over the last 2 to 3 weeks, is used in patients with thalassemia.[39] Diagnosis and treatment of this complication are the same as for the general population.

Hypoparathyroidism

Hypoparathyroidism is one of the less frequent endocrinopathies in patients with thalassemia.[17] It is supposed to be related to iron overload and to hormonal suppression induced by increased bone reabsorption consequent to chronic anemia. Often, clinically, signs are absent; but paresthesia, signs of latent tetany (Chvostek and Trousseau signs), or QT prolongation can be present. Laboratory data show hypocalcemia, hyperphosphatemia, and low levels of parathyroid hormone and 1,25 dihydroxy calcifediol. The therapy is represented by supplementation with 25-hydroxyvitamin D and calcium. If hyperphosphatemia persists, a therapy with phosphate binders can be associated.

Adrenal Insufficiency

The hypothalamic-pituitary-adrenal axis is generally considered to be an infrequent target of chronic iron toxicity. The reported prevalence of this complication is extremely variable, depending on the iron overload severity, available treatments, and diagnostic criteria.[40] The presence of high adrenocorticotropic hormone (ACTH) serum concentrations is consistent with direct damage to the adrenal glands, which can be confirmed by MRI.[41] ACTH levels lower than normal suggest secondary (central) adrenal insufficiency due to pituitary iron deposition, although combined central and peripheral impairments cannot be ruled out. Adrenal insufficiency develops gradually; symptoms, such as fatigue, may be nonspecific and overlapping with those of chronic anemia. The main risk of undetected disease is that it may present with a life-threatening acute crisis. Subclinical adrenal impairment may be more common than expected and revealed by conditions of stress.[42] An evaluation of basal adrenal function (ACTH and cortisol basal levels) must be performed every year in adult patients with thalassemia; considering that a normal basal function cannot rule out a reduced functional reserve, an ACTH stimulation test should be performed in selected cases. In case of adrenal insufficiency diagnosis, replacement therapy with cortisone acetate must be started; for patients with subclinical adrenal impairment, a replacement therapy should be implemented in case of stressful events.[43]

BONE DISEASE

Osteopenia and osteoporosis with a consequent increased risk of fractures are well known and important complications of patients with thalassemia, especially for their impact on quality of life. Bone disease, involving both TDT and NTDT, can be more severe in patients with NTDT. The physiopathology of osteopenia/osteoporosis is multifactorial involving direct iron toxicity on osteoblasts and endocrine diseases. Sexual hormones in both males and females have an important role on osteoblastic proliferation and differentiation and to prevent osteoclastic activity. Also iron chelation therapy with deferoxamine, in the past, had an impact on bone disease because it can block the DNA synthesis and, consequently, the osteoblastic and fibroblastic proliferation. In patients with NTDT, the chronic anemia is an important factor impacting on bone metabolism.

An additional negative influence may be due to the vitamin D–deficient state.[44]

Also hypercalciuria, often present in patients with thalassemia, is a subclinical contributor to low bone mass density and/or fragility fractures.

The gold standard for the classification of bone conditions is bone mineral density (BMD) as measured with bone densitometry. The Trabecular Bone Score (TBS) that can be obtained by reanalyzing spine densitometric images and converting them into a numeric value provides information on bone structure.[45] Several reports indicate a role of TBS, independent of BMD, in predicting fracture risk in postmenopausal and secondary osteoporosis.[46] The risk of fracture is higher when low bone quantity is associated with impaired bone quality.

The current treatment of patients with bone disease includes vitamin D and calcium supplementation and bisphosphonates therapy.

Bisphosphonates (oral or intravenous) represent the most widely used agents in the treatment of osteoporosis. The use of bisphosphonates, particularly intravenous, has been associated with the reduction of bone reabsorption, increase of BMD, reduction of back pain, and improved quality of life overtime[47–49]

Recently also denosumab[50] and anabolic therapy with teriparatide have been used in the treatment of osteoporosis in patients with thalassemia.

A good control in Hb values in both patients with TDT and patients with NTDT, the treatment of concurrent endocrinopathies and promotion of physical activity and smoking cessation are also part of the management of patients with thalassemia with bone disease.

HYPERCOAGULABILITY AND VASCULAR DISEASE

A hypercoagulable status has been identified in patients with thalassemia, especially in NTDT and even more in splenectomized patients.[51,52] The hypercoagulability in thalassemia is a multifactorial condition recognizing platelets abnormalities and pathologic red blood cells as key factors responsible for thrombotic events. Several other factors, such as endothelial injury, endocrine and hepatic dysfunction, and iron overload, may contribute to the increased risk of thrombosis in these patients. The prevalence of thrombotic events can reach up to 20% in patients with NTDT compared with less than 1% in patients with TDT. These events primarily occur in splenectomized patients with contributing factors represented by advanced age, total Hb level less than 9 g/dL, history of thrombotic or other vascular events and an elevated platelet count (>500 $\times$ 10^9/L) and nucleated blood cell count (>300 $\times$ 10^6/L).[52] Overt strokes have been documented in splenectomized patients with NTDT ranging between 5% and 9%[53]; however, a higher prevalence of silent cerebral ischemia is reported either in patients with NTDT or in patients with TDT with advanced age. A serious vascular complication that was found to occur at a relatively high frequency in patients with NTDT compared with TDT is PH.[54]

Pulmonary Hypertension

PH is defined as an increase in mean PAP (PAPm) of 25 mm Hg or greater, considering a normal PAPm at rest of 14 $\pm$ 3 mm Hg and an upper limit of normal of approximately 20 mm Hg, as assessed by right heart catheterization.[55]

PH has been recognized as the most significant cardiovascular finding and the main cause of heart failure in NTDT. Conversely, in TDT, PH is rare and mild, whereas left ventricular dysfunction prevails.[54–56]

The development of PH in thalassemia syndromes is multifactorial and includes endothelial dysfunction, increased vascular tone, inflammation, hypercoagulability, and finally vascular remodeling. Hemolysis seems to play a key role. It has been shown that chronic hemolysis leads to nitric oxide (NO) depletion due to NO scavenging, arginine catabolism, and endogenous NO synthesis inhibition.[57] Moreover, hemolysis and impaired NO bioavailability contribute to platelet activation, endothelial dysfunction, and increased oxidative stress, which result in tissue damage throughout the cardiovascular system.[58] Furthermore, splenectomy has been demonstrated to be a strong risk factor in the development of PH.[52]

No prospective randomized clinical trials in patients affected by NTDT are available to guide the treatment of these patients. The aforementioned higher prevalence of PH in NTDT compared with regularly transfused patients with thalassemia suggests a role for transfusion therapy. Indeed, transfusion therapy is associated with lower PH rates in NTDT.[18,52]

Data regarding the use of pulmonary vasodilator therapies in β-thalassemia are limited.

Sildenafil citrate, a potent inhibitor of cyclic guanosine monophosphate–specific phosphodiesterase-5, showed promising results for the management of PH in small studies in patients with β-thalassemia.[59] A multicenter trial on 10 patients with either TDT or TNTD showed that treatment with sildenafil resulted in a significant decrease in tricuspid regurgitant jet velocity by 13.3%, improved left ventricular end systolic/diastolic volume, and a trend toward an improved New York Heart Association functional class. No significant change in 6-minute walked distance was noted. The treatment was well tolerated.[57]

Bosentan, an endothelin receptor antagonist, and epoprostenol, a prostacyclin analogue, were also described to be effective in some cases.[60]

OTHER COMPLICATIONS

Some complications mainly due to the underlying pathophysiologic mechanisms involving chronic anemia, hemolysis, and bone marrow expansion are more common in patients with NTDT compared with regularly transfused patients with beta-thalassemia.[17,18] Ineffective erythropoiesis, which is the hallmark of untreated thalassemia, may force the expansion of the hematopoietic tissue leading to extramedullary masses. This complication is more common in patients with NTDT in whom the reported prevalence is around 20% compared with less than 1% in patients with TDT. Almost all body sites may be involved other than the liver and spleen. The paraspinal involvement, which accounts for approximately 11% to 15% of the manifestations, requires special attention because of the severe clinical consequences secondary to spinal cord compression. Transfusions, hydroxyurea, and, in some instances, radiation are the management approach to control extramedullary hematopoietic masses[61,62]

Cholelithiasis is a frequent complication in patients with NTDT due to the high degree of ineffective erythropoiesis, peripheral hemolysis not suppressed by regular transfusions, and older age.[3] The highest prevalence is observed in patients with the concomitant Gilbert syndrome genotype.[63] Ultrasonography is the most helpful tool to monitor cholelithiasis. Clinically, cholelithiasis results in gastrointestinal symptoms leading frequently to a cholecystectomy. Removal of the gallbladder during splenectomy is a common practice, especially if stones are symptomatic. This practice is particularly important, as acute cholecystitis can have serious consequences in splenectomized patients.[64]

Leg ulcers, although rare, are more common in patients with NTDT.[18] The risk of leg ulcers increases with advancing age, because the extremities skin is more thin due to reduced tissue oxygenation and the subcutaneous tissue is fragile, especially when exposed to minimal trauma. Higher rates of leg ulcers have also been reported in patients with NTDT with iron overload. Local iron overload is also thought to be a perpetuating factor causing chronicity of lesions, especially when the heme from degraded red blood cells accumulates locally and gives a dark hue.[65]

Although there is no sufficient evidence to recommend blood transfusion, iron chelation, or hydroxyurea therapy for the prevention of leg ulcers, once an ulcer has started to develop, regular blood transfusions may provide some relief in persistent cases.[18]

REFERENCES

1. Taher A, Weatherall DJ, Cappellini MD. Thalassaemia. Lancet 2017 [pii:S0140-6736(17)31822-6].
2. Borgna-Pignatti C, Rugolotto S, De Stefano P, et al. Survival and complications in patients with thalassemia major treated with transfusion and deferoxamine. Haematologica 2004;89:1187–93.
3. Musallam KM, Rivella S, Vichinsky E, et al. Non-transfusion dependent thalassemias. Haematologica 2013;98:833–44.
4. Carpenter JP, He T, Kirk P, et al. On T2* magnetic resonance and cardiac iron. Circulation 2011;123:1519–28.
5. Pennell DJ, Udelson JE, Arai AE, et al, on behalf of the American Heart Association Committee on Heart Failure and Transplantation of the Council on Clinical Cardiology and Council on Cardiovascular Radiology and Imaging. Cardiovascular function and treatment in beta-thalassemia major: a consensus statement from the American Heart Association. Circulation 2013;128:281–308.
6. Farmakis D, Triposkiadis F, Lekakis J, et al. Heart failure in haemoglobinophaties: pathophysiology, clinical phenotypes and management. Eur J Heart Fail 2017;19: 479–89.

7. Aessopos A, Farmakis D, Hatziliami A, et al. Cardiac status in well-treated patients with thalassemia major. Eur J Haematol 2004;73:359–66.

8. Aessopos A, Berdoukas V. Cardiac function and iron chelation in thalassemia major and intermedia: a review of the underlying pathophysiology and approach to chelation management. Mediterr J Hematol Infect Dis 2009;1(1):e2009002.

9. Di Odoardo LAF, Giuditta M, Cassinerio E, et al. Myocardial deformation in iron overload cardiomyopathy: speckle tracking imaging in a beta-thalassemia major population. Intern Emerg Med 2017;29:1670–4.

10. Kirk P, Roughton M, Porter JB, et al. Cardiac T2* magnetic resonance for prediction of cardiac complications in thalassemia major. Circulation 2009;120:1961–8.

11. Westwood MA, Anderson LJ, Maceira AM, et al. Normalized left ventricular volumes and function in thalassemia major patients with normal myocardial iron. J Magn Reson Imaging 2007;25:1147–51.

12. Cassinerio E, Roghi A, Orofino N, et al. A 5 year follow-up in deferasirox treatment. Improvement of cardiac and hepatic iron overload and amelioration in cardiac function in thalassemia major patients. Ann Hematol 2015;94:939–45.

13. Gammella E, Recalcati S, Rybinska I, et al. Iron induced damage in cardiomyopathy: oxidative-dependent and independent mechanisms. Oxid Med Cell Longev 2015;2015:230182.

14. Mariotti S, Loviselli A, Murenu S, et al. High prevalence of thyroid dysfunction in adult patients with beta-thalassemia major submitted to amiodarone treatment. J Endocrinol Invest 1999;22:55–63.

15. Mancuso L, Mancuso A, Bevacqua E, et al. Electrocardiographic abnormalities in thalassemia patients with heart failure. Cardiovasc Hematol Disord Drug Targets 2009;9:29–35.

16. Russo V, Rago A, Pannone B, et al. Dispersion of repolarization and beta-thalassemia major: the prognostic role of QT and JT dispersion for identifying the high-risk patients for sudden death. Eur J Haematol 2011;86:324–31.

17. Cappellini MD, Cohen A, Porter J, et al. Guidelines for the management of transfusion dependent thalassemia (TDT). 3rd edition. Nicosia, Cyprus: Thalassemia International Federation; 2014.

18. Taher A, Vichinsky E, Musallam K, et al. Guidelines for the management of non transfusion dependent thalassemia (NTDT). Nicosia, Cyprus: Thalassemia International Federation; 2013.

19. Angelucci E, Muretto P, Nicolucci A, et al. Effects of iron overload and hepatitis C virus positivity in determining progression of liver fibrosis in thalassemia following bone marrow transplantation. Blood 2002;100:17–21.

20. Brittenham GM. Iron-chelating therapy for transfusional iron overload. N Engl J Med 2011;364:146–56.

21. Singh H, Pradhan M, Singh RL, et al. High frequency of hepatitis B virus infection in patients with beta-thalassemia receiving multiple transfusions. Vox Sang 2003; 84:292–9.

22. Trepo C, Chan HL, Lok A. Hepatitis B virus infection. Lancet 2014;384:2053–63.

23. Prati D, Zanella A, Farma E, et al. A multicenter prospective study on the risk of acquiring liver disease in anti-hepatitis C virus negative patients affected from homozygous beta-thalassemia. Blood 1998;92:3460–4.

24. Di Marco V, D'Ambrosio R, Bronte F, et al. Dual therapy with peginterferon and ribavirin in thalassemia major patients with chronic HCV infection: is there still an indication? Dig Liver Dis 2016;48:650–5.

25. Di Marco V, Capra M, Angelucci E, et al. Management of chronic viral hepatitis in patients with thalassemia: recommendations from an international panel. Blood 2010;116:2875–83.
26. Jmakos E, Kountouras D, Kosmas J, et al. Treatment of chronic hepatitis C with direct-acting antiviral in patients with beta-thalassemia major and advanced liver disease. Br J Heamatol 2017;178:130–6.
27. Origa R, Ponti ML, Filosa A, et al. Treatment of hepatitis C virus infection with direct-acting antiviral drugs is safe and effective in patients with hemoglobinopathies. Am J Hematol 2017;92(12):1349–55.
28. Hezode C, Colombo M, Bourliere M, et al. Elbasvir/grazoprevir for patients with hepatitis C virus infection and inherited blood disorders: a phase III study. Hepatology 2017;66:736–45.
29. Borgna-Pignatti C, Garani MC, Forni GL, et al. Hepatocellular carcinoma in thalassaemia: an update of the Italian Registry. Br J Haematol 2014;167:121–6.
30. Moukhadder HM, Halawi R, Cappellini MD, et al. Hepatocellular carcinoma as an emerging morbidity in the thalassemia syndromes: a comprehensive review. Cancer 2017;123:751–8.
31. De Sanctis V, Elsedfy H, Ashraf T, et al. Endocrine profile of β-thalassemia major patients followed from childhood to advanced adulthood in a tertiary care center. Indian J Endocrinol Metab 2016;20:451–9.
32. Berkovitch M, Bistritzer T, Milone SD, et al. Iron deposition in the anterior pituitary in homozygous beta-thalassemia: MRI evaluation and correlation with gonadal function. J Pediatr Endocrinol Metab 2000;13(2):179–84.
33. De Sanctis V, Soliman AT, Elsedfy H, et al. Review and recommendations on management of adult female thalassemia patients with hypogonadism based on literature review and experience of ICET-a network specialists. Mediterr J Hematol Infect Dis 2017;9(1):e2017001.
34. De Sanctis V, Elsedfy H, Soliman AT, et al. Acquired hypogonadotropic hypogonadism (AHH) in thalassaemia major patients: an underdiagnosed condition? Mediterr J Hematol Infect Dis 2016;8(1):e2016001.
35. Cassinerio E, Baldini IM, Alamedine RS, et al. Pregnancy in patients with thalassemia major; a cohort study and conclusions for an adequate care management approach. Ann Hematol 2017;102:120–4.
36. Soliman AT, Khalafallah H, Ashour R. Growth and factors affecting it in thalassemia major. Hemoglobin 2009;33:S116–26.
37. Hantrakool S, Tantiworawit A, Rattarittamrong E, et al. Elevated serum ferritin levels are highly associated with diabetes mellitus and hypothyroidism in thalassemia patients. Blood 2012;120:5174–8.
38. Baldini M, Marcon A, Cassin R, et al. Beta-thalassaemia intermedia: evaluation of endocrine and bone complications. Biomed Res Int 2014;2014:174581.
39. Li MJ, Peng SS, Lu MY, et al. Diabetes mellitus in patients with thalassaemia major. Pediatr Blood Cancer 2014;61(1):20–4.
40. Huang KE, Mittelman SD, Coates TD, et al. A significant proportion of thalassemia major patients have adrenal insufficiency detectable on provocative testing. J Pediatr Hematol Oncol 2015;37(1):54–9.
41. Guzelbey T, Gurses B, Ozturk E, et al. Evaluation of iron deposition in the adrenal glands of β thalassemia major patients using 3-tesla MRI. Iran J Radiol 2016;13(3):e36375.
42. Scacchi M, Danesi L, Cattaneo A, et al. The pituitary–adrenal axis in adult thalassaemic patients. Eur J Endocrinol 2010;162(1):43–8.

43. Baldini M, Mancarella M, Cassinerio E, et al. Adrenal insufficiency: an emerging challenge in thalassemia? Am J Hematol 2017;92(6):E119–21.
44. Voskaridou E, Terpos E. New insights into the pathophysiology and management of osteoporosis in patients with beta-thalassaemia. Br J Haematol 2004;127: 127–39.
45. Baldini M, Forti S, Marcon A, et al. Endocrine and bone disease in appropriately treated adult patients with beta-thalassemia major. Ann Hematol 2010;89(12): 1207–13.
46. Bousson V, Bergot C, Sutter B, et al. Scientific committee of the Groupe de Recherche et d'Information sur les Ostéoporoses. Trabecular bone score (TBS): available knowledge, clinical relevance, and future prospects. Osteoporos Int 2012;23(5):1489–501.
47. Voskaridou E, Terpos E, Spina G, et al. Pamidronate is an effective treatment for osteoporosis in patients with beta-thalassaemia. Br J Haematol 2003;123(4): 730–7.
48. Voskaridou E, Anagnostopoulos A, Konstantopoulos K, et al. Zoledronic acid for the treatment of osteoporosis in patients with beta-thalassemia: results from a single- center, randomized, placebo-controlled trial. Haematologica 2006;91(9): 1193–202.
49. Forni GL, Perrotta S, Giusti A, et al. Neridronate improves bone mineral density and reduces back pain in beta-thalassaemia patients with osteoporosis: results from a phase 2, randomized, parallel-arm, open-label study. Br J Haematol 2012;158(2):274–82.
50. Yassin MA, Soliman AT, De Sanctis V, et al. Effects of the anti-receptor activator of nuclear factor kappa B ligand denusomab on beta thalassemia major-induced osteoporosis. Indian J Endocrinol Metab 2014;18(4):546–51.
51. Cappellini MD, Robbiolo L, Bottasso MB, et al. Venous thromboembolism and hyoercoagulabilty in splenectomized patients with thalassaemia intermedia. Br J Haematol 2000;111:467–73.
52. Taher AT, Musallam KM, Karimi M, et al. Overview on practices in thalassemia intermedia management aiming for lowering complication rates across a region of endemicity: the OPTIMAL CARE study. Blood 2010;115:1886–92.
53. Musallam KM, Taher AT, Karimi M, et al. Cerebral infarction in beta-thalassemia intermedia: breaking the silence. Thromb Res 2012;130:695–702.
54. Farmakis D, Aessopos A. Pulmonary hypertension associated with hemoglobin-opathies: prevalent but overlooked. Circulation 2011;123:1227–32.
55. Galie N, Humbert M, Vachiery JL, et al. 2015 ESC/ERS guidelines for the diagnosis and treatment of pulmonary hypertension: the Joint Task Force for the Diagnosis and Treatment of Pulmonary Hypertension of the European Society of Cardiology (ESC) and the European Respiratory Society (ERS): endorsed by: Association for European Paediatric and Congenital Cardiology (AEPC), International Society for Heart and Lung Transplantation (ISHLT). Eur Heart J 2016;37: 67–119.
56. Derchi G, Galanello R, Bina P, et al. Prevalence and risk factors for pulmonary arterial hypertension in a large group of beta thalassemia patients using right heart catheterization: a Webthal study. Circulation 2014;129:338–45.
57. Morris CR, Kim HY, Wood J, et al. Sildenafil therapy in thalassemia patients with Doppler-defined risk of pulmonary hypertension. Haematologica 2013;98: 1359–67.
58. Fraidenburg DR, Machado RF. Pulmonary hypertension associated with thalassemia syndromes. Ann New York Acad Sci 2016;1368:127–39.

59. Derchi G, Balocco M, Bina P, et al. Efficacy and safety of sildenafil for the treatment of severe pulmonary hypertension in patients with hemoglobinopathies: results from a long-term follow up. Haematologica 2014;99:e17–8.
60. Anthi A, Tsangaris I, Hamodraka ES, et al. Treatment with bosentan in a patient with thalassemia intermedia and pulmonary arterial hypertension. Blood 2012; 120:1531–2.
61. Rivella S. The role of ineffective erythropoiesis in non transfusion dependent thalassemias. Blood Rev 2012;26(suppl):S12–5.
62. Haidar R, Mhaidli H, Taher AT. Paraspinal extramedullary hematopoiesis in patients with thalassemia intermedia. Eur Spine J 2010;19:871–8.
63. Galanello R, Piras S, Barella S, et al. Cholelithiasis and Gilbert's syndrome in homozygous beta-thalassemia. Br J Haematol 2001;115:926–8.
64. Musallam KM, Taher AT, Rachmilewitz EA. Beta-thalassemia intermedia: a clinical perspective. Cold Spring Harb Perspect Med 2012;2:a013482.
65. Ackerman Z. Local iron overload in chronic leg ulcers. Isr Med Assoc J 2011;96: 1605–12.

Hypercoagulability and Vascular Disease

Ali T. Taher, MD, PhD, FRCP[a],*, Maria Domenica Cappellini, MD[b,c],
Rayan Bou-Fakhredin, BSc[d], Daniel Coriu, MD, PhD[e],
Khaled M. Musallam, MD, PhD[f]

KEYWORDS

• Thrombosis • Pulmonary hypertension • Cerebrovascular disease
• Hypercoagulable state

KEY POINTS

• Hypercoagulability in β-thalassemia is attributed to several factors, including the pro-thrombotic potential of red blood cells, activated platelets, and endothelial damage.
• Clinical thrombotic events are more commonly observed in splenectomized or nontrans-fused patients and include venous, arterial, and cerebrovascular events.
• Clinical trials to determine the best prevention or treatment approaches are absent and management should remain individualized, focusing on high risk patients.

INTRODUCTION

A hypercoagulable state has been identified in patients with β-thalassemias, especially in those with nontransfusion-dependent thalassemia (NTDT), which can be present since childhood.[1–3] This hypercoagulable state primarily results from abnormalities in pathologic red blood cells and platelets, ultimately leading to thrombosis or other types of vascular disease (**Fig. 1**).[4–9] This article summarizes current knowledge on such mechanisms and highlights available evidence on clinical sequelae and their management. Although hypercoagulability is thought to play a crucial role in the development of pulmonary hypertension in patients with β-thalassemia, other factors and disease dynamics are also involved and these will not be discussed in the scope of this review.

Conflicts of Interest: None to disclose.
[a] Department of Internal Medicine, Naef K. Basile Cancer Institute, American University of Beirut Medical Center, PO Box 11-0236, Beirut 11072020, Lebanon; [b] Department of Medicine, Ca' Granda Foundation IRCCS, Milan 20122, Italy; [c] Department of Clinical Science and Community, University of Milan, Milan 20122, Italy; [d] Department of Internal Medicine, American University of Beirut Medical Center, Beirut 11072020, Lebanon; [e] Department of Hematology, Fundeni Clinical Institute, University of Medicine and Pharmacy "Carol Davila", Bucharest 030167, Romania; [f] International Network of Hematology, London WC1V 6AX, UK
* Corresponding author.
E-mail address: ataher@aub.edu.lb

Hematol Oncol Clin N Am 32 (2018) 237–245
https://doi.org/10.1016/j.hoc.2017.11.001
0889-8588/18/© 2017 Elsevier Inc. All rights reserved.

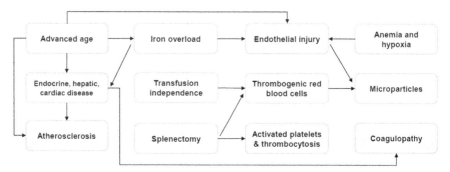

Fig. 1. Pathophysiologic and risk factors contributing to a hypercoagulable state and subsequent thrombotic and vascular events in β-thalassemia. Relevant associations between different factors are highlighted.

PATHOPHYSIOLOGY

Patients with β-thalassemia have enhanced platelet aggregation and chronically activated platelets,[10] as confirmed by the increased expression of CD62P (P-selectin) and CD63, which are markers of in vivo platelet activation.[11,12] β-thalassemia patients have been shown to have 4 to 10 times higher metabolites of thromboxane A2 and prostacyclin (PG I2), which are markers of hemostatic activity, than healthy individuals.[13] It has also been demonstrated that splenectomized patients have high platelet counts[14,15] but with a shorter life-span due to enhanced consumption.[16] One study showed that increased platelet adhesion is a finding that is commonly seen in splenectomized β-thalassemia patients. This is induced by mechanisms that involve both red blood cells and platelets, and is a strong contributor to occlusive thrombus formation in the carotid arteries of thalassemic mice.[17,18]

The role red blood cells play in the hypercoagulability of β-thalassemia has received great deal of attention. In thalassemia, the oxidation of globin subunits in erythroid cells leads to the formation of hemichromes,[19] which precipitate, prompting heme disintegration and the subsequent release of toxic iron species.[20] In turn, the free iron catalyzes the formation of reactive oxygen species, thereby leading to the oxidation of membrane proteins and the formation of red-cell senescence antigens such as phosphatidylserine,[21] which cause the red blood cells to aggregate and become rigid and deformed, resulting in premature cell removal.[22] Thalassemic red blood cells containing a high content of such negatively charged phospholipids often lead to an increase in thrombin generation,[23,24] as demonstrated by studies using annexin V, a protein with high specificity and affinity for anionic phospholipids.[24] Splenectomized patients have a considerably higher number of these negatively charged pathologic red blood cells and, as a result, higher thrombin generation is seen in these patients.[25,26] Compared with controls, β-thalassemia subjects were also found to have higher levels of procoagulant microparticles of red blood cell, leukocytic, and endothelial origins.[27]

The presence of other peripheral blood elements in patients with thalassemia, such as intercellular adhesion molecule-1, vascular cell adhesion molecule-1, E-selectin, and von Willebrand factor, shows that endothelial cell activation or injury may be an aspect of the disease itself, aiding in the recruitment of red and white blood cells, thus promoting thrombosis.[28,29] In fact, studies have revealed that red blood cells from β-thalassemia subjects often express an increased adhesion to cultured endothelial cells.[30] Although inherited thrombophilia does not play a role in the hypercoagulable state of β-thalassemia,[31,32] low levels of protein S, protein C, and antithrombin III have been documented.[33] Moreover, the presence of endocrine or hepatic dysfunction in older patients with severe iron overload may also be a factor that can contribute to hypercoagulability.[33]

Studies have shown that in a state of iron overload the presence of nontransferrin-bound iron can cause oxidative vessel injury.[34] Free radicals will act directly on the endothelial cells and closely interact with lipid peroxidation, which in turn will cause a modification of low-density lipoprotein and facilitate its deposition, with the subsequent formation of atherosclerotic plaques.[35] In fact, current studies support the notion that patients with β-thalassemia do indeed exhibit a proatherogenic biochemical phenotype.[36,37]

CLINICAL THROMBOSIS AND VASCULAR DISEASE

Data describing the incidence of thrombotic events in β-thalassemia patients are limited. One study that included 9 Italian pediatric thalassemia centers showed that 4% of 683 subjects with β-thalassemia major and 9.6% of 52 subjects with β-thalassemia intermedia experienced a thrombotic event.[38] In a cohort study that included 83 splenectomized β-thalassemia intermedia subjects that were followed up over 10 years, 29% of subjects experienced a venous thrombotic event.[26] Conventional risk factors for venous thrombosis were usually absent in such subjects,[39] further underlining the unique pathophysiology of hypercoagulability in β-thalassemia. Thrombotic events have also been documented in case series of pregnant women with β-thalassemia intermedia.[40] The largest study to date looked at data that were retrieved from 8860 subjects with thalassemia in the Mediterranean area and Iran, and found that thrombotic events, mostly venous, occurred 4.38 times more frequently in NTDT subjects (β-thalassemia intermedia) compared with regularly-transfused β-thalassemia major.[41] It was found that 14% of mortalities in the whole group were attributed to thrombotic events. The main risk factors for thrombosis in patients with β-thalassemia intermedia were identified as older than age 20 years, splenectomy, and personal or family history of thrombosis.[41]

The Overview on Practices in Thalassemia Intermedia Management Aiming for Lowering Complication Rates Across a Region of Endemicity (OPTIMAL CARE) study, which evaluated 584 β-thalassemia intermedia subjects at 6 comprehensive care centers (Lebanon, Italy, Iran, Egypt, United Arab Emirates, and Oman), showed that thrombotic disease, mostly venous, was the fifth most common complication, affecting about 14% of the subject population. The key independent risk factors for thrombotic events were splenectomy, iron overload (serum ferritin level ≥1000 ng/mL), age older than 35 years, and a hemoglobin level of less than 9 g/dL.[42] A substudy analysis of the OPTIMAL CARE was conducted. It determined that splenectomized β-thalassemia intermedia subjects who experience thrombosis are characterized by having high platelet counts (≥500 × 10⁹/l) and high nucleated red blood cell (≥300 × 10⁶/l),[43] further confirming the dual role of both red blood cells and platelets in this setting. The study additionally examined the time it took for a thrombotic event to develop following splenectomy and found the median time to thrombosis to be 8 years.[43] Other studies evaluating β-thalassemia intermedia subjects also showed that higher rates of thrombosis were observed with advancing age, severe ineffective erythropoiesis, and iron overload (liver iron concentration ≥5 mg iron per gram dry weight or serum ferritin level ≥800 ng/mL).[44–48]

The prevalence of overt strokes in NTDT patients with a history of thrombosis ranges between 5% and 9%.[41,43,49] In the literature, few case reports have described a frequent occurrence of overt strokes in β-thalassemia intermedia patients with moyamoya syndrome.[50–53] However, a higher prevalence of silent strokes has been consistently documented in this group of patients.[54] In 1999, 1 of the earliest studies was conducted and showed a 37.5% rate of ischemic lesions on brain MRI in 16 subjects with β-thalassemia intermedia (mean age 29 years) who were neurologically intact and had no conventional stroke-related risk factors.[55] More recently, a cross-sectional study in Lebanon using brain MRI was conducted on 30 splenectomized adults with β-thalassemia intermedia (mean age 32 years) who were selected from a larger cohort of subjects based on the absence of neurologic or gross cognitive signs or symptoms and any stroke-related risk factors. None of the subjects were receiving antiplatelet or anticoagulant therapy. Eighteen subjects (60%) showed evidence of 1 or more ischemic lesions, all involving the subcortical white matter. Most subjects showed evidence of multiple lesions. The frontal subcortical white matter was almost always involved, followed by the occipital and parietal subcortical white matter. About 94% of subjects had evidence of small to medium (<1.5 cm) lesions with only 1 subject showing evidence of a large lesion (>1.5 cm).[56] Increasing age and no transfusion history were both noted as independently associated with a higher occurrence and multiplicity of lesions.[56] Another Iranian cross-sectional study was conducted on 30 randomly selected β-thalassemia intermedia adults (mean age 24 years) who were splenectomized, and who had a platelet count greater than or equal to 500 times $10^9/l$ and a hemoglobin level greater than 7 g/dL. The investigators noted 8 subjects (26.7%) with silent ischemic lesions.[57] The harmful roles of splenectomy and thrombocytosis in this setting were confirmed in a more recent study.[58] The variability in the multiplicity and observed frequency of silent strokes in the currently available studies could be primarily attributed to the strength of the magnetic field used (Tesla units). Although these studies failed to include a control group, the incidence of silent strokes incidentally discovered on brain scans of healthy individuals of a similar age group (<50 years) ranged from 0% to a maximum of 11%, suggesting that the described changes are pathologic rather than normal variations.[56] It is important to note that similar observations were not observed in children with β-thalassemia intermedia.[59] Moreover, only 1 study assessed the prevalence of silent stroke in subjects with hemoglobin E/β-thalassemia (mean age 31 years), and the rate was also high (24%).[60] Most recently, a study conducted on regularly transfused β-thalassemia subjects showed that frequent transfusions and low platelet counts may not always be associated with a low frequency of silent strokes.[61]

Three independent studies evaluated the mechanism of intracranial blood flow velocity in neurologically asymptomatic subjects with β-thalassemia intermedia using transcranial Doppler Ultrasonography. They all showed that the mean flow velocities in the intracranial circulation of β-thalassemia intermedia subjects were higher than healthy controls but were lower than those associated with ischemic stroke risk in subjects with sickle cell disease (>2 m/s).[59,62,63] Studies using PET-computed tomography (PET-CT) and brain magnetic resonance angiography (MRA) have also been recently conducted in subjects with β-thalassemia intermedia. One study that included 29 asymptomatic, splenectomized adult subjects, revealed that 27.6% of subjects had evidence of arterial stenosis on MRA. Two subjects had more than 1 artery involved and the internal carotid artery was identified as the most commonly involved artery. Among the 12 identified stenotic lesions, 9 were mild (≤50% stenosis), 1 was moderate (51%–75% stenosis), and the remaining 2 were severe (>75% stenosis).[64] The risk of abnormality on MRA increased with declining hemoglobin level and increased nontransferrin-bound iron.[64] PET-CT scanning revealed that decreased neuronal function is also a common finding (63.3%) in this patient population. It is primarily left sided, multiple, and most commonly in the parietal and temporal lobes.[65] The risk of abnormality on PET-CT increased with higher liver iron concentration levels.[65]

There currently exist no data to determine whether the observed silent brain abnormalities in β-thalassemia intermedia patients are truly silent. In the general population and in sickle cell disease patients, silent strokes, arterial stenosis on MRA, and decreased neuronal function on PET-CT have all been associated with a subsequent risk of overt stroke and neurocognitive decline.[54]

PREVENTION AND MANAGEMENT

This delay in thrombotic events in splenectomized patients further emphasized that such a manifestation is a result of a chronic underlying process and emphasized the need for long-term preventive strategies.[43]

The role of blood transfusion in the primary or secondary prevention of thrombotic events patients with NTDT has not yet been evaluated in clinical trials. However, blood transfusions may control the hypercoagulability in NTDT patients by not only improving ineffective erythropoiesis but also decreasing the levels of pathologic red blood cells with thrombogenic potential.[66] Transfusion therapy may also explain the lower rates of thrombotic events that are seen in regularly transfused β-thalassemia major patients than in NTDT.[8,41,67] Data from observational studies conducted on subjects with β-thalassemia intermedia showed that transfusion therapy was associated with lower rates of silent strokes and thromboembolic events.[42,56] The success rate of transfusion therapy use for the prevention of silent strokes in subgroups of patients with sickle cell disease has also been established.[68]

Some observational studies have suggested that in subjects with NTDT there exists an independent association between iron overload and thrombotic disease.[42,44,45,69] However, further studies are necessary to confirm that such an observation is not confounded by the role of ineffective erythropoiesis. The role of iron chelation therapy has not yet been evaluated in this setting.

Hydroxyurea, a fetal hemoglobin inducer, was shown to decrease plasma markers of thrombin generation and coagulation activation in NTDT subjects by reducing phospholipid expression on the surface of red blood cells.[70] Hydroxyurea may also decrease hemostatic activation by its effect in decreasing the white blood cell count and, particularly, monocytes that express tissue factor.[6] In subjects with NTDT, the role of hydroxyurea in the prevention of thrombotic disease has not been evaluated. However, 1 study conducted on β-thalassemia intermedia subjects suggested an association between the use of hydroxyurea and lower rates of silent strokes.[58] A similar evaluation in subjects with sickle cell disease was not encouraging.[71]

There are currently no available results from clinical trials on the role of antiplatelet or anticoagulant therapy for the prevention of thrombotic or cerebrovascular disease in subjects with thalassemia. However, an association between high platelet counts and thrombosis, as well as a lower recurrence rate of thrombotic events in splenectomized β-thalassemia intermedia subjects who took aspirin after their first event, when compared with those who did not, suggest that aspirin could have a potential role in the prevention of thrombotic disease.[41,43] Furthermore, the high prevalence of silent strokes in splenectomized patients with elevated platelet counts also suggests a potential role for aspirin therapy.[57,58] It has been suggested by observations that, even in subjects with normal platelet counts, aspirin therapy could delay occlusive thrombus formation in carotid arteries of thalassemic mice.[17,18]

REFERENCES

1. Eldor A, Rachmilewitz EA. The hypercoagulable state in thalassemia. Blood 2002; 99(1):36–43.
2. Eldor A, Durst R, Hy-Am E, et al. A chronic hypercoagulable state in patients with beta-thalassaemia major is already present in childhood. Br J Haematol 1999; 107(4):739–46.
3. Cappellini MD, Musallam KM, Poggiali E, et al. Hypercoagulability in non-transfusion-dependent thalassemia. Blood Rev 2012;26(Suppl 1):S20–3.
4. Cappellini MD, Poggiali E, Taher AT, et al. Hypercoagulability in beta-thalassemia: a status quo. Expert Rev Hematol 2012;5(5):505–11 [quiz: 512].
5. Cappellini MD, Motta I, Musallam KM, et al. Redefining thalassemia as a hyper-coagulable state. Ann N Y Acad Sci 2010;1202:231–6.
6. Ataga KI, Cappellini MD, Rachmilewitz EA. Beta-thalassaemia and sickle cell anaemia as paradigms of hypercoagulability. Br J Haematol 2007;139(1):3–13.
7. Musallam KM, Taher AT. Thrombosis in thalassemia: why are we so concerned? Hemoglobin 2011;35(5–6):503–10.
8. Musallam KM, Rivella S, Vichinsky E, et al. Non-transfusion-dependent thalasse-mias. Haematologica 2013;98(6):833–44.
9. Musallam KM, Taher AT, Rachmilewitz EA. beta-thalassemia intermedia: a clinical perspective. Cold Spring Harb Perspect Med 2012;2(7):a013482.
10. Winichagoon P, Fucharoen S, Wasi P. Increased circulating platelet aggregates in thalassaemia. Southeast Asian J Trop Med Public Health 1981;12(4):556–60.
11. Del Principe D, Menichelli A, Di Giulio S, et al. PADGEM/GMP-140 expression on platelet membranes from homozygous beta thalassaemic patients. Br J Haematol 1993;84(1):111–7.
12. Ruf A, Pick M, Deutsch V, et al. In-vivo platelet activation correlates with red cell anionic phospholipid exposure in patients with beta-thalassaemia major. Br J Haematol 1997;98(1):51–6.
13. Eldor A, Lellouche F, Goldfarb A, et al. In vivo platelet activation in beta-thalassemia major reflected by increased platelet-thromboxane urinary metabo-lites. Blood 1991;77(8):1749–53.
14. Cappellini MD, Grespi E, Cassinerio E, et al. Coagulation and splenectomy: an overview. Ann N Y Acad Sci 2005;1054:317–24.
15. Atichartakarn V, Angchaisuksiri P, Aryurachai K, et al. In vivo platelet activation and hyperaggregation in hemoglobin E/beta-thalassemia: a consequence of splenectomy. Int J Hematol 2003;77(3):299–303.
16. Eldor A, Krausz Y, Atlan H, et al. Platelet survival in patients with beta-thalas-semia. Am J Hematol 1989;32(2):94–9.
17. Goldschmidt N, Spectre G, Brill A, et al. Increased platelet adhesion under flow conditions is induced by both thalassemic platelets and red blood cells. Thromb Haemost 2008;100(5):864–70.
18. Rachmilewitz E, Malyutin Z, Shai E, et al. Shorter carotid artery occlusion in a thal-assemic mouse model: a potential role for oxidative stress affecting both RBCs and platelets [abstract]. Haematologica 2012;97(S1):0943.
19. Rund D, Rachmilewitz E. Beta-thalassemia. N Engl J Med 2005;353(11):1135–46.
20. Hershko C, Graham G, Bates GW, et al. Non-specific serum iron in thalassaemia: an abnormal serum iron fraction of potential toxicity. Br J Haematol 1978;40(2): 255–63.
21. Kuypers FA, de Jong K. The role of phosphatidylserine in recognition and removal of erythrocytes. Cell Mol Biol (Noisy-le-grand) 2004;50(2):147–58.

22. Tavazzi D, Duca L, Graziadei G, et al. Membrane-bound iron contributes to oxidative damage of beta-thalassaemia intermedia erythrocytes. Br J Haematol 2001; 112(1):48–50.
23. Borenstain-Ben Yashar V, Barenholz Y, Hy-Am E, et al. Phosphatidylserine in the outer leaflet of red blood cells from beta-thalassemia patients may explain the chronic hypercoagulable state and thrombotic episodes. Am J Hematol 1993; 44(1):63–5.
24. Helley D, Eldor A, Girot R, et al. Increased procoagulant activity of red blood cells from patients with homozygous sickle cell disease and beta-thalassemia. Thromb Haemost 1996;76(3):322–7.
25. Atichartakarn V, Angchaisuksiri P, Aryurachai K, et al. Relationship between hypercoagulable state and erythrocyte phosphatidylserine exposure in splenectomized haemoglobin E/beta-thalassaemic patients. Br J Haematol 2002; 118(3):893–8.
26. Cappellini MD, Robbiolo L, Bottasso BM, et al. Venous thromboembolism and hypercoagulability in splenectomized patients with thalassaemia intermedia. Br J Haematol 2000;111(2):467–73.
27. Habib A, Kunzelmann C, Shamseddeen W, et al. Elevated levels of circulating procoagulant microparticles in patients with beta-thalassemia intermedia. Haematologica 2008;93(6):941–2.
28. Butthep P, Bunyaratvej A, Funahara Y, et al. Alterations in vascular endothelial cell-related plasma proteins in thalassaemic patients and their correlation with clinical symptoms. Thromb Haemost 1995;74(4):1045–9.
29. Butthep P, Bunyaratvej A, Funahara Y, et al. Possible evidence of endothelial cell activation and disturbance in thalassemia: an in vitro study. Southeast Asian J Trop Med Public Health 1997;28(Suppl 3):141–8A.
30. Hovav T, Goldfarb A, Artmann G, et al. Enhanced adherence of beta-thalassaemic erythrocytes to endothelial cells. Br J Haematol 1999;106(1): 178–81.
31. Zalloua PA, Shbaklo H, Mourad YA, et al. Incidence of thromboembolic events in Lebanese thalassemia intermedia patients. Thromb Haemost 2003;89(4):767–8.
32. Iolascon A, Giordano P, Storelli S, et al. Thrombophilia in thalassemia major patients: analysis of genetic predisposing factors. Haematologica 2001;86(10): 1112–3.
33. Taher AT, Otrock ZK, Uthman I, et al. Thalassemia and hypercoagulability. Blood Rev 2008;22(5):283–92.
34. Auer JW, Berent R, Weber T, et al. Iron metabolism and development of atherosclerosis. Circulation 2002;106(2):e7.
35. Aessopos A, Tsironi M, Andreopoulos A, et al. Heart disease in thalassemia intermedia. Hemoglobin 2009;33(Suppl 1):S170–6.
36. Hahalis G, Kalogeropoulos A, Terzis G, et al. Premature atherosclerosis in non-transfusion-dependent beta-thalassemia intermedia. Cardiology 2011;118(3): 159–63.
37. Lai ME, Vacquer S, Carta MP, et al. Thalassemia intermedia is associated with a proatherogenic biochemical phenotype. Blood Cells Mol Dis 2011;46(4):294–9.
38. Borgna Pignatti C, Carnelli V, Caruso V, et al. Thromboembolic events in beta thalassemia major: an Italian multicenter study. Acta Haematol 1998;99(2):76–9.
39. Gillis S, Cappellini MD, Goldfarb A, et al. Pulmonary thromboembolism in thalassemia intermedia patients. Haematologica 1999;84(10):959–60.

40. Nassar AH, Naja M, Cesaretti C, et al. Pregnancy outcome in patients with beta-thalassemia intermedia at two tertiary care centers, in Beirut and Milan. Haematologica 2008;93(10):1586–7.

41. Taher A, Isma'eel H, Mehio G, et al. Prevalence of thromboembolic events among 8,860 patients with thalassaemia major and intermedia in the Mediterranean area and Iran. Thromb Haemost 2006;96(4):488–91.

42. Taher AT, Musallam KM, Karimi M, et al. Overview on practices in thalassemia intermedia management aiming for lowering complication rates across a region of endemicity: the OPTIMAL CARE study. Blood 2010;115(10):1886–92.

43. Taher AT, Musallam KM, Karimi M, et al. Splenectomy and thrombosis: the case of thalassemia intermedia. J Thromb Haemost 2010;8(10):2152–8.

44. Musallam KM, Cappellini MD, Taher AT. Evaluation of the 5mg/g liver iron concentration threshold and its association with morbidity in patients with beta-thalassemia intermedia. Blood Cells Mol Dis 2013;51(1):35–8.

45. Musallam KM, Cappellini MD, Wood JC, et al. Elevated liver iron concentration is a marker of increased morbidity in patients with beta thalassemia intermedia. Haematologica 2011;96(11):1605–12.

46. Taher AT, Musallam KM, El-Beshlawy A, et al. Age-related complications in treatment-naive patients with thalassaemia intermedia. Br J Haematol 2010; 150(4):486–9.

47. Musallam KM, Taher AT, Duca L, et al. Levels of growth differentiation factor-15 are high and correlate with clinical severity in transfusion-independent patients with beta thalassemia intermedia. Blood Cells Mol Dis 2011;47(4):232–4.

48. Musallam KM, Cappellini MD, Daar S, et al. Serum ferritin level and morbidity risk in transfusion-independent patients with beta-thalassemia intermedia: the ORIENT study. Haematologica 2014;99(11):e218–21.

49. Karimi M, Khanlari M, Rachmilewitz EA. Cerebrovascular accident in beta-thalassemia major (beta-TM) and beta-thalassemia intermedia (beta-TI). Am J Hematol 2008;83(1):77–9.

50. Oberoi S, Bansal D, Singh P, et al. Stroke in a young boy with beta-thalassemia intermedia secondary to moyamoya syndrome. J Pediatr Hematol Oncol 2010; 32(7):568–70.

51. Goksel BK, Ozdogu H, Yildirim T, et al. Beta-thalassemia intermedia associated with moyamoya syndrome. J Clin Neurosci 2010;17(7):919–20.

52. Marden FA, Putman CM, Grant JM, et al. Moyamoya disease associated with hemoglobin Fairfax and beta-thalassemia. Pediatr Neurol 2008;38(2):130–2.

53. Sanefuji M, Ohga S, Kira R, et al. Moyamoya syndrome in a splenectomized patient with beta-thalassemia intermedia. J Child Neurol 2006;21(1):75–7.

54. Musallam KM, Taher AT, Karimi M, et al. Cerebral infarction in beta-thalassemia intermedia: breaking the silence. Thromb Res 2012;130(5):695–702.

55. Manfre L, Giarratano E, Maggio A, et al. MR imaging of the brain: findings in asymptomatic patients with thalassemia intermedia and sickle cell-thalassemia disease. AJR Am J Roentgenol 1999;173(6):1477–80.

56. Taher AT, Musallam KM, Nasreddine W, et al. Asymptomatic brain magnetic resonance imaging abnormalities in splenectomized adults with thalassemia intermedia. J Thromb Haemost 2010;8(1):54–9.

57. Karimi M, Bagheri H, Rastgu F, et al. Magnetic resonance imaging to determine the incidence of brain ischaemia in patients with beta-thalassaemia intermedia. Thromb Haemost 2010;103(5):989–93.

58. Karimi M, Haghpanah S, Bagheri MH, et al. Frequency and distribution of asymptomatic brain lesions in patients with beta-thalassemia intermedia. Ann Hematol 2012;91(12):1833–8.
59. Teli A, Economou M, Rudolf J, et al. Subclinical central nervous system involvement and thrombophilic status in young thalassemia intermedia patients of Greek origin. Blood Coagul Fibrinolysis 2012;23(3):195–202.
60. Metarugcheep P, Chanyawattiwongs S, Srisubat K, et al. Clinical silent cerebral infarct (SCI) in patients with thalassemia diseases assessed by magnetic resonance imaging (MRI). J Med Assoc Thai 2008;91(6):889–94.
61. Karimi M, Toosi F, Haghpanah S, et al. The frequency of silent cerebral ischemia in patients with transfusion-dependent beta-thalassemia major. Ann Hematol 2016;95(1):135–9.
62. Ashjazadeh N, Emami S, Petramfar P, et al. Intracranial blood flow velocity in patients with beta-thalassemia intermedia using transcranial doppler sonography: a case-control study. Anemia 2012;2012:798296.
63. Abboud MR, Maakaron JE, Khoury RA, et al. Intracranial blood flow velocities in patients with sickle cell disease and beta-thalassemia intermedia. Am J Hematol 2013;88(9):825.
64. Musallam KM, Beydoun A, Hourani R, et al. Brain magnetic resonance angiography in splenectomized adults with beta-thalassemia intermedia. Eur J Haematol 2011;87(6):539–46.
65. Musallam KM, Nasreddine W, Beydoun A, et al. Brain positron emission tomography in splenectomized adults with beta-thalassemia intermedia: uncovering yet another covert abnormality. Ann Hematol 2012;91(2):235–41.
66. Chen S, Eldor A, Barshtein G, et al. Enhanced aggregability of red blood cells of beta-thalassemia major patients. Am J Physiol 1996;270(6 Pt 2):H1951–6.
67. Taher A, Isma'eel H, Cappellini MD. Thalassemia intermedia: revisited. Blood Cells Mol Dis 2006;37(1):12–20.
68. DeBaun MR, Armstrong FD, McKinstry RC, et al. Silent cerebral infarcts: a review on a prevalent and progressive cause of neurologic injury in sickle cell anemia. Blood 2012;119(20):4587–96.
69. Musallam KM, Cappellini MD, Daar S, et al. Serum ferritin levels and morbidity in β-thalassemia intermedia: a 10-year cohort study [abstract]. Blood 2012;120(21):1021.
70. Singer ST, Vichinsky EP, Larkin S, et al. Hydroxycarbamide-induced changes in E/beta thalassemia red blood cells. Am J Hematol 2008;83(11):842–5.
71. Ware RE, Helms RW. Stroke with transfusions changing to hydroxyurea (SWiTCH). Blood 2012;119(17):3925–32.

Interaction of Transfusion and Iron Chelation in Thalassemias

John B. Porter, MA, MD, FRCP, FRCPath[a],*,
Maciej W. Garbowski, MD, PhD[b]

KEYWORDS

- Iron • Chelators • Iron overload • Transfusion • Erythropoiesis • Hepcidin
- Soluble transferrin receptor • Cardiosiderosis

KEY POINTS

- The goals of blood transfusion in thalassemias are to ameliorate anemia and decrease ineffective erythropoiesis and its associated erythron expansion.
- Low transfusion regimens increase residual erythropoiesis, allowing for apotransferrin-dependent clearance of non–transferrin-bound iron (NTBI) species otherwise destined for myocardium.
- Cardiac iron retention depends both on iron uptake via NTBI route and iron egress via cardiac ferroportin, which is sensitive to transfusion-dependent modulation of hepcidin.
- Iron chelation is a successful modality in prolonging life expectancy and decreasing morbidity in thalassemia but requires a dose balanced to the iron intake rate.
- A 24-hour per day exposure to chelation is required when transferrin nears saturation exceeding 70% to prevent extrahepatic NTBI uptake.

INTRODUCTION

The benefits of both transfusion and chelation when used together are well established for transfusion-dependent thalassemias (TDTs). With the advent of newer chelation regimens and monitoring techniques, and in light of recent data linking low erythron activity to increased risk of cardiosiderosis, a reappraisal of the optimal balance between transfusion rates and chelation may be warranted. In this article, current transfusion and

Disclosure Statement: Advisory Board and consultancy to Novartis, Cerus, Celgene, Anaylam (J.B. Porter). Advisory Board to Vifor (M.W. Garbowski). Dr J.B. Porter is supported by the BRC at UCL.
[a] Haematology Department, University College London, UCLH and Whittington Hospitals, UCL Cancer Institute, Paul O'Gorman Building, 72 Huntley Street, London WC1E 6BT, UK;
[b] Haematology Department, University College London, Cancer Institute, UCL Cancer Institute, Paul O'Gorman Building, 72 Huntley Street, London WC1E 6BT, UK
* Corresponding author.
E-mail address: j.porter@ucl.ac.uk

chelation practices are critically reviewed, with emphasis on how transfusion strategy affects iron distribution and the mechanisms through which this interaction occurs. The implications of this interaction for chelation strategy are also examined.

OBJECTIVES OF TRANSFUSION IN THALASSEMIAS

Blood transfusion in thalassemia aims to correct anemia so that physical and cognitive performances are close to healthy individuals, while preventing harmful or potentially disfiguring expansion of the erythron and not transfusing more blood and hence iron than necessary. Evidence for optimal hemoglobin (Hb) to achieve these goals was initially contradictory: some studies showed transfusion requirements remained constant at mean transfusion Hb levels of 10 g/dL to 14 g/dL (equivalent to pretransfusion Hb 8–12 g/dL),[1,2] whereas others showed that transfusion requirements were directly proportional to the mean Hb.[3,4] In a later study, transfusion requirement was measured in the same patients under 2 transfusion regimens[5]: those with mean pretransfusion Hb of 11.3 g/dL had mean annual transfusion of 137 mL/kg, but when the mean was subsequently lowered to Hb 9.4 g/dL, annual consumption decreased to 104 mL/kg/L and ferritin values fell.

Current guidelines recommend pretransfusion Hb values of 9.5 g/dL to 10.5 g/dL, thus keeping the mean Hb at approximately 12 g/dL with a post-transfusion Hb not above 14 g/dL.[6] This sweet spot for balancing considerations of iron loading and correction of anemia and ineffective erythropoiesis (IE) is based on a study of Italian patients[5] and may not be applicable to patients with different levels of effective erythropoiesis (discussed later). Under certain circumstances, higher Hb levels may be appropriate, for example, when some patients experience low back pain at Hb less than 10 g/dL to 11 g/dL, when the spleen size is expanding, or during pregnancy. The recommended frequency of transfusion every 2 weeks to 4 weeks has been determined to some extent by the convenience to patients and the availability of blood in some regions. Mathematical modeling suggested pretransfusion Hb of 9 g/dL with transfusions every 2 weeks rather than every 4 weeks would reduce requirements by 20% but no measurable effect was seen in a study comparing 3-week or 4-week intervals.[4]

Some populations are managed on lower pretransfusion Hb values: for example, in 464 Egyptian TDT patients aged 10 months to 31 years,[7] the mean pretransfusion Hb was 5.7 g/dL. In another study, the Hb values were significantly lower in patients from Cairo, Egypt (6.9 g/dL), than from Ismir, Turkey (Hb 8.9 g/dL) (Yesim Aydinok, MD, personal communication, 2017). The authors suggest that this variation in practice may account for differences in the proportion of patients with cardiosiderosis (discussed later).

Further considerations are whether and when to start transfusion, particularly for milder syndromes. Many patients with milder phenotypes may not require transfusion in the first few years of life, but as Hb values fall, particularly if there is failure to thrive, transfusion may become necessary. Guidelines generally suggest Hb values repeatedly less than 7 g/dL are suitable to begin transfusion but this approach may not be universally applicable, particularly in Eβ-thalassemia (haemoglobin E beta thalassaemia) syndromes, where the oxygen dissociation curve is right-shifted relative to β-thalassemia syndromes. For example, in a study where 109 Eβ-thalassemia patients from Sri Lanka were followed for 5 years, the untransfused group had Hb levels of 6.1 g/dL and, based on performance status, did not require starting transfusion, whereas in a second group with mean Hb values of 7.0 g/dL, 40% were able to stop transfusion without deleterious effects, despite the low Hb values.[8] These findings suggest that Eβ-thalassemia can be often managed without transfusion, even with low Hb levels.

BODY IRON CONTENT AND IMPACT OF TRANSFUSION

Thalassemia patients who are anemic but not receiving regular blood transfusion, so-called non–TDT (NTDT), absorb increased quantities of dietary iron, due to inappropriately low hepcidin relative to iron stores, that may not be balanced by insensible iron losses, so that iron overload gradually develops.[9] Excess iron absorption depends on the degree of IE, the extent of erythroid expansion, and the severity of anemia. Iron absorption rates determined with radioisotope markers, showing absorption of 5 times that of healthy controls were reported in β-thalassemia intermedia (range 3–10 times).[10] This was similar in Eβ-thalassemia, where studies also showed that iron absorption correlated with plasma iron turnover, transferrin saturation (TfSat), and liver iron concentration (LIC).[11] Iron absorption over 1 year has now been determined in larger populations, using MRI to measure changes in LIC[12] and hence calculate net iron absorption.[13] LIC and serum ferritin increased from baseline by 0.38 mg Fe/g dry weight and 115 ng/mL, respectively. This increase in LIC is equivalent to an average iron accumulation rate of 0.011 mg/kg/d.[12] Increased iron absorption is currently believed to result from inhibition of hepatic hepcidin synthesis by bone marrow–derived factors associated with IE that lead to inappropriately low hepcidin levels relative to iron stores.[9] Implicated factors have included growth differentiation factor (GDF)-15 in humans[14] and, more recently, erythroferrone in mice.[15] GDF-11 has also been identified as a factor associated with IE in a murine thalassemia model.[16] Iron overload in NTDT correlates with erythron expansion biomarkers (soluble transferrin receptor [sTfR], GDF-15, and nucleated red blood cell count), particularly in untransfused, such as Hb H, patients.[9] Plasma hepcidin correlates inversely with TfSat, NTBI, and labile plasma iron (LPI),[9] consistent with a link between iron absorption and depressed hepcidin levels. Hepcidin/serum ferritin ratios were also low, consistent with hepcidin suppression relative to iron overload.[9] Increased NTBI and, by implication, risk of extrahepatic iron distribution, were more likely in previously transfused, splenectomized and iron-overloaded NTDT patients with TfSat greater than 70%.[9]

The iron loading rate from blood transfusion in TDT is approximately 10 times the rate seen in NTDT or 20 mg/d to 35 mg/d in a 70-kg adult.[17] This is because of the high iron content in a unit of blood: a unit of red cells, processed from 420 mL of donor blood, contains approximately 200 mg of iron (or 0.47 mg/mL of whole donor blood equivalent to 1.16 mg/mL of pure red cells). The mean loading rate is approximately 0.4 mg/kg/d[17] equivalent to 28 mg/d of iron in 70-kg adult. Approximately 20% of patients receive less than 0.3 mg/kg/d, approximately 60% receive 0.3 to 0.5 mg/kg/d, and a further 20% greater than 0.5 mg/kg/d of iron. Without chelation therapy, LIC reaches 15 mg/dry weight after less than 5 years of blood transfusion. Average transfusion requirements are somewhat higher in unsplenectomized (0.43 mg/kg/d) TDT patients compared with splenectomized patients (0.33 mg/kg/d).[17] Thus, splenectomized patient receive the equivalent of 300 mL less of whole blood per kg per annum decreasing the annual iron loading by 39%. This is not sufficient reason to recommend splenectomy due the high complication rates and because modern chelation regimes can generally keep pace with this difference in iron accumulation. In patients who develop splenic enlargement, hypertransfusion can often diminish spleen size without the need for splenectomy.[18]

MECHANISMS OF BODY IRON DISTRIBUTION IN THALASSEMIAS

In the absence of blood transfusion, excess absorbed iron is found in the periportal hepatocytes in NTDT[19] and extrahepatic iron distribution is rare.[20,21] With blood transfusion in TDT, however, iron accumulates initially in the macrophage system after erythrophagocytosis of transfused red cells. Red cell heme is catabolized here by hemoxygenase with iron rapidly released through ferroportin channels for extracellular binding to transferrin. Alternatively, when hepcidin binding to membrane ferroportin degrades this molecule, more iron can be retained within macrophages as storage iron (ferritin or hemosiderin). The macrophage system is considered capable of storing approximately 10 g of iron (or approximately 50 units of transfused blood).

Once the macrophage system is replete, increasing proportions of storage iron are delivered to hepatocytes though diferric transferrin and/or through plasma iron species occurring when TfSat exceeds approximately 75%, the so-called plasma NTBI. Unlike transferrin-bound iron, which is targeted through transferrin receptors to the erythron or to hepatocytes, NTBI species are taken into endocrine system and myocardium, in addition to hepatocytes, probably though L-type voltage-dependent calcium channels into myocardium[22] and possibly also though Zip14 in the endocrine system.[23] The cells known to take up NTBI are similar to those tissues susceptible to the effects of transfusional iron overload (discussed later). Clinical conditions associated with high plasma NTBI, such as TDT and Diamond-Blackfan anemia (DBA), are associated with high NTBI levels. Conversely, conditions with low NTBI levels, even where severe iron overload co-exists, such as NTDT and sickle cell disease, have a low propensity to extrahepatic iron distribution.[24] Levels of NTBI are affected by several independent factors,[24] raised by iron overload but also raised when erythropoiesis is relatively inactive, such as in myeloablative chemotherapy, due to decreased clearance of transferrin-iron by the erythron[25] or when erythropoiesis is constitutively inactive, as in DBA.[24]

Cellular iron uptake from NTBI not only is dependent on plasma levels but also on its speciation.[26] NTBI is heterogeneous consisting largely of iron-citrate species where the molecular weight of the iron-citrate complex is determined by the ratio of constant plasma citrate concentrations to the variable concentrations of NTBI.[27] Recent work suggests that the makeup of iron-citrate species (their speciation) has a key impact on the iron uptake into tissues, such as myocardium.[26] Thus iron uptake in HL-1 cardiomyocytes and generation of intracellular reactive oxygen species occurred most rapidly when citrate exceeded iron (III) by more than 100:1. Such conditions favor kinetically labile monomer (monoferric) rather than oligomer citrate species. These same species are those detected by the LPI assay, which measures the redox-active component of NTBI.[28] Monoferric species also bind most rapidly to apo-transferrin, which therefore readily inhibits cellular iron uptake of these NTBI species.[26] Thus, apo-transferrin generated by high transferrin-iron utilization in an active bone marrow can inhibit NTBI tissue uptake by rapidly binding monoferric-citrate species (discussed later). Therefore, the activity of the erythron is critical to NTBI speciation and hence body iron distribution. This explains why patients who have iron overload but little utilization of transferrin-iron, such as DBA or heavily hypertransfused TDT patients, may be particularly susceptible to extrahepatic iron distribution.

The clinical consequences of this iron distribution, including cardiomyopathy, endocrinopathy, and bacterial infections, have been recently described and reviewed by the senior author.[29] The generation of reactive oxygen species by iron that redox-cycles between iron (II) and iron (III) is the major driver of oxidative tissue damage and iron chelation therapy has had a major impact on the frequency of these complications.[30]

EFFECT OF BLOOD TRANSFUSION REGIMEN ON IRON DISTRIBUTION
Effect of Cumulative Blood Transfusion on Iron Distribution

In the absence of regular transfusion in NTDT, a lack of cardiosiderosis has been consistently reported.[20,21] Once transfusion begins in TDT, however, there is a clear link between the risk of myocardial iron accumulation and the cumulative volume of blood transfused. This was clear in the prechelation era,[31] when interpretation was not muddied by chelation altering the relationship between liver and cardiac iron. Post mortem data on multitransfused patients with a variety of anemias showed that 100% of patients had evidence of increased cardiosiderosis after 200 transfused units.[31] The proportion fell as the number of transfused units decreased; thus, 60% of patients had increased heart iron after 100 units but only 10% after 25 units to 50 units.[31] Early MRI studies also reported that myocardial iron increased in myelodysplastic patients with the number of transfused blood units and with LIC.[32] In studies failing to show such a link,[33] interpretation has been confounded by recent chelation therapy, which perturbs the apparent relationship between liver and heart iron due to more rapid removal of liver than heart iron. It is important to examine trends of heart and liver iron over time, where a clear relationship between these has been shown in chelated patients with heart changes following those in the liver.[34]

Effect of Intensity of Transfusion Regimen on Iron Accumulation and Iron Distribution

The intensity of blood transfusion can be represented by the pretransfusion Hb combined with the frequency of transfusion, which contribute to mean Hb. The higher this is, the greater the suppression of endogenous erythropoiesis.[5] The most robustly studied marker of extrahepatic iron is myocardial T2*.[33] Little direct prospective information about its relationship to variables in blood transfusion regimens exists; however, several lines of evidence suggest a relationship. The first comes from the lack of cardiosiderosis in heavily iron-overloaded NTDT patients.[20,21] The next comes from surprising disparity in the frequency of cardiosiderosis between Middle Eastern and European countries. Baseline data from 11 countries of 925 patients, mainly with TDT (>99%),[35] found the frequency of cardiosiderosis (T2*<20 ms) was notably lower in the Middle East (28.5%) than in Europe (49.5%) or the Asia Pacific (40.9%).[35] This was despite the proportion of patients with LIC values greater than 15 mg/g dry weight higher in the Middle East (63%) than in Europe (51%). Similar observations have been reported in Egyptian patients.[36] The reason is not immediately obvious: genotypic regional differences in thalassemia mutations are unlikely to explain these findings because systematic differences in frequency of abnormal myocardial T2* have not been noted in migrants from these countries to Europe. In Oman, incidences of abnormal T2* are high (46%) compared with elsewhere in the Middle East, which is more likely due to difference in clinical management than to genetic differences from elsewhere in the Middle East region because the genotypes are highly heterogeneous.[37]

Could differences in chelation policy account for the low prevalence of abnormal myocardial T2* in the Middle East? Again, this is unlikely, Middle Eastern patients were generally poorly chelated, with high LIC and ferritin, and many patients had received little or no chelation and had spent highest proportions of their lives without any chelation than other regional groups.[35] Unfortunately, the pretransfusion Hb values were not given. The proportion of patients going more than 4 weeks between transfusions, however, was highest in the Middle Eastern patients (13%) compared with those from Europe (2.3%) or the Asia Pacific (5.5%), transfusion episodes being lowest in the Middle East. In Europe, transfusion regimens close to Thalassaemia

International Federation guidelines are generally followed, with pretransfusion Hb values of 9.5 g/dL to 10.5 g/dL, which would cause a significant suppression of endogenous erythropoiesis using the model of Cazzola and colleagues.[5] By contrast, reports from Egypt, for example, show pretransfusion Hb values of 7.5 g/dL or less. In another study, with more than 1700 patients, an analysis of transfusion and chelation policy by region (EPIC study)[38] showed lower annual volume of blood transfused in the Middle East than in Europe or the Asia Pacific.

Differences in the Activity of Erythron with Transfusion as Marked by Soluble Transferrin Receptors

The possibility that transfusion policy may have an impact on cardiosiderosis is strengthened by a recent study where the suppression of the erythron, as marked by sTfR, when combined with a high transfusion-iron loading rate was the greatest predictor of cardiosiderosis[26] (**Fig. 1**). In this study, a large number of risk factors for cardiosiderosis were examined in 73 patients. sTfR levels were significantly lower in patients with cardiosiderosis (odds ratio 21) and this risk increased further when the transfusion-iron loading was taken into account. When rates exceeded the erythroid transferrin uptake rate (derived from sTfR1)[26] by greater than 0.21 mg/kg/d, the odds ratio increased to 48. High levels of LIC, ferritin, and LPI were also risk factors but less strongly. High levels of bilirubin, reticulocyte counts, or low hepcidin were

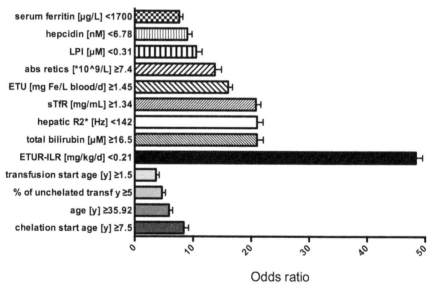

Odds ratio

Fig. 1. Statistically significant risk factors for cardiosiderosis in TDT. In 73 patients (half with cardiosiderosis) relevant factors were assessed for a relationship with cardiosiderosis. Thresholds protecting from cardiosiderosis are shown. ROC curves were constructed for every variable and a threshold protecting from cardiosiderosis for highest likelihood ratio was reported. Strength of association was expressed using an odds ratio. Factors not associated with cardiosiderosis were nucleated red blood cell count, total serum iron, weight, iron load rate (ILR), TfSat, GDF-15, NTBI, and years of transfusion dependence. abs retics, absolute reticulocyte; ETU, erythron transferrin uptake in μmol/litre of blood/day; ETUR, ethyron transferrin uptake rate in mg/iron/kg body wt/day; ILR, iron load rate from transfusion; transf, transfusion. (*Data from* Garbowski MW, Evans P, Vlachodimitropoulou E, et al. Residual erythropoiesis protects against myocardial hemosiderosis in transfusion-dependent thalassemia by lowering labile plasma iron via transient generation of apotransferrin. Haematologica 2017;102[10]:1640–49.)

associated with lower risk. A unifying mechanism for these risks, as discussed previously, is that unsaturated transferrin is generated by an active bone marrow, which in turn removes forms of NTBI, such as LPI that would otherwise be taken into myocardium. This suggests transfusion policy, in particular, the average Hb levels, estimated by pretransfusion Hb, have a key impact on the cardiosiderotic risk. The authors suggest that regional differences in risk may relate to differences in transfusion policy.

The sTfR-estimated erythropoietic expansion was also more predicated by the age of onset of transfusion dependence than by subsequent years of transfusion.[26] Other data, comparing 1266 TDT patients across 70 centers, support this, where sTfR levels relate to extramedullary hematopoiesis[39] and that where extramedullary hematopoiesis persists despite transfusion, patients do not develop cardiosiderosis.[40] Furthermore, in transfused sickle cell disease, the reduction of reticulocytes to less than 5% predicts future development of cardiosiderosis.[41] This points to a fundamental role for residual erythropoiesis in extrahepatic hemosiderosis. If residual erythropoiesis is maintained at a reasonable level (sweet spot), this constitutes a safety valve against toxic NTBI species and cardiosiderosis.[26]

Control of Iron Retention in Tissues Through Ferroportin-Hepcidin Interactions

Recent animal work provides novel insight into consequences of ferroportin-hepcidin interaction for the extrahepatic complications of TDT.[42–44] This work highlights the importance of cellular iron egress, rather than just uptake, to cardiomyocyte iron retention. The hemochromatotic model, resulting from a ferroportin mutation conferring resistance to hepcidin with unhindered ferroportin patency, causes fatal exocrine pancreatic failure due to iron overload of the acinar cells.[42] These never express ferroportin, so, unlike myocardium and endocrine system, are unable to export iron acquired from NTBI.[42] Hence cardiac-specific knockout of ferroportin, as confirmed elsewhere, results in cardiosiderosis.[43,44] Thus the authors predict that this under-recognized balance of NTBI uptake to ferroportin-mediated release is potentially important to net cardiosiderosis clinically.

Another mechanism by which a low transfusion regimen in TDT may result in decreased cardiosiderosis is, therefore, through decrease of hepcidin. The authors have shown that high plasma hepcidin is related to cardiosiderosis in TDT, although not as strongly as is low sTfR (low erythroid transferrin uptake rate).[26] The authors speculate that a low transfusion regime results in lower hepcidin because of less marrow suppression. Increased hepcidin, either post-transfusion[45,46] or as part of high transfusion regimes, is compounded by the switching off of the erythroid iron uptake (safety valve for LPI[26]), thus subjecting cardiomyocytes to a double impact of high LPI/NTBI exposure and limited cardiac iron exit via hepcidin-controlled ferroportin.

INTERACTION OF BLOOD TRANSFUSION AND CHELATABLE IRON POOLS

The structure, mechanisms of iron binding, pharmacokinetics, and clinical effects of the clinically licensed iron chelators—deferoxamine (DFO), deferiprone (DFP), and deferasirox (DFX) —have been described in detail recently by the senior author[30,47] and are not repeated in detail. This section focuses of the interaction of blood transfusion on iron chelation therapy.

Interaction of Transfusion with Chelatable Iron Pools

Early studies on DFO showed a relationship between blood transfusion and chelatable iron.[48] When DFO binds iron to form ferrioxamine (FO), the iron is derived from 2 key pools: first, the liver, and, second, from erythrocyte catabolism by macrophages in spleen, liver, and bone marrow. DFO is highly efficient at chelating liver iron because of rapid uptake into the hepatocytes.[49] FO can be eliminated in urine or in bile (feces) but is derived from 2 different sources. Urinary FO is derived from erythrocyte catabolism whereas fecal FO is mainly derived from hepatic iron. The proportion of endogenous red cells is higher pretransfusion than post-transfusion. This leads to increased peripheral hemolysis as well as more intramedullary IE, which in turn increases the magnitude of the chelatable iron pool from red cell catabolism. This iron pool is excreted in urine. Thus, at pretransfusion, at low Hb values, urinary iron excretion of FO (derived from erythrocyte catabolism) increases whereas fecal iron excretion is relatively unaffected or decreases slightly.

Factors affecting chelatable iron pools with DFP are less fully described than with DFO and even less is known about the effect of the transfusional iron loading rate. The authors, however, have examined iron pools that are chelatable with DFP by measuring concentrations of the DFP iron complex in plasma at the same time as measuring 24-hour urine iron excretion.[50] Chelated iron in the plasma compartment (forms ferriprone [FP], which is detected using the NTBI assay[50]) was greatest in patients with the highest LIC levels, as might be expected, but also greater in those with lowest transfusional iron loading rate, where hemolysis and/or IE is greater. Increments of plasma FP also correlate with total urine iron excretion and with decrements in LIC over the next year. Thus, blood transfusion decreases the iron available for chelation by DFP in the plasma compartment by decreasing IE and hemolysis. Conversely, high blood transfusion rate increases total body iron, which in turn increases the LIC-derived pool available for chelation.

Interaction of Blood Transfusion with Chelator Dose Needed for Iron Balance

Iron balance is simply the difference between iron input (from transfuson plus gastrointestinal iron absorption) and iron excretion from iron chelation (in urine plus faeces). From first principles, the dose of chelation needed under conditions of low transfusion would be better than at high transfusion rates. Body iron can be calculated from LIC using the Angelucci formula[13] and hence change in LIC can be used to calculate changes in body iron over time.

The interaction of transfusion rate with total iron excretion has been described using this approach for both DFO and DFX. With DFO, at typical transfusional iron loading rates (0.3–0.5 mg/kg/d), negative balance was achieved in 75% of patients prescribed subcutaneously 35 mg/kg/d to 49 mg/kg/d 5 d/wk, whereas at doses of 50 mg/kg/d or greater, response rates increased to 86%. At higher iron loading rates (>0.5 mg/kg/d), response was seen in only half of patients prescribed subcutaneously 35 mg/kg/d to 49 mg/kg/d 5 d/wk, but by increasing this dose to 50 mg/kg or greater, response increased to 89%.[17] With DFX, the importance of the blood transfusion rate to iron balance has also been shown using this approach. At low transfusion rates less than 0.3 mg/kg/d, 96% of patients have a negative iron balance at 30 mg/kg/d whereas at higher transfusion rates, only 82%.[17] The principle of adjusting dose to transfusional loading rate has been built into drug labeling and into the design of further studies of efficacy where serum ferritin was used to adjust dose even though this is a less precise marker of iron balance than LIC.

With DFP, data on the effects of transfusion rate on chelation efficacy are not as clear from prospective trials but useful data are available from retrospective analysis of LIC trends using superconducting quantum interference device biomagnetometry in 54 β-thalassemia major patients receiving DFP (75 mg/kg/d) or 51 patients receiving DFO.[51] Detailed contour plots of the interaction of transfusion with chelation dose were undertaken for both drugs. At 30 mg/kg/d of DFO (a low dose), negative iron balance was achieved when transfusion rates were less than 22 mg/d for total body iron stores exceeding 4 g or when transfusion rates were less than 17 mg/d for total body iron stores exceeding 1 g. With DFP at 75 mg/kg/d, negative iron balance was achieved when transfusion rates were less than 17 mg of iron per day for total body iron stores exceeding 1.8 g. Higher doses of both chelators could achieve negative iron balance when the transfusion rate was more than described. In conclusion, the successful dose for balancing input and output of iron of each form of monotherapy is critically dependent of the blood transfusion rate in the treatment group.

Other Factors Affecting Extrahepatic Iron Removal with Chelation Therapy

The authors do not regard blood transfusion as the sole factor affecting iron removal from extrahepatic tissues, simply that this factor may have been overlooked to some extent. Other factors are clearly important. For removing myocardial iron, which can be achieved with all chelators used alone or in combination,[30] removal of liver iron generally occurs at a much faster rate than from the heart, as shown elegantly by trajectory trends for myocardial and liver iron assessed by serial MRI.[34] Removing iron from the liver improves removal of myocardial iron: for example, in a subsidiary EPIC study on DFX, improvement of cardiac T2* was progressively better from 12 months to 36 months in patients who achieved LIC values less than 7 mg/g dry weight than those with LIC values greater than 15 mg/g dry weight.[52] Baseline, or pre-treatment, LIC values also seem to have an impact on success of removing cardiosiderosis. Thus in the CORDELIA DFX study, the percent improvement in cardiac T2* with DFX at 1 y was greater (17%) in patients with baseline LIC less than 7 mg/g compared with those with baseline LIC greater than 15 mg/g dry weight (9% improvement)[53] and this pattern was sustained at 2 years.[54]

Regimes where there is 24-hour presence of a chelator in plasma are preferable, because they provide continuous protection from NTBI or LPI uptake because these rebound rapidly after stopping treatment.[55,56] Not all forms of NTBI, available for uptake into cardiomyocytes, however, are equally inhibited.[26] The rate of access of the free chelator ligand and the rate of egress of the iron complex, determined by the size, charge, and lipid solubility,[57] are important to their ability to chelate intracellular iron pools. DFP, by virtue of its neutral charge and low molecular weight, has faster kinetic access to intracellular iron pools than DFO.[58] The interpretation of clinical studies, however, is somewhat problematic because randomized head-to-head comparison of DFP with DFO have used suboptimal low doses of DFO but relatively high doses of DFP,[59,60] and baseline LIC values often vary considerably between studies. The issue of combination of chelators providing a shuttling mechanism to enhance chelation rates is theoretically justified,[61–63] but the extent to which shuttling contributes to enhanced chelation, if the drugs are not given simultaneously, is questionable. Clinical benefit from sequential combinations is more likely to be a consequence of greater overall exposure to chelation, contributed to by improved adherence.

REFERENCES

1. Gabutti V, Piga A, Fortina P, et al. Correlation between transfusion requirement, blood volume and haemoglobin level in homozygous beta-thalassaemia. Acta Haematol 1980;64(2):103–8.

2. Gabutti V, Piga A, Nicola P, et al. Haemoglobin levels and blood requirement in thalassaemia. Arch Dis Child 1982;57(2):156–7.

3. Brunengo MA, Girot R. Transfusion requirements and mean annual hemoglobin level in thalassemia major. Nouv Rev Fr Hematol 1986;28(5):309–13 [in French].

4. Rebulla P, Modell B. Transfusion requirements and effects in patients with thalas-saemia major. Cooleycare Programme. Lancet 1991;337(8736):277–80.
5. Cazzola M, Borgna-Pignatti C, Locatelli F, et al. A moderate transfusion regimen may reduce iron loading in beta-thalassemia major without producing excessive expansion of erythropoiesis. Transfusion 1997;37(2):135–40.
6. Cappellini M-D, Cohen A, Porter J, et al. Guidelines for the management of trans-fusion dependent thalassaemia (TDT). Nicosia: Thalassaemia International Feder-ation; 2014.
7. Ragab LA, Hamdy MM, Shaheen IA, et al. Blood transfusion among thalassemia patients: a single Egyptian center experience. Asian J Transfus Sci 2013;7(1):33–6.
8. Premawardhena A, Fisher CA, Olivieri NF, et al. Haemoglobin E β thalassaemia in Sri Lanka. Lancet 2005;366(9495):1467–70.
9. Porter JB, Cappellini MD, Kattamis A, et al. Iron overload across the spectrum of non-transfusion-dependent thalassaemias: role of erythropoiesis, splenectomy and transfusions. Br J Haematol 2017;176(2):288–99.
10. Pippard MJ, Callender ST, Warner GT, et al. Iron absorption and loading in β-thal-assaemia intermedia. Lancet 1979;2(8147):819–21.
11. Pootrakul P, Kitcharoen K, Yansukon P, et al. The effect of erythroid hyperplasia on iron balance. Blood 1988;71(4):1124–9.
12. Taher AT, Porter J, Viprakasit V, et al. Deferasirox reduces iron overload significantly in nontransfusion-dependent thalassemia: 1-year results from a prospective, randomized, double-blind, placebo-controlled study. Blood 2012; 120(5):970–7.
13. Angelucci E, Brittenham GM, McLaren CE, et al. Hepatic iron concentration and total body iron stores in thalassemia major. N Engl J Med 2000;343(5):327–31.
14. Tanno T, Bhanu NV, Oneal PA, et al. High levels of GDF15 in thalassemia sup-press expression of the iron regulatory protein hepcidin. Nat Med 2007;13(9): 1096–101.
15. Kautz L, Jung G, Valore EV, et al. Identification of erythroferrone as an erythroid regulator of iron metabolism. Nat Genet 2014;46(7):678–84.
16. Dussiot M, Maciel TT, Fricot A, et al. An activin receptor IIA ligand trap corrects ineffective erythropoiesis in β-thalassemia. Nat Med 2014;20(4):398–407.
17. Cohen AR, Glimm E, Porter JB. Effect of transfusional iron intake on response to chelation therapy in β-thalassemia major. Blood 2008;111(2):583–7.
18. O'Brien RT, Pearson HA, Spencer RP. Transfusion-induced decrease in spleen size in thalassemia major: documentation by radioisotopic scan. J Pediatr 1972;81(1):105–7.
19. Origa R, Galanello R, Ganz T, et al. Liver iron concentrations and urinary hepcidin in beta-thalassemia. Haematologica 2007;92(5):583–8.
20. Taher AT, Musallam KM, Wood JC, et al. Magnetic resonance evaluation of hepatic and myocardial iron deposition in transfusion-independent thalassemia intermedia compared to regularly transfused thalassemia major patients. Am J Hematol 2010;85(4):288–90.
21. Roghi A, Cappellini MD, Wood JC, et al. Absence of cardiac siderosis despite hepatic iron overload in Italian patients with thalassemia intermedia: an MRI T2* study. Ann Hematol 2010;89(6):585–9.
22. Oudit GY, Sun H, Trivieri MG, et al. L-type Ca2+ channels provide a major pathway for iron entry into cardiomyocytes in iron-overload cardiomyopathy. Nat Med 2003;9(9):1187–94.
23. Pinilla-Tenas JJ, Sparkman BK, Shawki A, et al. Zip14 is a complex broad-scope metal-ion transporter whose functional properties support roles in the cellular

uptake of zinc and nontransferrin-bound iron. Am J Physiol Cell Physiol 2011; 301(4):C862–71.

24. Porter JB, Walter PB, Neumayr LD, et al. Mechanisms of plasma non-transferrin bound iron generation: insights from comparing transfused diamond blackfan anaemia with sickle cell and thalassaemia patients. Br J Haematol 2014;167(5): 692–6.

25. Bradley SJ, Gosriwitana I, Srichairatanakool S, et al. Non-transferrin-bound iron induced by myeloablative chemotherapy. Br J Haematol 1997;99(2):337–43.

26. Garbowski MW, Evans P, Vlachodimitropoulou E, et al. Residual erythropoiesis protects against myocardial hemosiderosis in transfusion-dependent thalassemia by lowering labile plasma iron via transient generation of apotransferrin. Haematologica 2017;102(10):1640–9.

27. Evans RW, Rafique R, Zarea A, et al. Nature of non-transferrin-bound iron: studies on iron citrate complexes and thalassemic sera. J Biol Inorg Chem 2008;13(1):57–74.

28. Esposito BP, Breuer W, Sirankapracha P, et al. Labile plasma iron in iron overload: redox activity and susceptibility to chelation. Blood 2003;102(7):2670–7.

29. Porter JB, de Witte T, Cappellini MD, et al. New insights into transfusion-related iron toxicity: implications for the oncologist. Crit Rev Oncol Hematol 2016;99: 261–71.

30. Porter JB. Treatment of systemic iron overload. In: Crichton RR, Ward RJ, Hider RC, editors. Metal chelation in medicine. London: Royal Society of Chemistry; 2016. p. 106–52.

31. Buja LM, Roberts WC. Iron in the heart. Etiology and clinical significance. Am J Med 1971;51(2):209–21.

32. Jensen PD, Jensen FT, Christensen T, et al. Relationship between hepatocellular injury and transfusional iron overload prior to and during iron chelation with desferrioxamine: a study in adult patients with acquired anemias. Blood 2003; 101(1):91–6.

33. Anderson LJ, Holden S, Davis B, et al. Cardiovascular T2-star (T2*) magnetic resonance for the early diagnosis of myocardial iron overload. Eur Heart J 2001;22(23):2171–9.

34. Noetzli LJ, Carson SM, Nord AS, et al. Longitudinal analysis of heart and liver iron in thalassemia major. Blood 2008;112(7):2973–8.

35. Aydinok Y, Porter JB, Piga A, et al. Prevalence and distribution of iron overload in patients with transfusion-dependent anemias differs across geographic regions: results from the CORDELIA study. Eur J Haematol 2015;95(3):244–53.

36. El Beshlawy A, El Tagui M, Hamdy M, et al. Low prevalence of cardiac siderosis in heavily iron loaded Egyptian thalassemia major patients. Ann Hematol 2014; 93(3):375–9.

37. Hassan SM, Harteveld CL, Bakker E, et al. Broader spectrum of β -thalassemia mutations in oman: regional distribution and comparison with neighboring countries. Hemoglobin 2015;39(2):107–10.

38. Viprakasit V, Gattermann N, Lee JW, et al. Geographical variations in current clinical practice on transfusions and iron chelation therapy across various transfusion-dependent anaemias. Blood Transfus 2013;11(1):108–22.

39. Ricchi P, Ammirabile M, Costantini S, et al. A useful relationship between the presence of extramedullary erythropoeisis and the level of the soluble form of the transferrin receptor in a large cohort of adult patients with thalassemia intermedia: a prospective study. Ann Hematol 2012;91(6):905–9.

40. Ricchi P, Meloni A, Spasiano A, et al. Extramedullary hematopoiesis is associated with lower cardiac iron loading in chronically transfused thalassemia patients. Am J Hematol 2015;90(11):1008–12.
41. Meloni A, Puliyel M, Pepe A, et al. Cardiac iron overload in sickle-cell disease. Am J Hematol 2014;89(7):678–83.
42. Altamura S, Kessler R, Groene HJ, et al. Resistance of ferroportin to hepcidin binding causes exocrine pancreatic failure and fatal iron overload. Cell Metab 2014;20(2):359–67.
43. Lakhal-Littleton S, Wolna M, Carr CA, et al. Cardiac ferroportin regulates cellular iron homeostasis and is important for cardiac function. Proc Natl Acad Sci U S A 2015;112(10):3164–9.
44. Lakhal-Littleton S, Wolna M, Chung YJ, et al. An essential cell-autonomous role for hepcidin in cardiac iron homeostasis. Elife 2016;5 [pii:e19804].
45. Jones E, Pasricha SR, Allen A, et al. Hepcidin is suppressed by erythropoiesis in hemoglobin e β-thalassemia and β-thalassemia trait. Blood 2015;125(5):873–80.
46. Pasricha SR, Frazer DM, Bowden DK, et al. Transfusion suppresses erythropoiesis and increases hepcidin in adult patients with β-thalassemia major: a longitudinal study. Blood 2013;122(1):124–33.
47. Porter J, Hershko C. The properties of clinically useful iron chelators. In: Anderson HJ, McLaren GD, editors. Iron physiology and pathophysiology in humans. New York: Humana Press; 2012. p. 591–630.
48. Pippard MJ, Callender ST, Finch CA. Ferrioxamine excretion in iron-loaded man. Blood 1982;60(2):288–94.
49. Porter JB, Rafique R, Srichairatanakool S, et al. Recent insights into interactions of deferoxamine with cellular and plasma iron pools: implications for clinical use. Ann N Y Acad Sci 2005;1054:155–68.
50. Aydinok Y, Evans P, Manz CY, et al. Timed non-transferrin bound iron determinations probe the origin of chelatable iron pools during deferiprone regimens and predict chelation response. Haematologica 2012;97(6):835–41.
51. Fischer R, Longo F, Nielsen P, et al. Monitoring long-term efficacy of iron chelation therapy by deferiprone and desferrioxamine in patients with beta-thalassaemia major: application of SQUID biomagnetic liver susceptometry. Br J Haematol 2003;121(6):938–48.
52. Porter J, Taher AT, Aydinok Y, et al. Impact of liver iron overload on myocardial T2* response in transfusion-dependent thalassemia major patients treated with deferasirox for up to 3 years. ASH Annu Meet Abstr. Blood 2013;122(21):1016.
53. Pennell DJ, Porter JB, Piga A, et al. A 1-year randomized controlled trial of deferasirox vs deferoxamine for myocardial iron removal in -thalassemia major (CORDELIA). Blood 2014;123(10):1447–54.
54. Pennell DJ, Porter JB, Piga A, et al. Sustained improvements in myocardial T2* over 2 years in severely iron-overloaded patients with beta thalassemia major treated with deferasirox or deferoxamine. Am J Hematol 2015;90(2):91–6.
55. Porter JB, Abeysinghe RD, Marshall L, et al. Kinetics of removal and reappearance of non-transferrin-bound plasma iron with deferoxamine therapy. Blood 1996;88(2):705–13.
56. Cabantchik ZI, Breuer W, Zanninelli G, et al. LPI-labile plasma iron in iron overload. Best Pract Res Clin Haematol 2005;18(2 SPEC. ISS.):277–87.
57. Porter JB, Gyparaki M, Burke LC, et al. Iron mobilization from hepatocyte monolayer cultures by chelators: the importance of membrane permeability and the iron-binding constant. Blood 1988;72(5):1497–503.

58. Cooper CE, Lynagh GR, Hoyes KP, et al. The relationship of intracellular iron chelation to the inhibition and regeneration of human ribonucleotide reductase. J Biol Chem 1996;271(34):20291–9.
59. Tanner MA, Galanello R, Dessi C, et al. A randomized, placebo-controlled, double-blind trial of the effect of combined therapy with deferoxamine and deferiprone on myocardial iron in thalassemia major using cardiovascular magnetic resonance. Circulation 2007;115(14):1876–84.
60. Pennell DJ. Randomized controlled trial of deferiprone or deferoxamine in beta-thalassemia major patients with asymptomatic myocardial siderosis. Blood 2006;107(9):3738–44.
61. Evans P, Kayyali R, Hider RC, et al. Mechanisms for the shuttling of plasma non-transferrin-bound iron (NTBI) onto deferoxamine by deferiprone. Transl Res 2010; 156(2):55–67.
62. Vlachodimitropoulou Koumoutsea E, Garbowski M, Porter J. Synergistic intracellular iron chelation combinations: mechanisms and conditions for optimizing iron mobilization. Br J Haematol 2015;170(6):874–83.
63. Vlachodimitropoulou E, Chen Y-L, Garbowski M, et al. Eltrombopag: a powerful chelator of cellular or extracellular iron(III) alone or combined with a second chelator. Blood 2017;130(17):1923–33.

Iron Chelation Therapy as a Modality of Management

Yesim Aydinok, MD

KEYWORDS

- Thalassemia major • Thalassemia intermedia • Transfusion-dependent thalassemia
- Non-transfusion dependent thalassemia • Chelation • Liver iron concentration
- Cardiac iron • Serum ferritin

KEY POINTS

- The monitoring of MRI-assessed liver and heart iron by using validated and standardized techniques has been the standard of care in management of iron chelation therapy in transfusion-dependent thalassemia and non-transfusion-dependent thalassemia.
- The transfusional iron intake, existing iron burden, and known compliance with chelation in a particular patient are crucial in response to prescribed chelation therapy.
- The accessibility of iron chelator to the different iron pools and efficiency for removing excess iron should be taken into account in chelator choice, dosing, and regimen based on the objective of iron chelation therapy.

INTRODUCTION

Iron chelation therapy is considered an essential component of thalassemia management. Body iron accumulation rate and distribution differ based on whether it develops as a consequence of the regular transfusion regimen that occurs in thalassemia major (TM),[1] or because of increased intestinal iron absorption and release of recycled iron from the reticuloendothelial system that occurs in thalassemia intermedia (TI).[2] It is estimated that 100 mL of pure concentrated packed red blood cells (with a hematocrit of 100%) contains 108 mg of iron, which is approximately 35 to 100 times more than the daily requirement.[3] Such extreme iron efflux by repeated transfusions in patients with transfusion-dependent thalassemia (TDT) results in an overwhelming carrying capacity of transferrin and the generation of harmful iron species, such as non-transferrin-bound iron and labile plasma iron (LPI) that is cleared preferentially by the liver, myocardium, and endocrine glands and that catalyses the formation of

Disclosure Statement: Receiving research grant funding, consulting fees, and lecture fees from Novartis Pharmaceuticals, research grant funding and lecture fees from Cerus, research grant funding from Celgene and Shire.
Department of Pediatric Hematology and Oncology, Ege University Children's Hospital, Bornova, Izmir 35100, Turkey
E-mail address: yesim.aydinok@yahoo.com

Hematol Oncol Clin N Am 32 (2018) 261–275
https://doi.org/10.1016/j.hoc.2017.12.002
0889-8588/18/© 2017 Elsevier Inc. All rights reserved.

hemonc.theclinics.com

free radicals leading to oxidative damage in these tissues.[4,5] In fact, when adequate transfusion regimens became the norm, transfusional iron overload became evident very early in the transfusion history, and iron-induced cardiac deaths replaced anemia as the most common cause of mortality in TM.[6] Although deferoxamine (DFO) chelation became the standard management modality in thalassemia and markedly improved prognosis of disease, since the 1980s,[7–9] iron-induced heart disease, including heart failure and arrhythmia, continued to be the leading cause of death in TM until 1999.[10] The improved efficiency of iron chelation therapy with the introduction of new oral iron chelators, in addition to the documentation of organ-specific siderosis by MRI technologies and appropriate intensification of iron chelation treatment, alongside other improvements in clinical care increased the probability of complication-free survival with normal life expectancy in the modern era.[10–12] On the other hand, iron overload resulting from increased intestinal iron absorption has been recognized as an important clinical challenge in patients with non-transfusion-dependent thalassemia (NTDT) beyond the ages of 10 to 15 years.[13,14] In never or minimally transfused TI patients, MRI assessed liver (R2) and cardiac (T2*) iron demonstrated no evidence of cardiac iron overload, whereas there may be significant hepatic iron accumulation,[15] predisposing patients to develop fibrosis[16] and hepatocellular carcinoma.[17] However, the use of frequent transfusion therapy within the wide severity range of TI likely predisposes to cardiac iron deposition as well. Therefore, iron levels should be regularly assessed, and iron chelation therapy should be initiated where appropriate in NTDT patients.

Quantifying Iron Overload

Although the same tools that are available for the assessment of iron burden are used in both TDT and NTDT, monitoring of iron loading should be initiated after 6 to 8 transfusions in newly diagnosed patients with TDT, whereas it can be postponed to up to 10 years of age by considering the slow kinetics of iron loading in NTDT.

Serum ferritin (SF) is the most commonly used measure for the diagnosis and monitoring of iron overload and still remains the only tool in many countries. Traditionally, iron chelation therapy is started when SF exceeds 1000 µg/L, and maintenance of SF between 500 and 1000 µg/L may be associated with additional beneficial effects on complication-free survival in TDT.[9,18] It has demonstrated that liver iron concentration (LIC) can reliably measure total body iron stores.[19] Although SF generally correlates with body iron stores, TM patients with identical SF show highly variable LIC.[20] Furthermore, the studies in TDT have consistently demonstrated that the predictive value of SF trends to forecast changes in LIC was not strong enough,[21,22] although it seems stronger when SF was less than 4000 (r^2 0.51) compared with greater than 4000 µg/L (r^2 0.37).[22] In the modern management of iron overload, noninvasive quantification of LIC by MRI is considered the standard of care where available and may be used on patients as young as 4 to 5 years of age without sedation. LIC exceeding 3 mg Fe/g dry weight (dw) has been recommended as an indication to start chelation therapy. Although the suggested LIC range, derived from clinical observations in genetic hemochromatosis, is between 3 and 7 mg Fe/g dw,[8,23] the long-term efficacy and safety of chelation regimens, that was carefully titrated to normalize LIC less than 1.5 mg Fe/g dw, have been reported in adult patients with thalassemia.[24] The ability of cardiac T2* MRI as a validated technique to assess myocardial siderosis has demonstrated little predictive value of LIC (as well as SF) for cardiac iron deposition in previously chelated patients[25,26] and has provided insights into the different kinetics of iron loading/unloading in liver and heart.[27] In fact, cardiac iron clearance was found to be nearly 4 times slower compared with hepatic iron removal.[28] In light of these observations, monitoring cardiac iron by T2* MRI has been an indispensable measure to detect cardiac risks resulted from myocardial siderosis and to accordingly initiate an appropriate management strategy using iron chelation therapy in TDT. Cardiac T2* MRI may be deferred in well-chelated children until 8 to 10 years of age when they are able to undergo MRI without anesthesia.[29] However, recent data have revealed that cardiac siderosis may occur even in younger children with high transfusion but poor chelation history.[30] Cardiac T2* of 20 ms and corresponding LIC of 1.16 mg/g dw are accepted as lower thresholds of normal.[25,31] Cardiac T2* of less than 20 ms has been associated with cardiac risk[25] and cardiac T2* of less than 10 ms has been strongly associated with heart failure and cardiac death.[32] Therefore, with the ability to recognize preclinical cardiac iron accumulation, clinicians were able to implement intensification of chelation therapy as a primary prevention strategy to save organ function in patients with TDT. A careful dose tailoring strategy on chelation therapy based on decreasing SF and/or LIC levels should be considered to avoid chelator toxicity. However, it is important not to cease chelation therapy in patients with TDT, even if their SF and LIC are well controlled because highly toxic LPI is continuously generated under regular transfusion regimen[33] and increased risk for endocrine and cardiac iron accumulation when chelator is not present in the circulation.[27]

Suppression of hepcidin levels in NTDT results in the release of recycled iron from the reticuloendothelial system and depletion of macrophage iron, which makes SF a less reliable tool of iron overload because SF more specifically reflects macrophage iron retention.[34,35] In NTDT, iron preferentially accumulates in hepatocytes, making LIC a reliable measure for the diagnosis and monitoring of iron overload. In patients with NTDT, LIC greater than 5 mg Fe/g dw is associated with increased morbidity,[36] supporting the initiation of lower intensity iron chelation therapy compared with TDT. In contrast to TDT, iron chelation therapy is suspended when LIC levels decrease to less than 3 mg Fe/g dw. In places where MRI is unavailable, it has demonstrated that SF thresholds of 800 μg/L and 300 μg/L correspond to LIC of 5 mg Fe/g dw and 3 mg Fe/g dw and appeared adequate to safely initiate and interrupt iron chelation therapy in NTDT.[37,38]

Table 1 summarizes the generally accepted SF and LIC thresholds for optimum management of iron chelation therapy in TDT and NTDT. Regardless of SF and LIC levels, cardiac T2* MRI should also be maintained greater than 20 ms, which is considered to be a lower limit of normal myocardial iron. SF assessments at 3 to 6 weekly intervals can provide the most rapid feedback with respect to patients' adherence and response to chelation therapy. Particularly, SF response can help predict LIC

Table 1
Recommended thresholds for iron chelation management in transfusion-dependent thalassemia and non-transfusion-dependent thalassemia

Metrics of Iron Stores	TDT			NTDT		
	Start Chelation	Maintain Chelation	Stop Chelation	Start Chelation	Maintain Chelation	Stop Chelation
SF (μg/L)	≥1000	500–1000	NR	>800	300–800	<300
LIC (mg Fe/g dw)	>3	1.5–3.0	NR	>5	3.0–5.0	<3

Abbreviation: NR, not recommended.

Data from Taher A, Vichinsky E, Musallam K, et al. Guidelines for the management of non-transfusion dependent thalassaemia (NTDT). Nicosia (Cyprus): Thalassaemia International Federation; 2013; and Cappellini MD, Cohen A, Porter J, et al. Guidelines for the management of transfusion dependent thalassaemia (TDT). 3rd edition. Nicosia (Cyprus): Thalassaemia International Federation; 2014.

response, but a lack of SF response should be interpreted with caution, and assessment of LIC should be prioritized for those with a lack of SF response.[22] However, whenever feasible, quantification of LIC is highly recommended in order to make appropriate chelation decisions and accurate conclusions regarding patients' adherence to chelation therapy.[21] Available guidelines recommend liver and cardiac iron examinations annually unless there is a clinical indication for more or less frequent assessments.[39,40] However, MRI is currently not universally available, and studies have highlighted the importance of using standardized and validated techniques to get an accurate LIC and cardiac T2*estimation in clinical practice[41,42] that should really be taken into account carefully in dissemination of the technology.

Properties of Iron Chelators in Clinical Use

Currently, the available iron chelators include parenteral DFO and oral tablet and syrup formulations of (deferiprone [DFP]) and dispersible tablets (DT) and film-coated tablet (FCT) formulations of deferasirox (DFX). The characteristics of these chelators are summarized in **Table 2** and are further discussed throughout the text.

Objectives of Iron Chelation Therapy in Thalassemia

The goal of iron chelation has shifted from treating to preventing iron overload in order to achieve a normal pattern of complication-free survival and quality of life. The key concepts of optimal chelation therapy include timely initiation, close monitoring, and continuous adjustment. Although the primary objective of iron chelation therapy is to maintain iron balance at safe levels, at all times, once iron is accumulated, the chelation therapy should be intensified appropriately to achieve a negative iron balance in order to accelerate unloading of tissue iron to safe levels during which suppression of LPI will be the key action that is necessary to avoid further organ toxicity and preserve organ functions.[59] The efficacy of different chelation regimens in maintaining the individual at low levels of exposure to LPI has been reviewed elsewhere.[43]

Prospective studies assessing the efficacy of iron chelation regimens have highlighted the importance of the rate of transfusional iron intake, the existing hepatic and extrahepatic (cardiac) iron burden, and the chelator dosing and regimen for appropriate management of iron overload.

The Impact of Transfusional Iron Intake on Chelation Efficacy

In a prospective, randomized study, comparing the efficacy of DFX and DFO during 1 year of treatment, the mean transfusional iron intake in TM was 0.4 mg/kg/d, but this varies considerably with 25% of patients taking less than 0.3 mg/kg/d, about 50% 0.3 to 0.5 mg/kg/d, and a further 25% greater than 0.5 mg/kg/d. It has clearly demonstrated that chelator dose and transfusional iron intake affected the proportion of patients achieving a negative iron balance depicted by a reduction in LIC during treatment of DFX or DFO.[16] This observation was confirmed in a large cohort study using DFX in which the investigators highlighted the importance of considering ongoing transfusional iron intake besides baseline body iron burden when selecting chelator dose and the need for a timely individual dose titration to achieve a therapeutic goal.[60]

The Importance of Existing Total Body Iron Burden on Choice of Chelator Dosing and Regimen

In standard practice, DFO is administered at the dose of 40 to 50 mg/kg, 8 to 12 hours of subcutaneous infusion 5 days a week.[61] In patients with TDT who become massively iron overloaded, prolonged infusions of higher doses of DFO (50–60 mg/kg/d) 5 to 7 days a week are recommended to reduce iron burden to safe levels.[62]

Table 2
Properties of iron chelators used in patients with transfusion-dependent thalassemia

	DFO	DFP	DFX	
			DT	FCT
Route	SC or IV infusion	Oral (tablet and syrup)	Oral	Oral
Usual dose	20–60 mg/kg/d over 8–24 h	75–100 mg/kg/d	20–40 mg/kg/d	14–28 mg/kg/d
Schedule	5–7 times weekly	3 times daily	Once daily	Once daily
Excretion	Urinary, with some fecal	Mainly urinary	Mainly fecal	Mainly fecal
Most frequent AEs	Injection-site reactions, Yersinia infections, HF hearing loss, retinopathy, poor growth, allergy	GI AEs (nausea, vomiting, abdominal pain), increased ALT levels, arthralgia, neutropenia	GI AEs (diarrhea, vomiting, nausea, abdominal pain), rash, increased ALT levels, increased serum creatinine	
Warnings		Agranulocytosis, neutropenia	Renal toxicity, hepatic toxicity, GI hemorrhage	
Depletion of LPI	Yes (if continuous infusion)	Yes (rebound between doses)	Yes	
Removal of hepatocellular iron	Yes	Less impressive	Yes	
Accessing LCI pool	Retard	Rapidly penetrate and bound	Rapidly penetrate and bound	
Clinical data; extracting LCI pool in cardiomyocytes	Benefits of 24 h IV infusion	Higher than standard DFO	Comparable with higher dose DFO	

Abbreviations: AE, adverse event; ALT, alanine aminotransferase; GI, gastrointestinal; HF, high frequency; IV, intravenous; LCI, labile cellular iron; SC, subcutaneous.
Data from Refs.[28,43–58]

It has been confirmed that a higher proportion of patients with TM receiving higher doses of DFO ($\geq$50 mg/kg/d, 5 d/wk) achieved a negative iron balance than standard practice in a more recent study.[16]

Accumulated data from prospective studies have provided strong evidence that oral DFX at a once-daily dose of 20 mg/kg and 30 mg/kg led to maintenance and a significant reduction in LIC, respectively,[63] whereas higher dose of DFX greater than 30 mg/kg/d up to 40 mg/kg/d may be required in heavily iron-loaded patients with TDT.[64–66]

The meta-analysis data of clinical trials involving the long-term use of DFP have shown that only 52% of the patients treated by standard doses (75 mg/kg/d) of DFP achieved a negative iron balance.[67] Because of the less impressive effect of DFP on decreasing body iron burden, combined use of DFP (a weak chelator with high cell penetration) and DFO (a strong chelator with poor cell penetration but efficient excretion) was tested in metabolic balance studies, and synergistic effects between the 2 compounds through iron shuttling were suggested.[68] However, an experimental study demonstrated that DFP promotes the excretion of storage iron from parenchymal iron stores but shows no advantage over DFO in promoting reticuloendothelial iron excretion. Simultaneous administration of DFO and DFP results in an increase in chelating effect that is additive but not synergistic.[69] In a prospective study, a higher dose of DFP (92 mg/kg/d) also revealed a less significant decrease in LIC than even relatively low dose of DFO (35 mg/kg/d, when normalized to a 7-day regimen).[50] A randomized prospective study demonstrated that combination therapy for daily DFP (75 mg/kg/d) plus twice weekly subcutaneous DFO (40–50 mg/kg/d) was as effective as DFO monotherapy (40–50 mg/kg, 5 days a week) and superior to DFP monotherapy (75 mg/kg/d) in lowering LIC.[70] In fact, in a randomized placebo controlled study, DFP (75 mg/kg/d) plus DFO (35 mg/kg, 5 days a week) showed a larger decrease in liver iron compared with DFO monotherapy (43 mg/kg, 5 days a week, 30 mg/kg/d, when normalized to a 7-day regimen).[71] Another attractive combination of DFX and DFO was evaluated in patients with severe transfusional liver (mean 33.4 $\pm$ 14.5 mg Fe/g dw) and myocardial siderosis (T2* 5 to <10 ms). In this 2-year study, the combined therapy protocol of DFX and DFO resulted in a very rapid decrease in LIC with clinically meaningful improvements in cardiac T2*. It has concluded that a combination of DFX and DFO may be useful when a rapid LIC reduction is required, regardless of myocardial iron.[72]

Cardiac Iron Clearance

Myocardial T2* has been transformative when it has recognized preclinical cardiac iron loading[25] and has been shown to be a strong prognostic value in prediction of cardiac complications in patients with cardiac T2* less than 10 ms.[32,73] Clinicians have focused on the administration of the most appropriate iron chelation therapies for achieving a faster cardiac unloading to avoid toxic cardiomyopathy related to myocardial siderosis.

All prospective single-arm and randomized control studies have demonstrated a decrease in cardiac iron in 1 year[50,51,71,74,75] and in longer-term studies.[52,76–78] Among them, the DFP-containing regimens (as either a monotherapy[50] or combined therapy for DFP and DFO,[71] see earlier discussion) have demonstrated the best improvement of cardiac T2* versus standard DFO,[50,71] and specifically, improvements in left ventricular ejection fraction (LVEF) within 1 year.[50,71,74] A prospective large cohort study of DFX in β-TM patients with mild to moderate (T2* 10 to <20 ms) and severe cardiac siderosis (T2* >5 to <10 ms) resulted in a significant and continued reduction of cardiac iron versus baseline levels at the start of the trial during which LVEF remained stable within the normal range and no cardiac death occurred over 3 years.[78] The results of a large randomized controlled trial confirmed the efficacy of DFX for removal of cardiac iron (with target dose of 40 mg/kg/d and mean actual dose of 36.7 mg/kg/d), with noninferiority of DFX compared with subcutaneous DFO infusion (40.7 mg/kg/d, when normalized to a 7-day regimen), but no change in LVEF. Notably, the patients included in this study were severely iron loaded without cardiac decompensation (LVEF $\geq$56%). DFX monotherapy resulted in improvements in myocardial siderosis irrespective of baseline iron burden for myocardial T2* (<10 ms vs >10 ms) LIC (<15 vs >15 mg Fe/g dw), highlighting the efficacy of an intensive DFX dosing regimen for myocardial iron removal across low and high iron burdens.[52] DFX has not been tested in TDT, which is characterized by severe myocardial siderosis and/or cardiac dysfunction.

The clinical experience for treating patients with the most severe levels of myocardial iron overload (T2* <6 ms) and those with depressed LVEF relies on the use of a combination regimen of DFO and DFP[73] or continuous intravenous DFO infusion 24 h/7 days a week.[28] A consensus report from the American Heart Association stated that acute decompensated heart failure in thalassemia is a medical emergency that requires immediate commencement of 24-hours per day continuous (uninterrupted) intravenous iron chelation treatment with DFO 50 mg/kg/d and introduction of DFP as soon as possible besides cardiac medication.[79]

Is There Any Impact of Hepatic Iron on Cardiac Iron Clearance?

Although lower hepatic iron concentrations do not guarantee noncardiac iron loading,[27] high liver iron exceeding 15 mg Fe/g dw appear to place patients at an increased cardiac risk.[8,80] A large cohort (n = 925) of transfusion-dependent patients, aged $\geq$10 years and screened for entry into a prospective study, revealed that 36.7% of patients had myocardial siderosis (T2* $\leq$20 ms). Despite this, of the 98.5% of the overall population that was receiving prior chelation, 64% of patients had severe liver iron overload (LIC $\geq$15 mg Fe/g dw). Most of those with noncardiac iron loading (58.5%) had a severe liver iron overload, indicating a group of patients with increased risk for cardiac iron loading.[81] This figure highlights the need for the optimization of effective and convenient iron chelation therapies for patients with severe hepatic and/or cardiac iron overload.

Prospective studies using DFX suggested that cardiac iron clearance is faster if liver iron is lower. In other words, cardiac iron may not be lowered unless liver iron is lowered, and in turn, less cardiac iron clearance occurs in the patients with higher LIC.[51,52,76] This hypothesis has not been tested in DFP studies because DFP studies have been conducted in patients with mild to moderate liver siderosis. Stratification for dosing and regimen of chelators based on different organ iron loading in TDT has been proposed in **Table 3**.

Iron Chelation Therapy for Prevention and Reversal of Endocrine Complications in Thalassemia

Despite the significant reduction in mortality from iron overload by awareness of cardiac risks and administration of effective chelation regimens, endocrinopathies still account for significant morbidity in TM.[82–87] Pancreatic iron loading (defined as MRI R2* >100 Hz) and severe pituitary iron deposition may develop during the first decade of life.[30,88] It has been shown that endocrine tissues have a very restricted regeneration capacity, and therefore, the therapeutic window between iron accumulation and organ damage should be used effectively. Normalization of body iron stores by intensive combination therapy for DFO and DFP has been associated with prevention

Table 3
Stratification proposal for dosing and regimen of chelators based on different organ iron loading in transfusion-dependent thalassemia patients

LIC (mg Fe/g dw)	1.5–3.0	3.0–7.0	7.0–15.0	>15.0
SF (μg/L)	500–1000	1000–2500	2500–4000	>4000
Cardiac T2* MRI >20 ms (normal LVEF)	Maintain existing therapy (DFX or DFP or DFO) with dose titration for not lowering LIC & SF further	Adjust chelation to the maximum doses of chelators (DFX 40 mg/kg/d or DFO 50–60 mg/kg, 5 dw or DFP 100 mg/kg/d)	DFX 40 mg/kg/d or combined therapy of DFX (40 mg/kg/d) & DFO (50–60 mg/kg, 5 dw) (if rapid reduction is required)	DFX 40 mg/kg/d or combined therapy of DFX (40 mg/kg/d) & DFO (50–60 mg/kg, 5–7 dw)
Cardiac T2* MRI 10–20 ms (normal LVEF)	Adjust chelation (DFX or DFP or DFO) to the maximum tolerable doses that may be applicable with no signs of chelator toxicity	DFX 40 mg/kg/d or combined therapy of DFP (100 mg/kg/d) & DFO (50–60 mg/kg, 5 dw)	DFX 40 mg/kg/d or combined therapy of DFP (100 mg/kg/d) & DFO (50–60 mg/kg, 5–7 dw)	DFX 40 mg/kg/d or combined therapy of DFP (100 mg/kg/d) & DFO (50–60 mg/kg, 5–7 dw)
Cardiac T2* MRI 6–10 ms (normal LVEF)	DFP 100 mg/kg/d (add DFO 40–50 mg/kg, 3–5 dw, if SF & LIC increase)	DFX 40 mg/kg/d or combined therapy of DFP (100 mg/kg/d) & DFO (50–60 mg/kg, 5–7 dw)	DFX 40 mg/kg/d or combined therapy of DFP (100 mg/kg/d) & DFO (50–60 mg/kg, 5–7 dw)	DFX 40 mg/kg/d or combined therapy of DFP (100 mg/kg/d) & DFO (50–60 mg/kg, 5–7 dw)
Cardiac T2* MRI <6 ms (normal LVEF)	Combined therapy of DFP (100 mg/kg/d) & DFO (40–50 mg/kg, 5–7 dw) with dose titration of DFO to maintain LIC & SF	Combined therapy of DFP (100 mg/kg/d) & DFO (50–60 mg/kg, 7 dw 24 h IV infusion)	Combined therapy of DFP (100 mg/kg/d) & DFO (50–60 mg/kg, 7 dw 24 h IV infusion)	Combined therapy of DFP (100 mg/kg/d) & DFO (50–60 mg/kg, 7 dw 24 h IV infusion)
HF	Combined therapy of DFP (100 mg/kg/d) & DFO (40–50 mg/kg, 7 dw 24 h IV infusion) with dose titration of DFO to maintain LIC & SF	Combined therapy of DFP (100 mg/kg/d) & DFO (50–60 mg/kg, 7 dw 24 h IV infusion)	Combined therapy of DFP (100 mg/kg/d) & DFO (50–60 mg/kg, 7 dw 24 h IV infusion)	Combined therapy of DFP (100 mg/kg/d) & DFO (50–60 mg/kg, 7 dw 24 h IV infusion)

and/or reversal of endocrinopathies.[24] In a recent multicenter retrospective cohort study, low prevalence of new endocrine disorders and stabilization of those preexisting during DFX therapy would suggest a protective role of DFX.[89]

Importance of Adherence

High levels of LPI may be the actual source of extrahepatic iron loading.[90] Poor compliance with iron chelation therapy, particularly in those with long-term excessive liver iron, may dramatically increase the risk for circulating LPI and appear to have negative prognostic value.[80]

It has been shown that noncompliance with iron chelation treatment is a major predictive factor for survival.[91] There has been clear evidence that high compliance to DFO was associated with stable ferritin levels over time, whereas poor compliance was strongly correlated with poor outcome.[91–93]

The results of comparative trials suggested lower adherence rates with subcutaneous DFO than with the oral iron chelators, either DFP or DFX.[94] Various factors may affect adherence to iron chelation therapy. Gastrointestinal side effects, such as abdominal pain, nausea, and vomiting, may create practical challenges to adherence with the oral iron chelators, although various measures can be helpful. Simplifying therapy and appropriate management of chelator-related adverse events when they occur may help adherence. Therefore, DFX may be beneficial, because it is a once-daily formulation. However, adherence to DFX DT may be affected by palatability and tolerability.[95,96] Recently, safety and tolerability of DFX FCT formulation has been compared with DFX (DT).[97] Because of the greater bioavailability of DFX (FCT) than DFX (DT), DFX (FCT) achieves the same chelation effect as DFX (DT) by 30% lower dose.[55–58] During the study, patients consistently found DFX (FCT) more palatable than DFX (DT).[97] The patients could swallow whole DFX (FCT) either on an empty stomach or with a light meal[57,58] and experienced less gastrointestinal adverse events than those receiving DFX (DT).[97]

However, the early identification of patients with poor adherence by regular inspection of trends in SF levels, LIC and myocardial T2* measurements, and appropriate counseling remains the key.

Chelation Therapy in Non-Transfusion-Dependent Thalassemia

Because iron overload has been recognized as an important clinical challenge in NTDT, all iron chelators have been used, but less insight has been gained about the efficacy and safety of DFO in NTDT. The relatively small, open-label and single-arm DFP studies reported that DFP was well tolerated in most patients and showed a decrease in SF and LIC.[98] The largest and first randomized placebo controlled study demonstrated that DFX therapy results in significant decrease in LIC compared with placebo with manageable safety profile at 1 year.[2] Another prospective study proposed a new treatment algorithm in NTDT patients based on baseline LIC in which the starting DFX dose was 10 mg/kg/d in all patients with LIC ≥ 5 mg Fe/g dw. Dose increment was allowed at week 4 (maximum dose of 20 mg/kg/d) and week 24 (maximum dose of 30 mg/kg/d). Dose was adjusted according to safety assessments to a minimum of 5 mg/kg/d. If repeated SF levels were less than 300 µg/L or LIC less than 3 mg Fe/g dw, treatment was suspended and then restarted at the previous effective dose (maximum 10 mg/kg/d) when SF increased to ≥ 300 ng/mL and LIC increased to ≥ 5 mg Fe/g dw. The investigators concluded that this treatment algorithm may guide in optimizing iron chelation therapy with DFX in NTDT patients by appropriate monitoring with either LIC or SF.[99]

REFERENCES

1. Cohen AR, Glimm E, Porter JB. Effect of transfusional iron intake on response to chelation therapy in beta-thalassemia major. Blood 2008;111(2):583–7.

2. Taher AT, Porter J, Viprakasit V, et al. Deferasirox reduces iron overload significantly in nontransfusion-dependent thalassemia: 1-year results from a prospective, randomized, double-blind, placebo-controlled study. Blood 2012;120(5): 970–7.

3. Porter JB. Practical management of iron overload. Br J Haematol 2001;115: 239–52.

4. Livrea MA, Tesoriere L, Pintaudi AM, et al. Oxidative stress and antioxidant status in beta-thalassemia major: iron overload and depletion of lipid-soluble antioxidants. Blood 1996;88(9):3608–14.

5. Hershko C. Pathogenesis and management of iron toxicity in thalassemia. Ann N Y Acad Sci 2010;1202:1–9.

6. Modell B, Khan M, Darlison M. Survival in β-thalassaemia major in the UK: data from the UK Thalassaemia Register. Lancet 2000;355(9220):2051–2.

7. Zurlo MG, De Stefano P, Borgna-Pignatti A, et al. Survival and causes of death in thalassaemia major. Lancet 1989;2:27–30.

8. Brittenham G, Griffith P, Nienhuis A, et al. Efficacy of deferoxamine in preventing complications of iron overload in patients with thalassemia major. N Engl J Med 1994;331(9):567–73.

9. Borgna-Pignatti C, Rugolotto S, De Stefano P, et al. Survival and complications in patients with thalassemia major treated with transfusion and deferoxamine. Haematologica 2004;89:1187–93.

10. Modell B, Khan M, Darlison M, et al. Improved survival of thalassaemia major in the UK and relation to T2* cardiovascular magnetic resonance. J Cardiovasc Magn Reson 2008;10(1):42.

11. Telfer P, Coen PG, Christou S, et al. Survival of medically treated thalassemia patients in Cyprus. Trends and risk factors over the period 1980-2004. Haematologica 2006;91(9):1187–92.

12. Borgna-Pignatti C, Cappellini MC, De Stefano P, et al. Cardiac morbidity and mortality in deferoxamine or deferiprone-treated patients with thalassemia major. Blood 2006;107:3733–7.

13. Taher AT, Musallam KM, El-Beshlawy A, et al. Age-related complications in treatment-naïve patients with thalassaemia intermedia. Br J Haematol 2010;150: 486–9.

14. Musallam KM, Cappellini MD, Daar S, et al. Serum ferritin level and morbidity risk in transfusion-independent patients with β-thalassemia intermedia: the ORIENT study. Haematologica 2014;99:e218–21.

15. Origa R, Barella S, Argiolas GM, et al. No evidence of cardiac iron in 20 never- or minimally-transfused patients with thalassemia intermedia. Haematologica 2008; 93(7):1095–6.

16. Musallam KM, Motta I, Salvatori M, et al. Longitudinal changes in serum ferritin levels correlate with measures of hepatic stiffness in transfusion-independent patients with β-thalassemia intermedia. Blood Cells Mol Dis 2012;49:136–9.

17. Maakaron JE, Cappellini MD, Graziadei G, et al. Hepatocellular carcinoma in hepatitis-negative patients with thalassemia intermedia: a closer look at the role of siderosis. Ann Hepatol 2013;12:142–6.

18. Telfer PT, Prestcott E, Holden S, et al. Hepatic iron concentration combined with long-term monitoring of serum ferritin to predict complications of iron overload in thalassaemia major. Br J Haematol 2000;110:971–7.
19. Angelucci E, Brittenham GM, McLaren CE, et al. Hepatic iron concentration and total body iron stores in thalassemia major. N Engl J Med 2000;343(5):327–31.
20. Aydinok Y, Bayraktaroglu S, Yildiz D, et al. Myocardial iron loading in patients with thalassemia major in Turkey and the potential role of splenectomy in myocardial siderosis. J Pediatr Hematol Oncol 2011;33(5):374–8.
21. Puliyel M, Sposto R, Berdoukas VA, et al. Ferritin trends do not predict changes in total body iron in patients with transfusional iron overload. Am J Hematol 2014; 89(4):391–4.
22. Porter JB, Elalfy M, Taher A, et al. Limitations of serum ferritin to predict liver iron concentration responses to deferasirox therapy in patients with transfusion-dependent thalassaemia. Eur J Haematol 2017;98(3):280–8.
23. Brittenham GM, Farrell DE, Harris JW, et al. Magnetic-susceptibility measurement of human iron stores. N Engl J Med 1982;307:1671–5.
24. Farmaki K, Tzoumari I, Pappa C, et al. Normalisation of total body iron load with very intensive combined chelation reverses cardiac and endocrine complications of thalassaemia major. Br J Haematol 2010;148:466–75.
25. Anderson LJ, Holden S, Davis B, et al. Cardiovascular T2-star (T2*) magnetic resonance for the early diagnosis of myocardial iron overload. Eur Heart J 2001;22(23):2171–9.
26. Wood JC, Tyszka JM, Ghugre N, et al. Myocardial iron loading in transfusion-dependent thalassemia and sickle-cell disease. Blood 2004;103(5):1934–6.
27. Noetzli LJ, Carson SM, Nord AS, et al. Longitudinal analysis of heart and liver iron in thalassemia major. Blood 2008;112(7):2973–8.
28. Anderson LJ, Westwood MA, Holden S, et al. Myocardial iron clearance during reversal of siderotic cardiomyopathy with intravenous desferrioxamine: a prospective study using T2*cardiovascular magnetic resonance. Br J Haematol 2004;127(3):348–55.
29. Wood JC, Origa R, Agus A, et al. Onset of cardiac iron loading in pediatric patients with thalassemia major. Haematologica 2008;93:917–20.
30. Berdoukas V, Nord A, Carson S, et al. Tissue iron evaluation in chronically transfused children shows significant levels of iron loading at a very young age. Am J Hematol 2013;88:E283–5.
31. Carpenter JP, He T, Kirk P, et al. On T2* magnetic resonance and cardiac iron. Circulation 2011;123:1519–28.
32. Carpenter JP, Roughton M, Pennell DJ, Myocardial Iron in Thalassemia (MINT) Investigators. International survey of T2* cardiovascular magnetic resonance in β-thalassemia major. Haematologica 2013;98(9):1368–74.
33. Porter JB, Abeysinghe RD, Marshall L, et al. Kinetics of removal and reappearance of non-transferrin-bound plasma iron with deferoxamine therapy. Blood 1996;88(2):705–13.
34. Cohen LA, Gutierrez L, Weiss A, et al. Serum ferritin is derived primarily from macrophages through a nonclassical secretory pathway. Blood 2010;116(9): 1574–84.
35. Origa R, Galanello R, Ganz T, et al. Liver iron concentrations and urinary hepcidin in beta-thalassemia. Haematologica 2007;92(5):583–8.
36. Musallam KM, Cappellini MD, Taher AT. Evaluation of the 5mg/g liver iron concentration threshold and its association with morbidity in patients with β-thalassemia intermedia. Blood Cells Mol Dis 2013;51:35–8.

37. Taher A, El Rassi F, Isma'eel H, et al. Correlation of liver iron concentration determined by R2 magnetic resonance imaging with serum ferritin in patients with thalassemia intermedia. Haematologica 2008;93:1584–6.

38. Taher A, Vichinsky E, Musallam K, et al. Guidelines for the management of non-transfusion dependent thalassaemia (NTDT). Nicosia (Cyprus): Thalassaemia International Federation; 2013.

39. Cappellini MD, Cohen A, Porter J, et al. Guidelines for the management of transfusion dependent thalassaemia (TDT). 3rd edition. Nicosia (Cyprus): Thalassaemia International Federation; 2014.

40. Musallam KM, Angastiniotis M, Eleftheriou A, et al. Cross-talk between available guidelines for the management of patients with beta-thalassemia major. Acta Haematol 2013;130(2):64–73.

41. He T, Kirk P, Firmin DN, et al. Multi-center transferability of a breath-hold T2 technique for myocardial iron assessment. J Cardiovasc Magn Reson 2008;10:11.

42. Garbowski MW, Carpenter JP, Smith G, et al. Biopsy-based calibration of T2* magnetic resonance for estimation of liver iron concentration and comparison with R2 Ferriscan. J Cardiovasc Magn Reson 2014;16:40.

43. Cabantchik ZI, Breuer W, Zanninelli G, et al. LPI-labile plasma iron in iron overload. Best Pract Res Clin Haematol 2005;18:277–87.

44. De Domenico I, Ward DM, Kaplan J. Specific iron chelators determine the route of ferritin degradation. Blood 2009;114(20):4546–51.

45. Hoffbrand AV, Cohen A, Hershko C. Role of deferiprone in chelation therapy for transfusional iron overload. Blood 2003;102(1):17–24.

46. Waldmeier F, Bruin GJ, Glaenzel U, et al. Pharmacokinetics, metabolism, and disposition of deferasirox in beta-thalassemic patients with transfusion-dependent iron overload who are at pharmacokinetic steady state. Drug Metab Dispos 2010;38(5):808–16.

47. Glickstein H, El RB, Shvartsman M, et al. Intracellular labile iron pools as direct targets of iron chelators: a fluorescence study of chelator action in living cells. Blood 2005;106(9):3242–50.

48. Glickstein H, El RB, Link G, et al. Action of chelators in iron-loaded cardiac cells: accessibility to intracellular labile iron and functional consequences. Blood 2006; 108(9):3195–203.

49. Davis BA, Porter JB. Long-term outcome of continuous 24-hour deferoxamine infusion via indwelling intravenous catheters in high-risk beta-thalassemia. Blood 2000;95(4):1229–36.

50. Pennell DJ, Berdoukas V, Karagiorga M, et al. Randomized controlled trial of deferiprone or deferoxamine in beta-thalassemia major patients with asymptomatic myocardial siderosis. Blood 2006;107:3738–44.

51. Pennell DJ, Porter JB, Piga A, et al. A 1-year randomized controlled trial of deferasirox vs deferoxamine for myocardial iron removal in β-thalassemia major (CORDELIA). Blood 2014;123(10):1447–54.

52. Pennell DJ, Porter JB, Piga A, et al. Sustained improvements in myocardial T2* over 2 years in severely iron-overloaded patients with beta thalassemia major treated with deferasirox or deferoxamine. Am J Hematol 2015;90(2):91–6.

53. Novartis Pharmaceuticals. Desferal® (deferoxamine) Basic Prescribing Information. 2011. Available at: http://www.pharma.us.novartis.com/product/pi/pdf/desferal.pdf. Accessed January 7, 2018.

54. Apotex. Ferriprox prescribing information. 2015. Available at: http://www.ferriprox.com/us/pdf/ferriprox_full_pi.pdf. Accessed January 7, 2018.

55. Novartis Pharmaceuticals. EXJADE® (deferasirox) US Prescribing Information. 2015. Available at: http://www.pharma.us.novartis.com/product/pi/pdf/exjade.pdf. Accessed January 7, 2018.
56. Novartis Pharmaceuticals UK Ltd. Summary of Product Characteristics - EXJADE 125 mg, 250 mg, 500 mg dispersible tablets. 2013. Available at: http://www.medicines.org.uk/emc/medicine/18805/SPC/. Accessed January 7, 2018.
57. Novartis Pharmaceuticals. Exjade film-coated tablets - summary of product characteristics. 2017. Available at: www.medicines.org.uk/emc/print-document?documentId=32428. Accessed January 7, 2018.
58. Novartis Pharmaceuticals. Jadenu (deferasirox) tablets and Jadenu Sprinkle (deferasirox) granules: US prescribing information. 2017. Available at: www.pharma.us.novartis.com/product/pi/pdf/jadenu.pdf. Accessed January 7, 2018.
59. Porter JB, Shah FT. Iron overload in thalassemia and related conditions: therapeutic goals and assessment of response to chelation therapies. Hematol Oncol Clin North Am 2010;24(6):1109–30.
60. Cappellini MD, Porter J, El-Beshlawy A, et al. Tailoring iron chelation by iron intake and serum ferritin: the prospective EPIC study of deferasirox in 1744 patients with transfusion-dependent anemias. Haematologica 2010;95(4):557–66.
61. Hoffbrand AV, Wonke B. Results of long-term subcutaneous desferrioxamine therapy. Baillieres Clin Haematol 1989;2:345–62.
62. Giardina PJ, Grady RW. Chelation therapy in beta-thalassemia: the benefits and limitations of desferrioxamine. Semin Hematol 1995;32:304–12.
63. Cappellini MD, Cohen A, Piga A, et al. A phase 3 study of deferasirox (ICL670), a once-daily oral iron chelator, in patients with beta-thalassemia. Blood 2006; 107(9):3455–62.
64. Cappellini MD, Bejaoui M, Agaoglu L, et al. Iron chelation with deferasirox in adult and pediatric patients with thalassemia major: efficacy and safety during 5 years' follow-up. Blood 2011;118:884–93.
65. Taher A, Elalfy MS, Al Zir K, et al. Importance of optimal dosing $\geq$ 30 mg/kg/d during deferasirox treatment: 2.7-yr follow-up from the ESCALATOR study in patients with beta-thalassaemia. Eur J Haematol 2011;87:355–65.
66. Porter JB, Elalfy MS, Taher AT, et al. Efficacy and safety of deferasirox at low and high iron burdens: results from the EPIC magnetic resonance imaging substudy. Ann Hematol 2013;92:211–9.
67. Addis A, Loebstein R, Koren G, et al. Meta-analytic review of the clinical effectiveness of oral deferiprone (L1). Eur J Clin Pharmacol 1999;55:1–6.
68. Grady RW, Giardina PJ. Iron chelation: rationale for combination therapy. In: Badman DG, Bergeron RJ, Brittenham GM, editors. Iron chelators: new development strategies. Ponte Vedra (FL): Saratoga Group; 2000. p. 293–310.
69. Link G, Konijn AM, Breuer W, et al. Exploring the "iron shuttle" hypothesis in chelation therapy: effects of combined deferoxamine and deferiprone treatment in hypertransfused rats with labeled iron stores and in iron-loaded rat heart cells in culture. J Lab Clin Med 2001;138(2):130–8.
70. Aydinok Y, Ulger Z, Nart D, et al. A randomized controlled 1-year study of daily deferiprone plus twice weekly desferrioxamine compared with daily deferiprone monotherapy in patients with thalassemia major. Haematologica 2007;92: 1599–606.
71. Tanner MA, Galanello R, Dessi C, et al. A randomized, placebo-controlled, double-blind trial of the effect of combined therapy with deferoxamine and deferiprone on myocardial iron in thalassemia major using cardiovascular magnetic resonance. Circulation 2007;115(14):1876–84.

72. Aydinok Y, Kattamis A, Cappellini MD, et al. Effects of deferasirox-deferoxamine on myocardial and liver iron in patients with severe transfusional iron overload. Blood 2015;125(25):3868–77.

73. Kirk P, Roughton M, Porter JB, et al. Cardiac T2* magnetic resonance for prediction of cardiac complications in thalassemia major. Circulation 2009;120(20): 1961–8.

74. Tanner MA, Galanello R, Dessi C, et al. Combined chelation therapy in thalassemia major for the treatment of severe myocardial siderosis with left ventricular dysfunction. J Cardiovasc Magn Reson 2008;10(1):12.

75. Pennell DJ, Porter JB, Cappellini MD, et al. Efficacy of deferasirox in reducing and preventing cardiac iron overload in beta-thalassemia. Blood 2010;115(12): 2364–71.

76. Wood JC, Kang BP, Thompson A, et al. The effect of deferasirox on cardiac iron in thalassemia major: impact of total body iron stores. Blood 2010;116:537–43.

77. Pennell DJ, Porter JB, Cappellini MD, et al. Continued improvement in myocardial T2* over two years of deferasirox therapy in β-thalassemia major patients with cardiac iron overload. Haematologica 2011;96(1):48–54.

78. Pennell DJ, Porter JB, Cappellini MD, et al. Deferasirox for up to 3 years leads to continued improvement of myocardial T2* in patients with b-thalassemia major. Haematologica 2012;97(6):842–8.

79. Pennell DJ, Udelson JE, Arai AE, et al. Cardiovascular function and treatment in beta thalassemia major: a consensus statement from the American Heart Association. Circulation 2013;128:281–308.

80. Wood JC, Glynos T, Thompson A, et al. Relationship between labile plasma iron, liver iron concentration and cardiac response in a deferasirox monotherapy trial. Haematologica 2011;96:1055–8.

81. Aydinok Y, Porter JB, Piga A, et al. Prevalence and distribution of iron overload in patients with transfusion-dependent anemias differs across geographic regions: results from the CORDELIA study. Eur J Haematol 2015;95(3):244–53.

82. Cunningham MJ, Macklin EA, Neufeld EJ, et al. Complications of beta-thalassemia major in North America. Blood 2004;104(1):34–9.

83. De Sanctis V, Elsedfy H, Soliman AT, et al. Endocrine profile of β-thalassemia major patients followed from childhood to advanced adulthood in a tertiary care center. Indian J Endocrinol Metab 2016;20(4):451–9.

84. Fung EB, Harmatz PR, Lee PD, et al. Increased prevalence of iron-overload associated endocrinopathy in thalassaemia versus sickle-cell disease. Br J Haematol 2006;135(4):574–82.

85. Toumba M, Sergis A, Kanaris C, et al. Endocrine complications in patients with thalassaemia major. Pediatr Endocrinol Rev 2007;5(2):642–8.

86. Vichinsky E, Butensky E, Fung E, et al. Comparison of organ dysfunction in transfused patients with SCD or beta thalassemia. Am J Hematol 2005;80(1):70–4.

87. Gamberini MR, De Sanctis V, Gilli G. Hypogonadism, diabetes mellitus, hypothyroidism, hypoparathyroidism: incidence and prevalence related to iron overload and chelation therapy in patients with thalassaemia major followed from 1980 to 2007 in the Ferrara centre. Pediatr Endocrinol Rev 2008;6(Suppl 1):158–69.

88. Noetzli LJ, Panigrahy A, Mittelman SD, et al. Pituitary iron and volume predict hypogonadism in transfusional iron overload. Am J Hematol 2012;87:167–71.

89. Casale M, Citarella S, Filosa A, et al. Endocrine function and bone disease during long-term chelation therapy with deferasirox in patients with β-thalassemia major. Am J Hematol 2014;89(12):1102–6.

90. Liu Y, Parkes JG, Templeton DM. Differential accumulation of nontransferrin-bound iron by cardiac myocytes and fibroblasts. J Mol Cell Cardiol 2003;35: 505–14.

91. Gabutti V, Piga A. Results of long-term iron-chelating therapy. Acta Haematol 1996;95:26–36.

92. Olivieri N, Nathan D, MacMillan J, et al. Survival in medically treated patients with homozygous β-thalassemia. N Engl J Med 1994;331:574–8.

93. Kattamis A, Dinopoulos A, Ladis V, et al. Variations of ferritin levels over a period of 15 years as a compliance chelation index in thalassemic patients. Am J Hematol 2001;68(4):221–4.

94. Delea TE, Edelsberg J, Sofrygin O, et al. Consequences and costs of noncompliance with iron chelation therapy in patients with transfusion-dependent thalassemia: a literature review. Transfusion 2007;47:1919–29.

95. Trachtenberg F, Vichinsky E, Pakbaz Z, et al. Iron chelation adherence to deferoxamine and deferasirox in thalassemia. Am J Hematol 2011;86:433–6.

96. Goldberg SL, Giardina PJ, Chirnomas D, et al. The palatability and tolerability of deferasirox taken with different beverages or foods. Pediatr Blood Cancer 2013; 60:1507–12.

97. Taher AT, Origa R, Perrotta S, et al. New film-coated tablet formulation of deferasirox is well tolerated in patients with thalassemia or lower-risk MDS: results of the randomized, phase II ECLIPSE study. Am J Hematol 2017;92:420–8.

98. Taher AT, Viprakasit V, Musallam KM, et al. Treating iron overload in patients with non-transfusion-dependent thalassemia (NTDT). Am J Hematol 2013;88:409–15.

99. Taher AT, Cappellini MD, Aydinok Y, et al. Optimising iron chelation therapy with deferasirox for non-transfusion-dependent thalassaemia patients: 1-year results from the THETIS study. Blood Cells Mol Dis 2016;57:23–9.

MRI for Iron Overload in Thalassemia

Juliano Lara Fernandes, MD, PhD, MBA

KEYWORDS

- MRI • Iron overload • Parametric map • T2* • Thalassemia

KEY POINTS

- MRI is an essential tool in the management of patients with thalassemia, given the limitations of current metrics to assess iron storage in different organs.
- The examination is simple, fast, and does not involve radiation or contrast, with most of the current installed base of scanners capable of performing the examination.
- The liver iron concentration can be accurately measured with T2* and T2 techniques, with high reproducibility and correlation.
- The myocardial iron concentration is determined with T2* measurements and has been shown to significantly impact the natural history of the disease.
- Improving access to MRI remains a challenge worldwide, with training and education efforts being the primary task to capacitate global centers.

INTRODUCTION

The use of MRI for the assessment of iron overload in thalassemia began its rapidly increasing use after the seminal work by Anderson and colleagues[1] in 2001. With an accelerated phase of development, simplification, and worldwide adoption, the significant clinical impact of MRI in thalassemia management has been shown by many authors,[2–5] and the examination has been incorporated by virtually all international guidelines on the subject.[6–10] In this review, we discuss why MRI plays such an important role in the diagnosis and follow-up of iron overload monitoring in thalassemia, the current techniques, and how MRI assesses iron overload in different organs, as well as practical aspects in the use of this tool in routine thalassemia management.

WHY MRI IS A CENTRAL PART OF IRON OVERLOAD DIAGNOSIS: LIMITATIONS OF ALTERNATIVE TOOLS

Monitoring iron overload has been a challenge since the initial follow-up of patients receiving regular transfusion therapy and chelation treatment.[11] Serum ferritin (SF) is

Disclosure Statement: The author discloses research grants from Siemens AG and speaker fees for Novartis AG.
Jose Michel Kalaf Research Institute, Radiologia Clinica de Campinas, Avenida Jose de Souza Campos 840, Campinas, São Paulo 13092-123, Brazil
E-mail address: jlaraf@terra.com.br

Hematol Oncol Clin N Am 32 (2018) 277–295
https://doi.org/10.1016/j.hoc.2017.11.012
0889-8588/18/© 2017 Elsevier Inc. All rights reserved.

hemonc.theclinics.com

the most widely available and inexpensive tool used to monitor body iron concentration, correlating with total body iron stores with long-term prognostic value.[12] It is included as an essential component in the regular monitoring of patients with thalassemia but, despite its many advantages, significant limitations prevent it from being an accurate form of following up with patients with iron overload (**Table 1**). The first main limitation is that, although SF reflects total body iron stores in the long run, short-term changes (up to months) can be difficult to track with this measurement. In 1 study, SF was shown to only reflect accurate changes in total body iron (as measured by liver iron concentration [LIC]) in 38% of measurements.[13] Not only that, in 26% of that cohort, SF actually showed an opposite direction to the assessment of iron changes in the liver. In a more recent study, more than one-half of the patients followed 1 year after chelation therapy did not show any SF decrease, despite a significant decrease of more than 1 mg/g of iron by LIC assessment making it difficult to differentiate responders and nonresponders to chelation based on SF alone.[14] Apart from its reduced short-term accuracy in reflecting iron concentration changes, SF has an inherent limitation of only measuring global iron storage and not reflecting individual organ concentrations. This particular limitation is of key pathologic interest because it is known that different diseases handle iron in diverse mechanisms and this is reflected in how each organ will be susceptible to iron overload.[15] In non–transfusion-dependent forms of thalassemia this has proved very important as lower levels of SF may not reflect low levels of LIC as measured by MRI.[16] In addition to this factor, different forms of iron will also be handled differently by each organ, reflecting the complexity of the mechanisms involved in iron metabolism, which cannot be depicted by looking only at the global iron burden by SF, but individually in each organ. Because the pathophysiologic pathway for iron entering the liver and heart are so distinct, one can understand the high proportion of cardiovascular deaths in patients with thalassemia with severe myocardial iron concentration (MIC) and apparently low or moderate SF or LIC before the advent of the ability to look at each organ separately.[2]

Another metric that has been suggested to may be useful for monitoring iron overload especially in extrahepatic tissues is non–transferrin-bound iron and its redox fraction labile plasma iron. Both appear in the circulation when the capacity of common iron buffers in the body are exceeded (mainly liver and transferrin), with a correlation with outcomes.[17] Despite its possible importance in the pathophysiology of iron overload and closest link to heart disease, measuring non–transferrin-bound iron and labile plasma iron is fairly complicated and much less validated than other methods, with a wide variability in results,[15] and limited number of sites having it available clinically. Non–transferrin-bound iron measurements also suffer from limitations of very short-term variations in values, including a great influence by recent chelation therapy, without any studies showing the validity of serial follow-up for this metric in guiding therapeutic strategies.[18]

Apart from laboratory variables, other modalities have also been shown to be able to identify iron overload in different organs. Biomagnetic susceptometry measured by special devices called superconducting quantum interference devices were developed to allow for the assessment of liver iron overload.[19] Based on the effects of iron on a magnetic field created by these devices, the LIC can be determined with a fair correlation with current MRI measurements.[20] The main limitations of this method are restricted worldwide availability and limitation to assess iron overload only in the liver and spleen. Computed tomography has also recently emerged as an imaging modality that can track iron content with accuracy and reproducibility.[21] However, very few studies have been conducted with this modality to

Table 1
Strengths and limitations of different tools for monitoring iron overload

	Cost	Availability	Short Term Follow-up Accuracy	Reflects Global Iron Storage	Reflects Individual Organ Storages	Influenced by Other Factors (Inflammation, Infection, etc)	Standardized Measurement	Shown in RCTs to Guide Management to Improve Outcomes
Serum ferritin	Low	High	Poor	Partially	No	Yes	Yes	No
NTBI/LPI	High	Low	Poor	No	No	Yes	No	No
SQUID	High	Low	Good	Yes	Liver and Spleen only	No	Yes	No
Echocardiography/ ultrasound/CT	Low to moderate	High (echocardiography)	Low	Yes (CT)	Yes	No	No	No
MRI	High	Moderate	Good (mo)	Yes	Yes	No (only at very low levels of iron)	Yes	Yes

Abbreviations: CT, computed tomography; LPI, labile plasma iron; NTBI, non–transferrin-bound iron; RCT, randomized, controlled trial; SQUID, superconducting quantum interference devices.

date, because the techniques developed depend on dual energy scanners with limited availability, which are the most accurate for higher concentrations of iron in the liver only, and are associated with repeated doses of ionizing radiation in a particular vulnerable population of reduced age.[22] In the heart, echocardiography has always been pursued for deriving a metric that would reflect myocardial iron storages accurately given its wide availability, low cost, and lack of radiation. Despite these advantages, even with newer and more accurate techniques such as speckle tracking imaging, there has been consistent failure in demonstrating that any echocardiographic parameter robustly correlates to MICs, making this method inappropriate for the follow-up of patients with thalassemia for this purpose.[23]

PRINCIPLES OF MRI
General Principles

Given the limitations of other methods to diagnose and serially follow changes in iron concentration, MRI has emerged as a tool that overcomes most of the previously mentioned restrictions. The technique is based on a scanner that generates a strong magnetic field measured in Tesla units, commonly presenting at strengths of 1.5 and 3.0 T.[24] All images are generated based on the different magnetic properties of each tissue in the body, measured by the differences in hydrogen proton density and interactions. The hydrogen proton is most commonly used owing to its abundance in the human body, but other elements such as sodium, phosphorus, carbon, and fluor can also be measured. When outside the magnetic field, all of the body's protons suffer a constant spin, but with random alignments to each other. Inside the magnet, the field strength creates a more homogeneous environment that permits alignment of these spins and, when an outside source of energy produced by specific radiofrequency waves is generated by gradients, this alignment is displaced momentarily. When the energy source is turned off, the spins return to their original position while transmitting back a signal captured by coils placed around the segment of interest in the body. The amount and intensity of these signals depend on the type of tissue and hydrogen concentration, represented by the created gray scale images. Different types of images can be generated based on the design of the radiofrequency waves emitted to the body, a programmable feature that generates pulse sequences, which are series of instructions for different energy waves that allow for tissue differentiation.

Because the magnetic field and radiofrequency waves used to generate images work outside the range of ionizing radiation (at 1.5 T the frequency is roughly 64 MHz and at 3.0 T 128 MHz, very close to frequency modulation radio that uses the 87.5–108.0 MHz spectrum), there is minimum biological hazard to undergoing multiple serial examinations, both in adults and children.[25,26] Complications in patients undergoing noncontrast MRI scans are extremely rare and most adverse events are correlated with the baseline disease itself and not the procedure.[26] Claustrophobia is the most common adverse reaction to the MRI examination and can occur in 1% to 2% of the population, but generally can be managed with nonpharmacologic strategies, although sedation may be used in extreme cases.[27] Because the MRI environment requires a constantly active magnetic field, care must be taken in patients with metallic implants, with absolute contraindications for the examination in patients with pacemakers, ferromagnetic cerebral aneurysm clips, and cochlear implants (although some newer MRI conditional devices are bending this rule). A complete list with all MRI safe and MRI conditional medical devices that can be scanned can be searched online at www.mrisafety.com.

How Does MRI Measure Iron?

During an MRI examination for iron overload assessment, the images generated are not measuring the iron molecule directly, but mostly through the indirect effect that iron produces in the local hydrogen protons. In **Fig. 1**, a graphical representation of this effect is shown with different iron concentrations. As mentioned, outside the magnet the hydrogen molecules present themselves with aleatory spin vector directions (red arrows) producing no signal (black box). When entering a magnetic field, these spins can then be aligned in the Z direction governed by the scanner magnetic vector (purple arrows), potentially carrying all signal (white box; see **Fig. 1A**). To produce the image, a radiofrequency wave is produced and a time is set to wait for the corresponding energy signal to be captured by the coils, called the echo time (TE). As the duration of TE increases, in a normal tissue without iron as pictured in **Fig. 1**B, more spins lose their coherence and the image is progressively darker. In other words, the longer the TE time, the smaller amount of signal is produced owing to a dephasing effect. When we image a tissue that has a mild concentration of iron within it, the iron molecules affect the homogeneous field created by the MRI and disrupts the signal, therefore generating less signal within the same TE time as in normal tissue. As seen in **Fig. 1**C, at the same TE of 5 ms the tissue with iron is darker than the same tissue without iron at the same TE time owing to the effect of iron in disarranging more hydrogen protons (red arrows). Because this effect is proportional to the amount of iron, as we increase its quantity as in **Fig. 1**D, the darkening effect is intensified accordingly. In summary, the higher the concentration of iron, the more rapidly the image will become darker at progressively shorter TEs. By quantifying a decay curve with many signal intensities at different TEs or by comparing an iron overloaded tissue signal intensity with a normal tissue, we can estimate the concentration of iron within most organs of interest. This principle applies to the liver, heart, and all other endocrine organs that can be imaged using MRI.

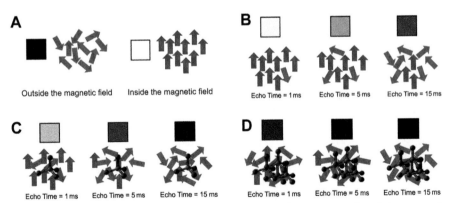

Fig. 1. MRI measures iron indirectly through its effect on the homogeneity of the magnetic field. (*A*) The protons spin randomly (*red arrows*) producing no image (*black signal box*) outside the magnetic field; inside the magnet, spins are aligned (*purple arrows*) and signal may be produced in full (*white signal box*). (*B*) The effect of prolonging echo times (TE) in the image is observed as the signal gets darker at longer TEs in a normal tissue. (*C*) As we insert iron in the tissue, the signal gets darker for the same TE time and this is proportional to the iron concentration (*D*) where the signal is much darker than the comparative normal tissue. The reason for this is shown by the amount of incoherency that iron adds to the local tissue, as is pictured by the increase in red arrows as opposed to the aligned purple arrows.

ASSESSMENT OF IRON OVERLOAD IN THE LIVER

The basic principles explained herein can now be applied to understanding the implementation of MRI for assessment of iron overload in the liver. For the liver, there are 3 main different techniques to measure iron: a signal intensity ratio method and 2 relaxometry methods based on quantification of T2 and T2* times.

The Signal Intensity Ratio Technique

The signal intensity ratio technique was one of the first techniques to be used clinically to quantify LIC by comparing results obtained by MRI to direct quantification of iron through liver biopsies.[28] The technique relies on correlating the signal intensity obtained in 3 different locations in the liver with the signal obtained in a skeletal muscle within the same field of view, a tissue that is not influenced by iron overload.[29] The sequences used for obtaining the images are routine and standardized in scanners across multiple field strengths (1.0, 1.5, and 3.0 T). The interpretation of these images and the quantification of the LIC can be performed using a downloadable open source JAVA-based software or through an online portal (both at https://imagemed.univ-rennes1.fr/en/mrquantif/overview). Although the technique can be used widely, some limitations of the signal intensity ratio method reduce its applicability for patients with thalassemia. The first limitation refers to the current range in which the method reliably estimates LIC, with an upper level of around 15 mg/g at 1.5 T. This cutoff value represents the transition from moderate to severe LIC and in some regions of the world more than 80% of patients will present with levels above this cutoff.[30] Second, the correlation of MRI results with levels of iron measured by biopsy are more variable than relaxometry methods and the curves used originally by Gandon and colleagues have been challenged by alternative authors.[31,32] Some technical limitations also may apply to this technique, because body habitus, choice of sequence, and coil position may introduce additional variation to the measurements.[33] Finally, to our knowledge, no chelation randomized controlled trial has used this method as their method of choice, limiting the applicability of this technique in a more generalized clinical scenario.

Relaxometry Methods: T2 and T2*

To overcome the initial limitations presented by the signal intensity ratio technique, relaxometry methods were introduced, in which there is no need for comparison of the signal intensity obtained by the MRI with a different normal tissue. To determine the amount of iron in the liver using these methods, multiple TEs are obtained in single or multiple breath holds and decay curves are generated by a universal exponential decay formula (**Fig. 2**). T2* and T2 represent the spin–spin relaxation times expressed in the curve and represent the exponential loss of signal as we elongate the TEs, measured in milliseconds. From that principle, it is implied that the faster the curve decreases (ie, the smaller T2* and T2 times), the greater amount of iron in the tissue and the darker the images as we progressively increase TEs, as presented in **Fig. 1**. T2 is usually longer than T2* and is generated using a spin echo sequence versus the gradient echo pulse sequence used for generating T2* images. Both values can be converted to their reciprocals R2 and R2* by the simple application of the mathematical formula $R2 = 1000/T2$ and $R2* = 1000/T2*$, emphasizing the fact that T2/R2 and T2*/R2* are essentially the same, just expressed either in time (ms) or rate constant (Hz), respectively.

The T2/R2 measurements have been standardized routinely by different authors and a commercially available option is available for clinical use (Ferriscan, Resonance

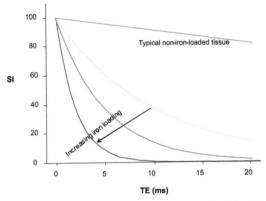

Fig. 2. Exponential decay curve representing relaxometry methods in which with elongating echo times (TEs) the signal intensity (SI) decreases. T2 and T2* represent how fast the decay occurs. In green, a normal tissue with no iron has a slower decay (ie, longer T2/T2* times); as the concentration of iron increases, the decay is faster as represented in the yellow, orange, and red lines.

Health, Burswood, Australia).[34,35] The commercial solution uses a proprietary method where images are obtained locally and interpretation is performed by a third-party company for a fee. Validation of the method and correlation of T2 values to LIC have been reproduced in a multicenter fashion and the method has been used in clinical trials.[36,37] The main advantage of the technique is the strong quality control ensured by the commercial company with the interpretation always performed by experienced readers; limitations include the relatively high cost, especially for the bulk of countries where most of the patients with thalassemia reside, and the longer scan times needed for image acquisition.

T2*/R2* images of the liver were also developed to assess LIC accurately. Like the T2 method, T2* images rely on correlation curves obtained between MRI values and biopsy-obtained samples. For this purpose, 3 extensively validated studies have proposed different curves to correlate T2*/R2* with the LIC with small differences among them, mostly accounted by curve fitting methods, technique to obtain the signal intensity in the liver, and the relatively large coefficient of variation of liver biopsy samples themselves.[36,38–40] Although the upper limit of LIC used in the studies was as high as 41 mg/g, most data were limited to patients with up to 30 mg/g, with only a few outliers above this limit. Interstudy, interreader, and interscanner reproducibility of T2* measurements is high, with coefficients variation in the order of 4% to 7%.[36,41,42] Efficiency for serial analyses for both T2* and T2 to determine the LIC were considered superior than regular biopsies, with T2* demonstrating the most robust estimates up to a 24-week interval.[43] An example of T2* images of the liver is shown in **Fig. 3**.

Comparing both relaxometry techniques, at least 5 studies have shown that the LIC obtained by both T2 and T2* are equally effective in the evaluation of patients with iron overload up to the higher ranges expressed by T2* LIC, with coefficients of determination of $r^2 = 0.93$ to 0.95.[37,40,44–46] Importantly, although the correlation among the 2 methods was consistently high, individual LIC estimates had wide limits of agreement, which increased especially after an LIC of greater than 10 mg/g, making swap of methods for a single patient not recommended during follow-up. Both sequences can be programmed or imported to most 1.5 T scanners

Liver with normal iron levels

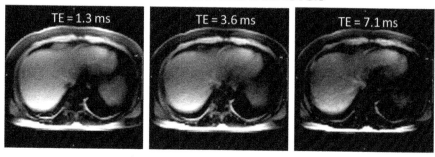

T2* = 15.7 ms or R2* = 63.7 Hz or LIC = 1.96 mg/g

Liver with severe iron overload

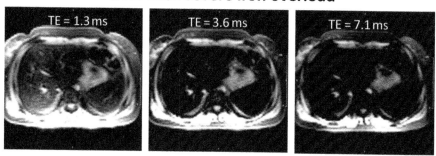

T2* = 1.1 ms or R2* = 909 Hz or LIC = 29.0 mg/g

Fig. 3. T2* images representing a normal (*upper row*) and severely overloaded liver (*lower row*). In the normal liver, the signal intensity does not change significantly as the echo times (TEs) increase, observed by the bright or gray color in all images. In comparison, a severely overloaded liver is dark even in the initial TE of 1.3 ms and completely black in the subsequent TEs. Without any calculations, one can already qualitatively assess that the lower images represent severe iron overload. A visual interpretation is always recommended along the calculated values when performing the examination to ensure that measurements are in accordance to that inspection. LIC, liver iron concentration.

and T2* can be used to assess liver iron at 3.0 T, but with approximately one-half of the upper range and much less validation.[47] Although T2 interpretation of data basically relies on commercial outsourcing, T2* analysis has been integrated into many US Food and Drug Administration- and European Commission-validated analysis software and can also be performed with free tools that have scientific validation but no specific government agency commercial credentialing.[48–51] The greatest limitation of independent analysis of T2* data compared with T2 images is the strict quality and expert-based reading controls exerted when using the commercial option versus the knowledge required to understand the limitations and pitfalls of interpreting T2* images, with both approved analysis software and open source tools. Because of the more rapid decay in signal, T2* images have to be acquired with a very small first TE and with high LIC values a plateau is created in the decay curve requiring either truncation of data or the use of an offset parameter correction factor.[52,53] Failure to recognize this limitation either by using high initial TE values or not correcting the decay curve can occur with any software used to analyze T2* image and result in grossly wrong interpretations (thus, the importance of concurrent visual inspection of the raw images). Because of the identified difficulty in teaching qualified centers across the world to correctly perform independent analysis, many authors have improved the interpretation by adding automatic steps that would allow for the avoidance of these mistakes, either with automated correction or the use of newer sequences with very short TE times.[49,54,55] Even further, new T2* sequences are now available where no offline postprocessing is needed at all, and T2* values are already color coded with inline technology, allowing for accurate and robust results.[56] An example of such automatically generated T2* liver maps is shown in **Fig. 4.**

ASSESSMENT OF IRON OVERLOAD IN THE HEART

For the heart, T2* imaging with MRI is the key technique to detect early iron deposition and to allow for therapeutic changes that significantly impact the natural history of the disease.[2] For imaging the heart, T2* images are obtained in the same way as the T2* method is performed in the liver but with the addition of electrocardiogram gating and focusing on the short axis of the left ventricle (**Fig. 5**).[1] All modern 1.5-T scanners that have electrocardiogram-gating capabilities are, in principle, capable of acquiring myocardial T2* images. Because the severe pathologic concentration of iron in the heart is more than 5 times lower than in the liver (severe LIC >15 mg/g; severe MIC >2.7 mg/g), myocardial T2* is usually easier to analyze, although correction for low signal images and initial lower TEs also should be observed.[57] As with liver T2*, interstudy, interscanner, and intercenter reproducibility have been established with a coefficient of variation around 8% for techniques that use bright blood images and 4% for black blood methods.[42,58–60]

The acquisition of myocardial T2* images can be performed in the same examination when liver iron imaging is being done. Initially, the technique required multiples breath-holds, but almost all centers currently acquire the set of images in a single breath-hold.[61] More recently, new techniques have allowed for the acquisition of myocardial images in a free-breathing manner either using traditional T2* sequences or new hybrid pulse sequences.[62,63] Most centers acquire and analyze only a single-slice midventricular image, using the septum as the segment in which to quantify iron, because it has been shown in biopsies that the septum iron accurately reproduces the global myocardial iron distribution.[64] Other factors such as fibrosis, fat, or oxygen level of the myocardium do not seem to interfere with the measurements at ranges of T2* of less than 30 ms.[65,66] Nevertheless, some investigators prefer to cover multiple slices, because there is a concern that the distribution of iron along the myocardial may be heterogeneous and one might miss greater MICs in other segments of the myocardium apart from the septum.[67,68] Along with this more holistic approach, some centers also seek to search for myocardial scars in patients with thalassemia, a finding that has been show in biopsies not to correlate directly with iron, but that might add increased prognostic information to the examination, despite the need for the use of contrast agents.[69–71] Given the simplicity, practicality, lower cost, and yet completely proven addition of clinical impact for more complex protocols, performing myocardial assessment with a single slice and septum analysis seems to be currently the most cost-effective clinical strategy for routine use.

One important but frequently overlooked detail in the analysis of myocardial images is the presentation of data in T2* values in comparison with the use of LIC for hepatic data. The major reason for this discrepancy stems from the fact that the conception of

T2*   R2*

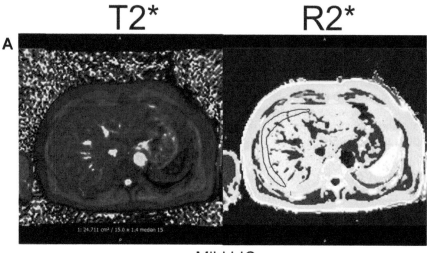

Mild LIC

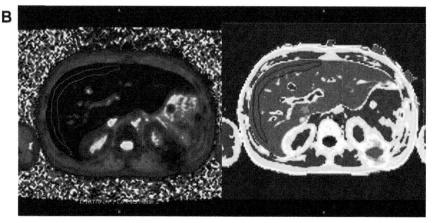

Severe LIC

Fig. 4. Automated in-line generated T2* maps of the liver, without the need for any off-line postprocessing and with respiratory motion correction. (*A*) An example of a liver with mild elevation of the liver iron concentration (LIC) with the T2* map on the left and the corresponding R2* image on the right. Using a region of interest in the right lobe of the liver (*blue line*) with values obtained directly from the image with no manual calculation, the T2* was measured at 15.0 ms, corresponding with an R2* of 66.7 Hz and LIC of 2.05 mg/g (mild elevation above the normal threshold of 2.0 mg/g). (*B*) A liver with severe iron overload and a T2* = 1.6 ms, R2* = 625 Hz, and LIC 19.8 mg/g (severe elevation). The automated processing already corrects for images with low signal-to-noise ratio and plateaus in the decay curve, limiting the potential for any human error in measurements. (*Courtesy of* P. Kellman, PhD, Bethesda, MD.)

iron liver imaging—the correlation of MRI data with direct iron values obtained by routine liver biopsies—was rather straightforward. This was not the case with direct iron quantification in the heart, which was performed first in animal models and then finally in humans.[64,72] With those studies, the correlation of myocardial T2* with the

TE = 4.0   TE = 9.0   TE = 15.0

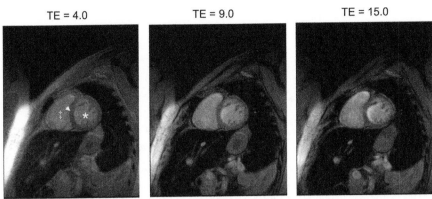

T2* = 22.8 ms or R2* = 43.9 Hz or MIC = 0.99 mg/g

TE = 4.0   TE = 9.0   TE = 15.0

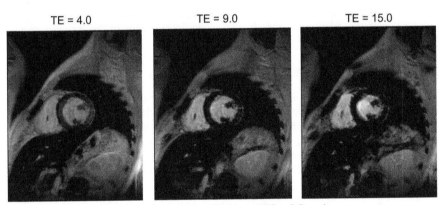

T2* = 5.2 ms or R2* = 192 Hz or MIC = 6.0 mg/g

Fig. 5. As with liver T2*, myocardial T2* is performed with multiple echo times (TEs) but with electrocardiography triggering and in a different slice location, focusing in a midventricular short axis view of the heart. In the upper row, a normal heart with the calculated T2*, R2*, and corresponding myocardial iron concentration (MIC) values. In the first TE image, the left ventricle (*asterisk*) and right ventricle (*double dagger*) are identified along with the septum where commonly the T2* values are read (*arrowhead*). In the lower row, an example of a severely overloaded heart with a very high MIC. Visual analysis shows that the myocardium is much darker than the images on the upper row at the same TE times, in agreement with the calculated values.

MIC was established and now we can report all myocardial data in MIC, as is done with LIC. This development provided a significant advantage for following patients serially, because the correlation between T2* and iron concentration in both heart and liver are nonlinear and small changes in T2* can signify different variations in absolute iron concentrations (**Fig. 6**).

Besides T2*, newer studies in the field are now looking at another parametric map of the heart by measuring its T1 values, corresponding with the longitudinal relaxation time of protons. In some patients with apparently normal T2* ranges, T1 values have been shown to already be reduced, although the clinical applicability of these data remain to be understood.[73,74] For routine clinical use, however, T2* remains the best MRI metric correlating with therapeutic changes.

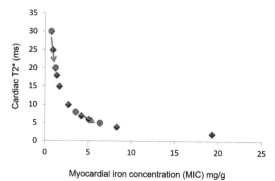

Myocardial iron concentration (MIC) mg/g

Fig. 6. The myocardial T2* and myocardial iron concentration (MIC) are not related linearly, and this factor may limit how one interprets changes in values in the serial follow-up of patients. In this figure, a graph showing the T2* versus MIC correlation is shown. In the *top arrow*, a large decrease in T2* of 10 ms corresponds to a change in MIC of only 0.71 mg/g to 1.16 mg/g (+0.45 mg/g). At the same time, in the *lower arrow*, a small change of 3 ms from a T2* of 8 ms to 5 ms corresponds with a significant change in the absolute amount of MIC from 3.6 mg/g to 6.3 mg (+2.7 mg/g).

ASSESSMENT OF IRON OVERLOAD IN OTHER ORGANS

Although liver and myocardial imaging are the central part of iron assessment with MRI, other organs have also been subject of investigation and can be included in the same MRI examination if needed. The third organ most frequently studied by MRI has been the pancreas, which can be imaged using the same T2* sequence as used for the liver.[75,76] Some studies have shown the correlation of glucose dysregulation and increased pancreatic iron whereby MRI evaluation of iron could identify high-risk patients before irreversible functional damage occurred.[77] Pancreatic iron also seems to precede the accumulation of iron in the heart and can serve as a gatekeeper for centers that can perform only liver and pancreatic abdominal T2* imaging, but do not have electrocardiogram-gating capabilities in their scanner.[78]

Other endocrine organs such as the pituitary gland have also been investigated with MRI and results have shown a discrepancy between iron overload and gland volume with a potential window for treatment before definitive hypogonadism may ensue.[79] Because intensive chelation seems to allow for the reversal of endocrine complications in patients with thalassemia, exploring both pancreatic and pituitary with MRI can prove to be a successful clinical strategy in the future, although not yet fully explored.[80] Finally, renal iron overload imaging has also been possible with MRI, but the correlation of the findings seems to be more linked to hemolysis than transfusion iron overload and its clinical application more suitable for patients with sickle cell disease and not as much for thalassemia.[81,82]

INTERPRETING MRI RESULTS: A PRACTICAL APPROACH TO FIRST USE OF MRI AND FOLLOWING PATIENTS

The first recommendation to perform an MRI study varies in different guidelines, but is usually reserved until patients can understand the procedure and lay down still in the scanner table. Although the liver accumulates iron early, iron accumulation in the heart is often only observed after 10 years of age if a patient is undergoing adequate chelation.[83] However, as is observed in many countries where chelation is irregular or begun late after transfusions starts, children may develop severe forms of myocardial iron overload even as early as 7 years of age.[84] It is, therefore, recommended that the first MRI scan is based not only on these cutoff thresholds for the heart, but earlier if irregular chelation is suspected or if liver analysis is needed for clinical purposes.

The most current MRI protocols today are very short (<20 minutes), especially if only using T2* imaging for the liver and the heart with a focus on the information regarding iron overload and not a more comprehensive cardiac examination with functional imaging, anatomic evaluations, and so on. Different centers have applied accelerated protocols where the goal is to have the examination last for less than 10 minutes with the same data integrity as previous longer examinations, effectively decreasing dropping the cost for the study and increasing its accessability.[85,86] Sedation is rarely necessary in routine examinations, even in very young children, and no contrast is injected for the purpose of iron analysis. Although breath-holding can be sometimes difficult for some patients, despite being relatively short (<10 seconds), liver images for both T2 and T2* can be obtained free-breathing with routine sequences and myocardial T2* free-breathing sequences are starting to gain routine use as new scanner installations take place.[62,63] Although claustrophobia can occur, as mentioned, newer scanners are now produced with wide bores (60–70 cm) and smaller lengths (125–150 cm), making the examination a bit more comfortable. Parents can always stay inside the MRI room and this also adds to easing the procedure for children, because the noise produced by the changing gradients in the scanner are quite loud (around 100–110 dB).

Once a patient performs the first MRI, follow-up studies are usually repeated on a yearly basis for monitoring both liver and heart iron concentrations, but a range of 6 months to 2 years is acceptable depending on the clinical scenario and MRI availability. Loading and unloading of iron in the liver and heart occur through different mechanisms and at different speeds, with LIC observing earlier and more dynamic changes than the ones seen in MIC.[87] Serial changes can sometimes be difficult to interpret if one uses myocardial T2* values rather than the final MIC (see **Fig. 6**), a problem not dealt with liver values, which are most always expressed in LIC derived either from T2 or T2*. A general recommendation reporting MRI examinations should be to include the information of the scan values used to generate the data, the final iron concentration in each organ, and a qualitative classification for the finding with cutoffs established based on previous clinical observations of risk and complications (**Table 2**). A

Table 2
Reference values for liver and myocardial iron concentrations for MRI

T2* (ms) 1.5 T	R2* (Hz) 1.5 T	T2* (ms) 3.0 T	R2* (Hz) 3.0 T	MIC/LIC (mg/g dw)	Classification
Myocardium					
≥20	≤50	≥12.6	≤79	≤1.16	Normal
10–20	51–100	5.8–12.6	80–172	>1.16–2.71	Mild to moderate
<10	>100	<5.8	>172	>2.71	Severe
Liver					
≥15.4	≤65	≥8.4	≤119	≤2.0	Normal
4.5–15.4	66–224	2.3–8.4	120–435	>2.0–7.0	Mild
2.1–4.5	225–475	1.05–2.3	436–952	>7.0–15	Moderate
<2.1	>475	<1.05	>952	>15	Severe

Abbreviations: LIC, liver iron concentration; MIC, myocardial iron concentration.
    Data from Refs.[40,47,64]

graph demonstrating the decay curve and the fitted coefficient of determination used to generate T2/T2* numbers should also be included if possible for the clinician to evaluate the quality of the data generating the calculations with ideal coefficients of greater than 0.98.[54]

As mentioned, although both T2 and T2* for the liver allow for robust serial follow-up of LIC, one should not exchange one value for the other, because the confidence interval for paired results are wide. When using the same method for follow-up, changes greater than the coefficient of variation of 4% to 8% for both the liver and the heart should be considered significant. In the heart, these changes are best followed using MIC and, when using T2* values, should be interpreted carefully in values that are greater than 30 ms, because other factors apart from iron may interfere with high T2* numbers in the myocardial.[88] Finally, because myocardial T2* values reflect mostly chronically deposited iron stores within lysosomes, acutely decompensated patients may sometimes rapidly improve clinically when treated with intensive chelation and heart failure support drugs, whereas very small changes in T2* will be observed owing to the predominant clearance of labile plasma iron first, which has small effects on this MRI metric.[89]

SUMMARY

MRI is an essential tool today to precisely manage individual organ iron stores and guide chelation therapy in patients with thalassemia. Through the development of faster and easier to perform protocols, cost effectiveness is increasing rapidly, along with the availability of centers performing the examination worldwide. More than the focus on specific techniques, improvement in the field will come from training and educating MRI centers on how to correctly perform and interpret these examinations. Quality assurance and accurate results can only be provided through continuous training while newer tools are developed to facilitate and automate MRI iron analysis, guaranteeing examination access to patients with thalassemia all across the globe.

REFERENCES

1. Anderson LJ, Holden S, Davis B, et al. Cardiovascular T2-star (T2*) magnetic resonance for the early diagnosis of myocardial iron overload. Eur Heart J 2001;22(23):2171–9.
2. Modell B, Khan M, Darlison M, et al. Improved survival of thalassaemia major in the UK and relation to T2* cardiovascular magnetic resonance. J Cardiovasc Magn Reson 2008;10:42.
3. Musallam K, Cappellini MD, Taher A. Challenges associated with prolonged survival of patients with thalassemia: transitioning from childhood to adulthood. Pediatrics 2008;121(5):e1426–9.
4. Voskaridou E, Ladis V, Kattamis A, et al. A national registry of haemoglobinopathies in Greece: deducted demographics, trends in mortality and affected births. Ann Hematol 2012;91(9):1451–8.
5. Chouliaras G, Berdoukas V, Ladis V, et al. Impact of magnetic resonance imaging on cardiac mortality in thalassemia major. J Magn Reson Imaging 2011;34(1):56–9.
6. Angelucci E, Barosi G, Camaschella C, et al. Italian Society of Hematology practice guidelines for the management of iron overload in thalassemia major and related disorders. Haematologica 2008;93(5):741–52.

7. Cogliandro T, Derchi G, Mancuso L, et al. Guideline recommendations for heart complications in thalassemia major. J Cardiovasc Med (Hagerstown) 2008;9(5): 515–25.
8. Musallam KM, Angastiniotis M, Eleftheriou A, et al. Cross-talk between available guidelines for the management of patients with beta-thalassemia major. Acta Haematol 2013;130(2):64–73.
9. Pennell DJ, Udelson JE, Arai AE, et al. Cardiovascular function and treatment in beta-thalassemia major: a consensus statement from the American Heart Association. Circulation 2013;128(3):281–308.
10. Verissimo MP, Loggetto SR, Fabron Junior A, et al. Brazilian thalassemia association protocol for iron chelation therapy in patients under regular transfusion. Rev Bras Hematol Hemoter 2013;35(6):428–34.
11. Propper RD, Cooper B, Rufo RR, et al. Continuous subcutaneous administration of deferoxamine in patients with iron overload. N Engl J Med 1977;297(8):418–23.
12. Olivieri NF, Nathan DG, MacMillan JH, et al. Survival in medically treated patients with homozygous beta-thalassemia. N Engl J Med 1994;331(9):574–8.
13. Puliyel M, Sposto R, Berdoukas VA, et al. Ferritin trends do not predict changes in total body iron in patients with transfusional iron overload. Am J Hematol 2014; 89(4):391–4.
14. Porter JB, Elalfy M, Taher A, et al. Limitations of serum ferritin to predict liver iron concentration responses to deferasirox therapy in patients with transfusion-dependent thalassaemia. Eur J Haematol 2017;98(3):280–8.
15. Porter JB, Walter PB, Neumayr LD, et al. Mechanisms of plasma non-transferrin bound iron generation: insights from comparing transfused diamond blackfan anaemia with sickle cell and thalassaemia patients. Br J Haematol 2014;167(5): 692–6.
16. Taher A, El Rassi F, Isma'eel H, et al. Correlation of liver iron concentration determined by R2 magnetic resonance imaging with serum ferritin in patients with thalassemia intermedia. Haematologica 2008;93(10):1584–6.
17. Brissot P, Ropert M, Le Lan C, et al. Non-transferrin bound iron: a key role in iron overload and iron toxicity. Biochim Biophys Acta 2012;1820(3):403–10.
18. de Swart L, Hendriks JC, van der Vorm LN, et al. Second international round robin for the quantification of serum non-transferrin-bound iron and labile plasma iron in patients with iron-overload disorders. Haematologica 2016;101(1):38–45.
19. Brittenham GM, Farrell DE, Harris JW, et al. Magnetic-susceptibility measurement of human iron stores. N Engl J Med 1982;307(27):1671–5.
20. Sharma SD, Fischer R, Schoennagel BP, et al. MRI-based quantitative susceptibility mapping (QSM) and R2* mapping of liver iron overload: comparison with SQUID-based biomagnetic liver susceptometry. Magn Reson Med 2017;78(1): 264–70.
21. Luo XF, Xie XQ, Cheng S, et al. Dual-energy CT for patients suspected of having liver iron overload: can virtual iron content imaging accurately quantify liver iron content? Radiology 2015;277(1):95–103.
22. Wood JC, Mo A, Gera A, et al. Quantitative computed tomography assessment of transfusional iron overload. Br J Haematol 2011;153(6):780–5.
23. Di Odoardo LAF, Giuditta M, Cassinerio E, et al. Myocardial deformation in iron overload cardiomyopathy: speckle tracking imaging in a beta-thalassemia major population. Intern Emerg Med 2017;12(6):799–809.
24. Wood JC. Use of magnetic resonance imaging to monitor iron overload. Hematology Oncology Clin North Am 2014;28(4):747–64, vii.

25. Holland SK, Altaye M, Robertson S, et al. Data on the safety of repeated MRI in healthy children. Neuroimage Clin 2014;4:526–30.
26. Shellock FG, Crues JV. MR procedures: biologic effects, safety, and patient care. Radiology 2004;232(3):635–52.
27. Murphy KJ, Brunberg JA. Adult claustrophobia, anxiety and sedation in MRI. Magn Reson Imaging 1997;15(1):51–4.
28. Gandon Y, Guyader D, Heautot JF, et al. Hemochromatosis: diagnosis and quantification of liver iron with gradient-echo MR imaging. Radiology 1994;193(2):533–8.
29. Gandon Y, Olivié D, Guyader D, et al. Non-invasive assessment of hepatic iron stores by MRI. Lancet 2004;363(9406):357–62.
30. Aydinok Y, Porter JB, Piga A, et al. Prevalence and distribution of iron overload in patients with transfusion-dependent anemias differs across geographic regions: results from the CORDELIA study. Eur J Haematol 2015;95(3):244–53.
31. Rose C, Vandevenne P, Bourgeois E, et al. Liver iron content assessment by routine and simple magnetic resonance imaging procedure in highly transfused patients. Eur J Haematol 2006;77(2):145–9.
32. Alustiza Echeverria JM, Castiella A, Emparanza JI. Quantification of iron concentration in the liver by MRI. Insights Imaging 2012;3(2):173–80.
33. Sirlin CB, Reeder SB. Magnetic resonance imaging quantification of liver iron. Magn Reson Imaging Clin N Am 2010;18(3):359–81, ix.
34. St Pierre TG, Clark PR, Chua-anusorn W, et al. Noninvasive measurement and imaging of liver iron concentrations using proton magnetic resonance. Blood 2005;105(2):855–61.
35. St Pierre TG, El-Beshlawy A, Elalfy M, et al. Multicenter validation of spin-density projection-assisted R2-MRI for the noninvasive measurement of liver iron concentration. Magn Reson Med 2014;71(6):2215–23.
36. Wood JC, Enriquez C, Ghugre N, et al. MRI R2 and R2* mapping accurately estimates hepatic iron concentration in transfusion-dependent thalassemia and sickle cell disease patients. Blood 2005;106(4):1460–5.
37. Wood JC, Zhang P, Rienhoff H, et al. R2 and R2* are equally effective in evaluating chronic response to iron chelation. Am J Hematol 2014;89(5):505–8.
38. Wood JC. Estimating tissue iron burden: current status and future prospects. Br J Haematol 2015;170(1):15–28.
39. Hankins JS, McCarville MB, Loeffler RB, et al. R2* magnetic resonance imaging of the liver in patients with iron overload. Blood 2009;113(20):4853–5.
40. Garbowski MW, Carpenter JP, Smith G, et al. Biopsy-based calibration of T2* magnetic resonance for estimation of liver iron concentration and comparison with R2 Ferriscan. J Cardiovasc Magn Reson 2014;16:40.
41. Tanner MA, He T, Westwood MA, et al. Multi-center validation of the transferability of the magnetic resonance T2* technique for the quantification of tissue iron. Haematologica 2006;91(10):1388–91.
42. Westwood MA, Anderson LJ, Firmin DN, et al. Interscanner reproducibility of cardiovascular magnetic resonance T2* measurements of tissue iron in thalassemia. J Magn Reson Imaging 2003;18(5):616–20.
43. Wood JC, Zhang P, Rienhoff H, et al. Liver MRI is more precise than liver biopsy for assessing total body iron balance: a comparison of MRI relaxometry with simulated liver biopsy results. Magn Reson Imaging 2015;33(6):761–7.
44. Wood JC, Pressel S, Rogers ZR, et al. Liver iron concentration measurements by MRI in chronically transfused children with sickle cell anemia: baseline results from the TWiTCH trial. Am J Hematol 2015;90(9):806–10.

45. Chan WC, Tejani Z, Budhani F, et al. R2* as a surrogate measure of Ferriscan iron quantification in thalassemia. J Magn Reson Imaging 2014;39(4):1007–11.
46. Clarke L, Kidson-Gerber G, Moses D, et al. T2* MRI correlates with R2 liver iron concentration in transfusion dependent thalassaemia. J Hematol Blood Disord 2016;2(1):102.
47. Storey P, Thompson AA, Carqueville CL, et al. R2* imaging of transfusional iron burden at 3T and comparison with 1.5T. J Magn Reson Imaging 2007;25(3): 540–7.
48. Fernandes JL, Sampaio EF, Verissimo M, et al. Heart and liver T2 assessment for iron overload using different software programs. Eur Radiol 2011;21(12):2503–10.
49. Git KA, Fioravante LA, Fernandes JL. An online open-source tool for automated quantification of liver and myocardial iron concentrations by T2* magnetic resonance imaging. Br J Radiol 2015;88(1053):20150269.
50. Mavrogeni S, Bratis K, van Wijk K, et al. The reproducibility of cardiac and liver T2* measurement in thalassemia major using two different software packages. Int J Cardiovasc Imaging 2013;29:1511–6.
51. Bacigalupo L, Paparo F, Zefiro D, et al. Comparison between different software programs and post-processing techniques for the MRI quantification of liver iron concentration in thalassemia patients. Radiol Med 2016;121(10):751–62.
52. He T, Gatehouse PD, Smith GC, et al. Myocardial T2* measurements in iron-overloaded thalassemia: an in vivo study to investigate optimal methods of quantification. Magn Reson Med 2008;60(5):1082–9.
53. Ghugre NR, Enriquez CM, Coates TD, et al. Improved R2* measurements in myocardial iron overload. J Magn Reson Imaging 2006;23(1):9–16.
54. He T, Zhang J, Carpenter JP, et al. Automated truncation method for myocardial T2* measurement in thalassemia. J Magn Reson Imaging 2013;37(2):479–83.
55. Doyle EK, Toy K, Valdez B, et al. Ultra-short echo time images quantify high liver iron. Magn Reson Med 2017. [Epub ahead of print].
56. Alam MH, He T, Auger D, et al. Validation of T2* in-line analysis for tissue iron quantification at 1.5 T. J Cardiovasc Magn Reson 2016;18(1):23.
57. Wood JC, Noetzli L. Cardiovascular MRI in thalassemia major. Ann N Y Acad Sci 2010;1202:173–9.
58. Hartge MM, Unger T, Kintscher U. The endothelium and vascular inflammation in diabetes. Diab Vasc Dis Res 2007;4(2):84–8.
59. Westwood MA, Firmin DN, Gildo M, et al. Intercentre reproducibility of magnetic resonance T2* measurements of myocardial iron in thalassaemia. The Int J Cardiovasc Imaging 2005;21(5):531–8.
60. Kirk P, He T, Anderson LJ, et al. International reproducibility of single breathhold T2* MR for cardiac and liver iron assessment among five thalassemia centers. J Magn Reson Imaging 2010;32(2):315–9.
61. Westwood M, Anderson LJ, Firmin DN, et al. A single breath-hold multiecho T2* cardiovascular magnetic resonance technique for diagnosis of myocardial iron overload. J Magn Reson Imaging 2003;18(1):33–9.
62. Jin N, da Silveira JS, Jolly MP, et al. Free-breathing myocardial T2* mapping using GRE-EPI and automatic non-rigid motion correction. J Cardiovasc Magn Reson 2015;17:113.
63. Kellman P, Xue H, Spottiswoode BS, et al. Free-breathing T2* mapping using respiratory motion corrected averaging. J Cardiovasc Magn Reson 2015;17(1):3.
64. Carpenter JP, He T, Kirk P, et al. On T2* magnetic resonance and cardiac iron. Circulation 2011;123(14):1519–28.

65. Meloni A, Pepe A, Positano V, et al. Influence of myocardial fibrosis and blood oxygenation on heart T2* values in thalassemia patients. J Magn Reson Imaging 2009;29(4):832–7.

66. Kirk P, Smith GC, Roughton M, et al. Myocardial T2* is not affected by ageing, myocardial fibrosis, or impaired left ventricular function. J Magn Reson Imaging 2010;32(5):1095–8.

67. Positano V, Pepe A, Santarelli MF, et al. Multislice multiecho T2* cardiac magnetic resonance for the detection of heterogeneous myocardial iron distribution in thalassaemia patients. NMR Biomed 2009;22(7):707–15.

68. Meloni A, Restaino G, Borsellino Z, et al. Different patterns of myocardial iron distribution by whole-heart T2* magnetic resonance as risk markers for heart complications in thalassemia major. Int J Cardiol 2014;177(3):1012–9.

69. Casale M, Meloni A, Filosa A, et al. Multiparametric cardiac magnetic resonance survey in children with thalassemia major: a multicenter study. Circ Cardiovasc Imaging 2015;8(8):e003230.

70. Kirk P, Sheppard M, Carpenter JP, et al. Post-mortem study of the association between cardiac iron and fibrosis in transfusion dependent anaemia. J Cardiovasc Magn Reson 2017;19(1):36.

71. Pepe A, Meloni A, Rossi G, et al. Prediction of cardiac complications for thalassemia major in the widespread cardiac magnetic resonance era: a prospective multicentre study by a multi-parametric approach. Eur Heart J Cardiovasc Imaging 2017. [Epub ahead of print].

72. Wood JC, Otto-Duessel M, Aguilar M, et al. Cardiac iron determines cardiac T2*, T2, and T1 in the gerbil model of iron cardiomyopathy. Circulation 2005;112(4): 535–43.

73. Krittayaphong R, Zhang S, Saiviroonporn P, et al. Detection of cardiac iron overload with native magnetic resonance T1 and T2 mapping in patients with thalassemia. Int J Cardiol 2017;248:421–6.

74. Alam MH, Auger D, Smith GC, et al. T1 at 1.5T and 3T compared with conventional T2* at 1.5T for cardiac siderosis. J Cardiovasc Magn Reson 2015;17:102.

75. Au WY, Lam WW, Chu W, et al. A T2* magnetic resonance imaging study of pancreatic iron overload in thalassemia major. Haematologica 2008;93(1):116–9.

76. Noetzli LJ, Coates TD, Wood JC. Pancreatic iron loading in chronically transfused sickle cell disease is lower than in thalassaemia major. Br J Haematol 2011; 152(2):229–33.

77. Noetzli LJ, Mittelman SD, Watanabe RM, et al. Pancreatic iron and glucose dysregulation in thalassemia major. Am J Hematol 2012;87(2):155–60.

78. Meloni A, Restaino G, Missere M, et al. Pancreatic iron overload by T2* MRI in a large cohort of well treated thalassemia major patients: can it tell us heart iron distribution and function? Am J Hematol 2015;90(9):E189–90.

79. Noetzli LJ, Panigrahy A, Mittelman SD, et al. Pituitary iron and volume predict hypogonadism in transfusional iron overload. Am J Hematol 2012;87(2):167–71.

80. Farmaki K, Tzoumari I, Pappa C, et al. Normalisation of total body iron load with very intensive combined chelation reverses cardiac and endocrine complications of thalassaemia major. Br J Haematol 2010;148(3):466–75.

81. Vasavda N, Gutierrez L, House MJ, et al. Renal iron load in sickle cell disease is influenced by severity of haemolysis. Br J Haematol 2012;157(5):599–605.

82. Schein A, Enriquez C, Coates TD, et al. Magnetic resonance detection of kidney iron deposition in sickle cell disease: a marker of chronic hemolysis. J Magn Reson Imaging 2008;28(3):698–704.

83. Wood JC, Origa R, Agus A, et al. Onset of cardiac iron loading in pediatric patients with thalassemia major. Haematologica 2008;93(6):917–20.

84. Fernandes JL, Fabron A Jr, Verissimo M. Early cardiac iron overload in children with transfusion-dependent anemias. Haematologica 2009;94(12):1776–7.

85. Fernandes JL. Use of an accelerated protocol for rapid analysis of iron overload in the heart and liver: the All Iron Detected (AID) Multicenter Study. J Cardiovasc Magn Reson 2015;17(Suppl 1):O62.

86. Abdel-Gadir A, Vorasettakarnkij Y, Ngamkasem H, et al. Ultrafast magnetic resonance imaging for iron quantification in thalassemia participants in the developing world: the TIC-TOC study (Thailand and UK International Collaboration in Thalassaemia Optimising Ultrafast CMR). Circulation 2016;134(5):432–4.

87. Noetzli LJ, Carson SM, Nord AS, et al. Longitudinal analysis of heart and liver iron in thalassemia major. Blood 2008;112(7):2973–8.

88. Wacker CM, Hartlep AW, Pfleger S, et al. Susceptibility-sensitive magnetic resonance imaging detects human myocardium supplied by a stenotic coronary artery without a contrast agent. J Am Coll Cardiol 2003;41(5):834–40.

89. Wood JC, Enriquez C, Ghugre N, et al. Physiology and pathophysiology of iron cardiomyopathy in thalassemia. Ann N Y Acad Sci 2005;1054:386–95.

Fertility and Pregnancy in Women with Transfusion-Dependent Thalassemia

Katie T. Carlberg, MD*, Sylvia T. Singer, MD,
Elliott P. Vichinsky, MD

KEYWORDS

- Thalassemia major • Fertility • Pregnancy • NIPT • Iron chelation

KEY POINTS

- Hypogonadism and ovulation abnormalities are still common, ranging from 30% to 80% in adult women with transfusion-dependent thalassemia.
- Discussion of fertility preservation and the importance of optimizing chelation therapy should occur early, with the prepubescent girl and her family.
- Prenatal multidisciplinary evaluation should include assessment of fertility, iron burden, liver and cardiac function, glucose tolerance, thrombotic risk, infection screening, and extended red blood cell phenotyping.
- Pregnancy in women with transfusion-dependent thalassemia should be considered high risk, and close monitoring is needed to maintain hemoglobin over 10 g/dL, assess for gestational diabetes, and reevaluate the need for chelation therapy should cardiac symptoms or rapid increase in ferritin develop.
- The development of earlier and safer prenatal screening is under way and has the potential to open new therapeutic windows during the perinatal period.

In the not so distant past, pregnancy for women with transfusion-dependent thalassemia (TDT) was considered very high risk and often not recommended. As management of these patients has evolved, pregnancy in recent decades has proved not only possible but also increasingly safe, with marked improvements in maternal and fetal survival. What has become evident, however, is the high rate of fertility problems, mostly attributed to hypogonadism, which affects 40% to 90% of patients with TDT.[1–4] As the pathophysiology of the reproductive issues in these women is beginning to be understood, the general perception and even official recommendations seemed to have lagged behind the clinical evidence. Although many case reports depict successful pregnancies in the past 2 decades, the most recent American College of

Disclosure Statement: No disclosures.
Hematology Oncology, UCSF Benioff Children's Hospital Oakland, 747 52nd Street, Oakland, CA 94609, USA
* Corresponding author.
E-mail address: KCarlberg@mail.cho.org

Hematol Oncol Clin N Am 32 (2018) 297–315
https://doi.org/10.1016/j.hoc.2017.11.004
0889-8588/18/© 2017 Elsevier Inc. All rights reserved.
hemonc.theclinics.com

Obstetricians and Gynecologists recommendations from 2007 remain restrictive in terms of those for whom they recommend pregnancy.[5] Moreover, there is a disparity between the methods of expanding reproductive options available for women with infertility and the knowledge and resources accessible to TDT women striving to achieve this goal. Women with TDT have a wide array of complications beyond the reproductive axis that can affect infertility treatment outcomes and pregnancy course. These need to be addressed by a multidisciplinary approach when patients are consulted for family planning. This article reviews these topics and addresses clinical recommendations for optimizing pregnancy outcomes for women with TDT.

IRON TOXICITY AND THE FEMALE REPRODUCTIVE SYSTEM
Mechanisms

Physiologic decline in female fertility and follicle aging results from oxidative stress. Mechanisms include an increase in reactive oxygen species production, reduced enzymatic antioxidant defense mechanisms, mitochondrial flaws, a compromised microenvironment, and a decline in granulosa cell production of estradiol.[6] Iron-induced disruption of reproductive tissue in women with TDT is believed to occur via mechanisms similar to those evidenced by increased levels of redox activity in the follicular fluid and deposition of hemosiderin in endometrial glandular epithelium of iron overloaded TM women.[7,8] Extensive iron deposition may impair oocyte function and has been implicated as a cause of ovarian failure and failure of in vitro fertilization (IVF) attempts.[8,9] Furthermore, the ovarian volume in TDT women (mean age of 30.3 years) was significantly reduced to the range of that seen in postmenopausal women.[10] This effect was believed secondary to lack of gonadotropin stimulation and possible iron deposition within ovarian tissue. The pathophysiology of a compromised reproductive system in women with TDT and iron overload has been extensively reviewed by Roussou and colleagues.[8]

Despite this, ovarian function is typically preserved in women with TDT, even those suffering from primary or secondary amenorrhea, as evidenced by pregnancies after hormonal stimulation. Data on frequency of failure of ovulation induction or timeline to a successful pregnancy, however, are limited. Given the frequent successful results of ovulation induction, infertility is generally attributed to pituitary siderosis disrupting the pituitary-gonadal axis.[10,11]

Iron-induced damage to the anterior pituitary results in defective gonadotropins secretion, a condition also known to occur in patients with iron overload due to genetic hemochromatosis.[12] The anterior pituitary has increased transferrin receptor expression, perhaps making it particularly vulnerable to siderosis, and significant loading has been suggested secondary to increased gland activity during puberty.[13] Standard iron burden measures and intensity of chelation have been used for association with gonadal dysfunction; however, they cannot reliably assess pituitary hormone secretion capacity and reproductive potential.[14,15] MRI technology for pituitary iron quantitation brought about significant progress in determining the intensity of pituitary siderosis, the relation to total body iron, and detection of early-stage endocrinopathies.[16] Pituitary iron deposition was observed in TDT patients younger than 10 years of age whereas clinically significant effects and pituitary volume loss were observed during the second decade of life. Both pituitary iron overload and gland shrinkage were independently predictive of hypogonadism.[17]

Evaluation

Although luteinizing hormone/follicle-stimulating hormone and estradiol along with pubertal development can define hypogonadism in thalassemia,[3] they have poor predictive values of female reproductive potential. Antimüllerian hormone (AMH)[10] and antral follicle counts (AFC) have been suggested alternatives. AMH is produced by the granulosa cells of the preantral and antral follicles and has little gonadotropin-induced intercycle and intracycle variability, making it an ideal biomarker for this patient population. In a study of 36 TDT women, 60% (n = 22) showed diminished reserve as assessed by AFC and AMH levels.[18] Both AMH and AFC have an inverse relationship to ferritin levels in women with TDT and decline more rapidly in this patient population than in normal age-matched women (**Fig. 1**).[1,10,19]

Beyond the severity and duration of iron overload affecting fertility, the age at which a woman attempts pregnancy is another important consideration. Early introduction of the topic and clinical evaluation, even before young women are contemplating having a child, is important and can assist in attaining pregnancy when relevant. Education programs and counseling for fertility preservation are scarce. Still, physicians taking care of thalassemia patients must address reproduction and family planning.

PREGNANCIES IN WOMEN WITH TRANSFUSION-DEPENDENT THALASSEMIA

Since the first account in 1969,[27] more than 400 pregnancies in TDT women have been reported; most delivered healthy term babies. From the literature between 2000 and 2017, the authors reviewed 17 publications, which described 417 pregnancies (**Table 1**). Of these 417 pregnancies, there were 2 maternal deaths (0.48%). Complications in this patient population include intrauterine growth retardation, low birth weight, prematurity, and multiple gestations. Although higher rates of miscarriage

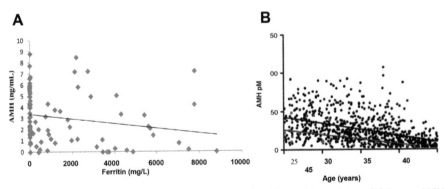

A

AMH (ng/mL) vs Ferritin (mg/L)

B

AMH pM vs Age (years)

Fig. 1. Correlation of Anti-Müllerian hormone Levels with Ferritin and Age. (*A*) Serum AMH and ferritin levels in women with TM (n = 43) and normal controls (n = 44). AMH levels were significantly lower in women with TM (median = 1.77 ng/mL; interquartiles range 3.29 ng/mL) compared with those in controls (median = 3.52 ng/mL; interquartile range: 3.53 ng/mL; *P* = .002). Ferritin levels for women with TM were significantly higher (median = 2287 mg/L) than in controls (median = 13.0 mg/L; *P*≤.001). (*B*) AMH levels in TM women, 25 years and older (*n = 23, red circles*), were compared with normo-ovulatory controls (*n = 759, black circles*), showing that the slopes of the regression lines against age were not statistically different (*P* = .56). The slope was significant for the normal controls (*P*<.001; 95% CI, −1.867 to −1.406) and for the thalassemia patients (*P*<.03; 95% CI, −2.323 to −0.1142), implying an association with age. There was a 5.0 pM (95% CI, 13.4–26.8) difference between the group means. The levels in the thalassemia women were in the low range of normal and dropped below normal levels in women older than 30 years. pM; picomolar. (*Adapted from* [*A*] Uysal A, Alkan G, Kurtoğlu A, et al. Diminished ovarian reserve in women with transfusion-dependent beta-thalassemia major: is iron gonadotoxic? Eur J Obstet Gynecol Reprod Biol 2017;216:72; with permission.)

Table 1
Successful pregnancies (n=417) reported in transfusion-dependent thalassemia women (2000–2017)

Number of Pregnancies	Maternal Age (y)	Number (%) Received Ovulation Induction	Sets of Multiples	Ferritin (Mean or Range) ug/L		Maternal Parameters		Delivery by CS (%)	Fetal Complications (%)			Reference, Year
				Pre-pregnancy	Post-pregnancy	Liver	Cardiac	Non-Cardiac Complications During Pregnancy		Preterm	SGA	Spontaneous Miscarriage/ Stillbirth	
3	23.6	0	0	736–1412	708–1160	—	Echos at 4 time points (pre, 24th week, 33rd week, 37th week)	None	1 (33)	0	0	0	Perniola et al,[37] 2000
86	25.5–28.5	23 (27)	—	2000	2750	—	9 had serial echos: all had transient increase in LV EDD, minimal change in LV ESD, and increase EF - all of which returned to pre-pregnancy values following delivery	None	28 (32)	13.3 (1/2 were multiples)	4.5	6.8	Skordis et al,[32] 2004
24	19–38	12 (50)	2 twins	1,000–11,000	—	Some patients with increasing LFTs	None	18 (75)	16.7	— (mean BW 3240 g)	6.9	Tuck,[38] 2005
1	28	0	0	3,800	5,800	—	Normal echo pre-pregnancy	None	1 (100)	0	0	0	Buttwick,[49] 2005
62	—	0	1 twin	—	—	Monitored hepatic parameters pre-, during, and post-pregnancy	5 with cardiac problems (1 dysarrythmia, 1 RV dysfunction, 3 failures), 27 with no cardiac problems	None	12/45 (26)	8.1	— (mean BW 2678.43 g, range 1500–3850 g)	19	Ansari,[28] 2006

Echos at 4 time points row: "worsened in all parameters worsened in all 3, 1 required digoxin" (Perniola row Cardiac continued)

Tuck row Non-Cardiac Complications: "2 deaths; 10 days and 9 months post delivery"

1	38	0	0	—	67	1,583	LIC pre-pregnancy: 1 mg/g dw, LIC post-pregnancy: 11.3 mg/g dw	T2* MRI pre-pregnancy: 34 ms, T2* MRI post-pregnancy: 27 ms	None	—	—	—	0	Farmaki et al,[15] 2008
5	31 ± 3.5	3 (60)	0	—	770–2,100	—	—	Cardiac evaluation pre-pregnancy and then once per trimester: 1 arrhythmia	1 GD, 1 renal colic	4 (80)	20	40	—	Mancuso et al,[20] 2008
158 (88TM, 12TI)	—	—	—	7 twins, 1 triplet	—	—	—	9 patients had serial echos: 1 patient with triplets developed CHF and recovered	—	—	13.3 (1/2 were multiples)	2.5 (mean BW 2700 g)	6.8	Toumba et al,[31] 2008
11	—	11 (100)	0	2 twins, 1 triplet	2,000	5,000	Liver MRI used to monitor but no data provided	Cardiac MRI used to monitor - no data other than "no significant cardiac complications were encountered"	1 TE episode, premature labor	7 (63)	Preterm labor and growth restriction were 3 fold higher than background population	No data		Bajoria and Chatterjee,[18] 2009
58	29.5 ± 4.5	33 (57)	0	5 twins, 1 triplet	1,463 ± 1,306	2,692 ±1,629	Pre-pregnancy SQUID or MRI but no data provided	No significant change in LVEF, transient increase in LVEDD and HR, both returned to normal post delivery. T2* MRI available for 2 patients (10.2 and 12.0 ms and 16.9 and 8.4 ms)	None	52 (89)	32.8	17.2 of total, 8.9% of singletons	6.9	Origa et al,[4] 2010
1	34	1 (100)	0	—	—	—	—	—	None	1 (100)	0	0	0	Anastasi et al,[21] 2011

(continued on next page)

Table 1 (continued)

Number of Pregnancies	Maternal Age (y)	Number (%) Received Ovulation Induction	Sets of Multiples	Ferritin (Mean or Range) ug/L		Maternal Parameters			Delivery by CS (%)	Fetal Complications (%)			Reference, Year
				Pre-pregnancy	Post-pregnancy	Liver	Cardiac	Non-Cardiac Complications During Pregnancy		Preterm	SGA	Spontaneous Miscarriage/ Stillbirth	
5	23-29	1 (20)	0	500–1,000	—	All had transaminases rise	Normal echos pre-pregnancy	None	5 (100)	0	0	0	Pafumi et al,[22] 2011
1	35	0	0	2,430	2,260	—	Normal echos during	1 GD	1 (100)	0	0	0	Vini,[23] 2011
28	27	22 (78)	—	—	—	—	4 with complications: Afib during labor, peripartum LVD (n=2), LA enlargement - all were transient	4 GD	—	12	—	12.4	Thompson et al,[24] 2013
4	27.9 ± 3.7	1 (25)	0	236 ± 1,258	336 ± 3,054	Minimal iron overload pre-pregnancy and all patients had an increase in liver iron overload post-pregnancy	T2* MRI showed no significant change pre- or post-pregnancy	None	3 (75)	0	0	25	Al-Riyami,[25] 2014

2	27	0	1 twin	417	1,196	—	"Cardiac function was monitored by a cardiologist and remained stable throughout pregnancy"	None	0	100 (twins)	0	50	Merchant et al,[26] 2015
37	30 ± 4	20 (54)	7 twins	409–5,724	836–6,918	LIC significant increase: 3.37 ± 2.11 mg/g dw pre-pregnancy and 9.06 ± 5.75 dw post-pregnancy	T2* MRI were stable: 35.94 ± 8.90 ms pre pregnancy and 31.06 ± 13.26 ms	1 hypertension and proteinuria (in all 3 of her pregnancies), 2 rupture of membranes, 1 placenta accreta, 1 placenta previa, 1 placental abruption, 2 postpartum subfascial hematoma, 2 postdelivery htn, 1 polyhydramnios	35/37 (95)	10	—	—	Cassinerio et al,[29] 2017

Abbreviations: Afib, atrial fibrillation; BW, birth weight; CHF, congestive heart failure; CS, cesarean section; echos, echocardiograms; EF, ejection fraction; GD, gestational diabetes; HR, heart rate; htn, hypertension; LA, left atrium; LFT, liver function test; LIC, liver iron concentration; LV ESD, left ventricular end systolic dimension; LVEDD, left ventricular end diastolic dimension; LVEF, left ventricular ejection fraction; RV, right ventricle; SGA, small for gestational age; SQUID, superconducting quantum interference device; TE, thromboembolic; TI, thalassemia intermedia; TM, thalassemia major.

have also been reported,[4,28] the rate in women with TDT was comparative to that of the general population in a large Italian study.[4] The other complications can be attributed to hormonal stimulation or IVF and the resulting higher rates of multiples, which ranges from 1.6% to 18.9%.[4,28–32] If only accounting for the singleton gestations, the rate of intrauterine growth retardation in pregnancies of women with thalassemia decreased to 8.9%, similar to the rate of 8% within the general Italian population.[4] Cesarean section is most often the chosen delivery method due to concerns of cephalopelvic disproportion resulting from maternal short stature and skeletal deformities.

Planning for Pregnancy: Considerations Prior to and During Pregnancy

Counseling and planning are essential to minimize risk to the mother and fetus. Testing the partner for β-globin gene mutations is imperative. Cardiac disease; endocrinopathies, including diabetes mellitus and hypothyroidism; liver disease; and chronic viral infections, increase the risk during pregnancy. Ideally, a multidisciplinary team composed of a hematologist, reproductive medicine specialist, obstetrician, and cardiologist should be involved. Psychological care is recommended to support the prospective parents.

Cardiac

The maternal cardiovascular system undergoes dramatic adjustments during the course of a pregnancy secondary to increased metabolic demand and blood volume. These include myocardial hypertrophy, chamber enlargement, and mild functional multivalvular regurgitation. Benign arrhythmias are also common. These changes are typically transient, with parameters returning to baseline within weeks of delivery. Patients with TDT, however, may have decreased cardiac reserve because iron deposition in the myocytes, in particular the labile iron fraction of non-transferrin bound iron, results in cellular injury.[33] Chronic anemia and an increased systemic vascular resistance can also lead to left ventricular dysfunction and in some patients right-sided strain may be present due to pulmonary hypertension. Cardiac complications remain the primary cause of death in TDT, making close cardiac monitoring throughout pregnancy imperative. Pregnant women with TDT may experience complications, such as dysrhythmia, right ventricular dysfunction, and cardiac failure, reported in 1.1% to 15.6%.[28,34] Complicating this picture is the common clinical practice of withholding chelation therapy during pregnancy, which can worsen cardiac function in those patients with marginal myocardial function or siderosis.

In a recent study, 2 of 17 women (12%) who had had normal prepregnancy global heart T2* values (>20 ms) showed development of myocardial iron on their postpartum imaging.[35] Similar results were depicted in another study in which 3 of 16 patients (19%) had evidence of new iron overload on postpregnancy imaging.[29] Liver iron concentration (LIC) increased significantly in a majority of these women in both studies. Minimal transient cardiac function changes have been shown in a large report.[4] The increase in left ventricular end-diastolic diameter and left-ventricular end-systolic diameter in TDT women is more pronounced than seen in normal pregnancies.[28,36,37] Additional observable changes include fall in ejection and shortening fractions. Two cases of overt heart failure and subsequent death have been reported.[38]

All women with thalassemia should have a thorough evaluation of their cardiac function prior to pursuing a pregnancy. This includes an ECG, echocardiogram, 24-hour Holter monitor, T2* MRI, and evaluation by a cardiologist. Ideally a prepregnancy T2* of greater than or equal to 20 ms should be achieved, and patients with evidence of significant cardiac iron overload (T2* MRI ≤10 ms) or cardiac dysfunction should be discouraged from planning a pregnancy at that time.

Thrombotic risk

Pregnancy induces a hypercoagulable state with physiologic increases in fibrin and coagulation factors and concomitant decreases in fibrinolytic activity and protein S levels. Additionally, there is reduction in venous flow velocity during gestation. Thalassemia, in particular for those patients who are nontransfused and splenectomized, is also a hypercoagulable state, the pathophysiology of which has been well described and involves interactions of disrupted thalassemic red blood cell membrane surfaces, platelets, and endothelium.[34,39,40]

The recommendations, therefore, are to keep women who are at higher risk (prior splenectomy, nontransfused thalassemia intermedia [TI], and prior recurrent miscarriages) on prophylaxis during pregnancy and during the postpartum period. No specific regimen or guidelines have been established; however, both low-molecular-weight heparin[41] and aspirin[4] have been used.

Infection

The immune system of pregnant women with thalassemia is compromised due to the elevated estrogen levels of pregnancy, the variable state of iron overload, and absence of a spleen in some. Antibodies to transfusion-related viral infections that could affect pregnancy should be checked (**Box 1**). Therapy should be recommended for women with HIV and/or hepatitis C virus (HCV).[42] HCV treatment with interferon or ribavirin should be discontinued 6 months prior to pregnancy. Patients who have been splenectomized should be on penicillin prophylaxis.[43]

Liver disease

Prior to pregnancy, all women should have their liver iron load assessed. Goal LIC should be less than 7 mg/g dry weight.[42] If significantly elevated, intensified chelation should be administered to optimize liver health prior to conception. Ultrasound (US) should be obtained of the gallbladder given increased risk of gallstones, especially in TI.[44] In patients with evidence of sludge or stones, cholecystectomy can be considered prior to pregnancy.

Endocrine

Osteopenia and osteoporosis are common in TDT.[45] Assessment of bone mineral density with dual-energy x-ray absorptiometry (DEXA) should occur when planning pregnancy and regular supplementation with vitamin D and calcium before and during pregnancy is recommended to optimize bone health.[42] Although regular supplementation of vitamin D with 1000 IU to 16000 IU (25–40 mg/d) is used to maintain optimal levels, the levels of 25-hydroxyvitamin D and dose of vitamin D to be targeted and used during pregnancy are not yet clear. Vitamin D is recommended not only for bone health but also to minimize risk of gestational diabetes.[46] Women on bisphosphonates should discontinue use at least 6 months prior to conception.

For patients with diabetes, optimal glucose control should be stressed to improve chances of conception. Because hemoglobin A_{1C} cannot be used for transfusion-dependent patients,[47] fructosamine concentrations can be followed with a goal of less than 300 nmol/L for a minimum of 3 months prior to conception.[42]

Other considerations

One study describes a higher rate neural tube defects in this population[48] and subsequent recommendations include a higher dose of folic acid than is typically recommended for pregnancy (5 mg daily rather than 1 mg daily).[34,49]

Box 1
Recommendations for the clinical management of pregnant women with transfusion-dependent thalassemia

Prepregnancy evaluation

- Fertility: to be discussed and assessed early (prepubertal): menstrual history (PA or SA), AMH, AFC, US of uterus and ovaries. Discussion should include option of cryopreservation where applicable.

- Multidisciplinary care team (obstetrician, cardiologist, psychologist, endocrinologist, and hematologist)

- Assessment of iron burden
  ○ Ferritin: intensification of chelation to achieve ≤l000 ng/mL
  ○ Cardiac: echocardiogram, ECG, 24-h Holter monitor, T2* MRI
  ○ Liver: LFTs and US or MRI. Target LIC prior to conception: ≤7 mg/g dry weight

- If not previously obtained, extended red blood cell phenotyping, genotyping as needed

- Infection screening: HIV, HCV, HBV, rubella, toxoplasmosis, CMV, human parvovirus B19, syphilis

- US of gallbladder to assess need for cholecystectomy

- Assessment for endocrinopathies: thyroid function, glucose tolerance test (fructosamine <300 nmol/L × 3 months prior to conception), vitamin D levels, DEXA scan

- Thrombotic risk assessment: clinical history (splenectomy) and family history of thrombophilia, prior miscarriages)

- Screen for red blood cell antibodies

- Medication review
  ○ To be stopped: chelators, bisphosphonates, ACE inhibitor, interferon, ribavirin, hydroxyurea, vitamin C, oral hypoglycemic agents
  ○ To be started: folic acid, calcium, vitamin D, transition to insulin if previously on oral hypoglycemic agent

Management and monitoring during pregnancy

Maternal
- Frequent assessment of iron burden
  ○ Ferritin each month, echocardiogram each trimester
- Indications to restart chelation (SQ DFO)
  ○ Development of cardiac symptoms, rapid increase in ferritin
- Liver functions each trimester
- Endocrine
  ○ Thyroid function monitored each trimester
  ○ Testing for gestational diabetes at 16 weeks and, if normal, again 28 weeks
- Blood pressure
- Transfuse to keep Hgb greater than 10 g/dL
- Prophylactic anticoagulation with aspirin or LMWH for women considered at high risk

Fetal
- In addition to first (18th–21st weeks) and second (11th–14th weeks) trimester US, serial US starting at 24 weeks should occur monthly to monitor fetal growth

Perinatal considerations

- Assess for cephalopelvic disproportion and need for cesarean section, especially in women with evidence of cardiac dysfunction or iron overload

- Postpartum prophylactic anticoagulation with LMWH for women at high risk

- Reinitiation of chelation therapy with DFO as soon as possible (2–3 weeks postdelivery)

Abbreviations: ACE, angiotensin converting enzyme; AFC, antral follicle count; AMH, anti-müllerian hormone; CMV, cytomegalovirus; DFO, Deferoxamine; HBV, hepatitis B virus; Hgb, hemoglobin; LFT, liver function test; LMWH, low molecular weight heparin; PA, primary amenorrhea; SA, secondary amenorrhea; SQ, subcutaneous; US, ultrasound.

Overall, proper pregnancy planning is essential; establishing an individualized approach and collaboration of specialists decrease the risk of complications during pregnancy, thus reducing couples' anxiety and providers' uncertainties on treatment specifics.

Attaining Pregnancy

Despite improvements in management of iron overload, abnormalities of ovulation occur for 30% to 80% of adult women.[11,50–52] Although a majority of patients with hypogonadotrophic hypogonadism no longer have pulsatile gonadotropins, induction of ovulation in women has been highly successful. In 1 study with 36 patients, ages 20 years to 39 years, ovulation was achieved for 80% of patients.[18] The high rate of success suggests a degree of ovarian protection from damage resulting in sufficient reserve.[53] A variety of induction regimens exist and monitoring parameters should include AMH, estradiol levels, and transvaginal US to monitor size of follicles.[29] There are no data on harmful effects of iron chelation therapy during hormonal stimulation therapy. Although some women are able to become pregnant spontaneously or with ovulation induction, others require further treatments with assisted reproductive technology (ART) that involves manipulation of eggs or embryos in vitro, paired with fertility drugs.[4,29] Indications for ART in patients with thalassemia are not well established and consideration for early referral should be taken, in particular for patients over 30 years old or with comorbidities.

Given the risk for ovarian insufficiency, especially in older TDT women, elective cryopreservation of oocytes or ovarian tissue should be considered while these tissues are still attainable. Such methods are also relevant to TDT women planning hematopoietic stem cell transplant (HSCT), which involves hematotoxic treatment and has shown to be successful.[30,54]

MANAGEMENT DURING PREGNANCY AND PERINATAL PERIOD
Transfusions

For women who were transfusion-dependent prior to pregnancy, regular transfusions should continue with a pretransfusion hemoglobin goal of greater than 10 g/dL. Some patients require more frequent low-volume transfusions due to the increased metabolic stress of pregnancy as well as to support adequate fetal oxygenation. Women with thalassemia intermedia (TI) may develop a transfusion requirement during pregnancy due to the dilutional drop in hemoglobin, which occurs naturally; 13.3 g/dL pre-pregnancy to 11.0 g/dL by the 36th week of gestation.[55] Caution should be used when considering initiation of transfusions given the potential risk of alloimmunization and hemolysis leading to worsening anemia in the fetus.

All thalassemia women should have extended phenotyping and in some cases genotyping at the outset of pregnancy if they have not had such testing in the past. If initiation of transfusions is deemed necessary, phenotypically matched units should be used. If unavailable, matching for Rh and Kell has been shown to decrease alloimmunization by 53%.[34]

Iron Chelation

The use of chelation therapy and choice of best chelation agent during pregnancy have not been addressed in clinical studies and remain controversial. The current standard of practice is to discontinue chelation therapy as soon as pregnancy is established and hold throughout the course of pregnancy due to the concern of teratogenicity. Fetal malformations, including skeletal anomalies, were reported in the offspring of rats after deferoxamine (DFO) exposure. Decreased offspring viability and increased renal anomalies were reported in animal studies after deferasirox exposure. Case reports of women who had become pregnant while taking deferasirox,[56] however, all of whom discontinued chelation on discovery of pregnancy at various time points, report no teratogenicity. Similarly, reports depicting the use of DFO during the second and third trimesters did not report any fetal toxicities.[57,58] Holding chelation for 9 months might have deleterious long-term consequences on cardiac function. Some investigators support chelation, mostly with DFO, in the second and third trimesters,[29,42,57,59,60] when the benefits outweigh the risks, such as for women who had developed either impaired cardiac function or increasing transfusion requirements with rising ferritins. DFO has been the agent of choice during pregnancy, its larger molecular size prohibiting it from crossing the placenta. No clinical trials have addressed this topic and specific recommendations are needed.

Cardiac, Endocrine, and Gastroenterology Evaluation

Echocardiograms and laboratory tests to assess thyroid and liver function should be obtained once each trimester. Screening for gestational diabetes should occur at 16 weeks' gestation and again at 28 weeks if the initial check at 16 weeks is normal. This population is at higher risk of developing gestational diabetes given their low reserve.

Perinatal

For women with prior evidence of cardiac iron overload or dysfunction, continuous infusion of DFO during labor may be considered to minimize the risk of cardiac decompensation or arrhythmias in the setting of acidosis associated with labor: 2 g intravenous over 24 hours during labor.[42]

Skeletal pathologies common in women with TDT have significant implications during childbirth. Approximately 80% of these women require cesarean section, often due to cephalopelvic disproportion. There are, however, case series comprised of well-transfused and chelated women that report cesarean section rates as low as 19%.[28]

For anesthesia, regional blockade is preferred to general anesthesia given the prevalence of maxillofacial deformities. The anatomic changes associated with marrow expansion can complicate intubation and securing the airway. Placement of a spinal epidural must also be carefully considered, because scoliosis and osteoporosis are common. Osteoporosis, present in 40% to 50%[61] of patients with TDT, can lead to reduced height of the vertebral bodies displacing the conus caudally.[62]

Postnatal Considerations

In the procoagulant states of pregnancy and thalassemia, cesarean section and ART add to the risk of venous thromboembolism. No clear guidelines exist regarding postpartum thromboprophylaxis. One study recommended managing women who are at high risk (nontransfused TI, splenectomized, or history of recurrent abortions) with low-molecular-weight heparin for 7 days after a vaginal delivery and for 6 weeks after a cesarean section.[42] Antibiotic treatment is recommended after delivery due to the higher risk of infections, particularly in splenectomized patients.[29,63] Initiation of chelation therapy shortly after delivery is critical. Recent reports suggest that use of DFO during breastfeeding is safe but study on its transmission through breast milk is limited.[64,65] Breastfeeding should be encouraged in all women except in those who are at risk of vertical transmission: women who are hepatitis C RNA positive and/or are hepatitis B surface antigen positive.

Options for contraception are limited in patients with TDTs. Intrauterine devices should be avoided given the increased risk of infection. Estrogen-containing oral contraception may further increase the risk of thromboembolism. Progestin-only oral contraceptive pills are most commonly recommended.

Social/Psychological/Ethical Considerations

The ability to create a family, traditionally by bearing children, has a significant impact on and is often seen as a measurement of an individual's quality of life. The approach to counseling a couple regarding the maternal and fetal risks for a woman with TDT may vary based on culture. In some regions, the influence of a strong societal expectation for family development may play a significant role in a provider's decision to support a couple as they pursue a pregnancy. In the United States, the conversation may place more weight on couples to decide based on their own beliefs and goals, with a medical team providing information to help inform a couple's decision. One topic that is difficult but important to discuss is that of shortened life span. Although the projected life expectancy for individuals with TDT has improved, studies depict that it remains significantly shorter than expected for the general population.[66] How this may have an impact on a couple's decision cannot be known until the conversation is had. Evaluation and counseling prepregnancy and during gestation as part of a multidisciplinary approach are strongly recommended.

Careful planning of care prior to and during pregnancy, involving various specialists, can result in a good outcome of a pregnant TDT woman. Strict monitoring of the parameters listed previously is crucial, in particular, cardiac function and considerations of initiation of chelation.

ATTAINING A FAMILY: OTHER OPTIONS

For at-risk couples, preimplantation genetic diagnosis (PGD) is a method for reducing the risk of having an affected fetus. Embryo biopsy after IVF allows for the selection of unaffected embryos for implantation. One study assesses the implantation rates for 20 couples in which both partners were β-thalassemia carriers who underwent PGD when biopsies occurred at 1 of 2 stages: blastomere or blastocyst. The rate of implantation was found to be slightly increased when biopsies were taken at the blastocyst stage: 26.7% and 47.6%, respectively.[67] The rate of successful pregnancy after PGD is only 30% in couples of thalassemia carriers.[68] PGD for HLA typing is increasingly becoming an option for at-risk couples with children affected by thalassemia and considering HSCT.[69]

For couples in which both partners have TI or thalassaemia major (TM), counseling should be offered regarding third-party reproduction as well as adoption. Third-party reproduction involves IVF using donor gametes and allows a couple to have offspring genetically related to 1 of the partners. The use of either a donor egg or donor sperm is a viable option, although sperm may be preferred given the cost and ease of collection. The feasibility of gamete donation varies between countries.[70] Similarly, access to and eligibility for adoption vary.

PRENATAL SCREENING FOR THALASSEMIA: AN UPDATE

The motivations for determining disease status once a pregnancy is established range from termination of an affected pregnancy, providing information to help family and providers prepare for a child's needs, and, in the case of α-thalassemia, therapeutic options, such as intrauterine transfusion and recently in utero HSCT. Each of these options benefits from early diagnosis. Current methods of prenatal diagnosis involve invasive procedures, such as chorionic villus sampling and amniocentesis, which can be offered no earlier than at 10 weeks' and 15 weeks' gestations, respectively, and pose risks that include miscarriage, limb reduction, infection, and Rh sensitization.[71,72]

FUTURE METHODS OF PRENATAL DIAGNOSIS

The discovery of cell-free fetal DNA in maternal plasma[73] and advances in next-generation sequencing have recently made possible safer, noninvasive prenatal testing (NIPT), which could feasibly be carried out as early as 7 weeks of gestation. NIPT utilizing cell-free fetal DNA is currently used to detect aneuploidies and paternally inherited autosomal-dominant disorders.[74] Diagnosing autosomal recessive disorders, such as thalassemia, however, has proved more challenging because a definitive diagnosis requires the determination of which maternal allele has been transmitted. Unlike the paternal allele, qualitatively determining the maternal allele is complicated because cell-free DNA (cfDNA) is inherently 50% identical to the background of maternally derived cfDNA. This obstacle has led to several investigational approaches:

1. One way in which placental DNA varies from maternal DNA is a slight difference in fragment size.[75] Through size selection, the fetal fraction can be enriched and thereby the sensitivity of a given test for detecting a mutation increased.[76,77]
2. Another method of differentiating maternal from fetal cfDNA is through epigenetic markers, such as DNA methylation.[78] The placenta-derived DNA is hypomethylated or hypermethylated relative to the maternal-derived DNA.[79] Again, this feature could be used to enrich the fetal component in the maternal plasma.
3. A different strategy is to indirectly determine which maternal allele has been inherited by a fetus. This can be done by detecting minute increases in the frequencies of single-nucleotide polymorphism (SNP) alleles for a given locus or haplotype. This approach is termed, *relative mutant dosage* or *relative haplotype dosage*, and has been reported in small series for diseases, such as spinal muscular atrophy,[80] β-thalassemia,[81] and a few others. The specific approaches vary and have different limitations: prior knowledge of parental haplotypes, presence of linked SNPs, and gender-specific application.

There are no clinically available assays for autosomal recessive disorders currently. The possibility of curing thalassemia and other autosomal recessive diseases, however, prior to the birth of an affected child provides compelling motivation. There are several groups working on developing an NIPT for autosomal recessive disorders, including the thalassemias, and such testing likely will be available in the near future.

In summary, as more women with TDT are seeking pregnancy, ensuring the best outcomes for both mother and baby require concerted, collaborative efforts between practitioners and must include the family. With proactive counseling, early fertility evaluation, optimal management of iron overload, and recent advances in reproductive technology and prenatal screening, healthy outcomes have become the expectation. Topics that require further study include management that allows fertility preservation, the use of chelation therapy during pregnancy, and indications and duration of anticoagulation.

REFERENCES

1. Uysal A, Alkan G, Kurtoglu A, et al. Diminished ovarian reserve in women with transfusion-dependent beta-thalassemia major: is iron gonadotoxic? Eur J Obstet Gynecol Reprod Biol 2017;216:69–73.
2. Galanello R, Origa R. Beta-thalassemia. Orphanet J Rare Dis 2010;5:11.

3. Borgna-Pignatti C, Rugolotto S, De Stefano P, et al. Survival and complications in patients with thalassemia major treated with transfusion and deferoxamine. Haematologica 2004;89(10):1187–93.
4. Origa R, Piga A, Quarta G, et al. Pregnancy and beta-thalassemia: an Italian multicenter experience. Haematologica 2010;95(3):376–81.
5. ACOG practice bulletin No. 78: hemoglobinopathies in pregnancy. Obstet Gynecol 2007;109(1):229–37.
6. Tarin JJ. Potential effects of age-associated oxidative stress on mammalian oocytes/embryos. Mol Hum Reprod 1996;2(10):717–24.
7. Birkenfeld A, Goldfarb AW, Rachmilewitz EA, et al. Endometrial glandular haemosiderosis in homozygous beta-thalassaemia. Eur J Obstet Gynecol Reprod Biol 1989;31(2):173–8.
8. Roussou P, Tsagarakis NJ, Kountouras D, et al. Beta-thalassemia major and female fertility: the role of iron and iron-induced oxidative stress. Anemia 2013;2013:617204.
9. Reubinoff BE, Simon A, Friedler S, et al. Defective oocytes as a possible cause of infertility in a beta-thalassaemia major patient. Hum Reprod 1994;9(6):1143–5.
10. Singer ST, Vichinsky EP, Gildengorin G, et al. Reproductive capacity in iron overloaded women with thalassemia major. Blood 2011;118(10):2878–81.
11. Allegra A, Capra M, Cuccia L, et al. Hypogonadism in beta-thalassemic adolescents: a characteristic pituitary-gonadal impairment. The ineffectiveness of long-term iron chelation therapy. Gynecol Endocrinol 1990;4(3):181–91.
12. Olivieri NF, Brittenham GM. Management of the thalassemias. Cold Spring Harb Perspect Med 2013;3(6):1–14.
13. Cetincakmak MG, Hattapoglu S, Menzilcioglu S, et al. MRI-based evaluation of the factors leading to pituitary iron overload in patients with thalassemia major. J Neuroradiol 2016;43(4):297–302.
14. Papadimas J, Goulis DG, Mandala E, et al. beta-thalassemia and gonadal axis: a cross-sectional, clinical study in a Greek population. Hormones (Athens) 2002;1(3):179–87.
15. Farmaki K, Tzoumari I, Pappa C, et al. Normalisation of total body iron load with very intensive combined chelation reverses cardiac and endocrine complications of thalassaemia major. Br J Haematol 2010;148(3):466–75.
16. Lam WW, Au WY, Chu WC, et al. One-stop measurement of iron deposition in the anterior pituitary, liver, and heart in thalassemia patients. J Magn Reson Imaging 2008;28(1):29–33.
17. Noetzli LJ, Panigrahy A, Mittelman SD, et al. Pituitary iron and volume predict hypogonadism in transfusional iron overload. Am J Hematol 2012;87(2):167–71.
18. Bajoria R, Chatterjee R. Hypogonadotrophic hypogonadism and diminished gonadal reserve accounts for dysfunctional gametogenesis in thalassaemia patients with iron overload presenting with infertility. Hemoglobin 2011;35(5–6):636–42.
19. Chang HH, Chen MJ, Lu MY, et al. Iron overload is associated with low anti-mullerian hormone in women with transfusion-dependent beta-thalassaemia. BJOG 2011;118(7):825–31.
20. Mancuso A, Giacobbe A, De Vivo A, et al. Pregnancy in patients with beta-thalassaemia major: maternal and foetal outcome. Acta haematologica 2008;119(1):15–7.
21. Anastasi S, Lisi R, Abbate G, et al. Absence of teratogenicity of deferasirox treatment during pregnancy in a thalassaemic patient. Pediatric endocrinology reviews: PER 2011;8(Suppl 2):345–7.

22. Pafumi C, Leanza V, Coco L, et al. The reproduction in women affected by cooley disease. Hematology reports 2011;3(1):e4.

23. Vini D, Servos P, Drosou M. Normal pregnancy in a patient with beta-thalassaemia major receiving iron chelation therapy with deferasirox (Exjade(R)). European journal of haematology 2011;86(3):274–5.

24. Thompson AA, Kim HY, Singer ST, et al. Pregnancy outcomes in women with thalassemia in North America and the United Kingdom. American journal of hematology 2013;88(9):771–3.

25. Al-Riyami N, Al-Khaduri M, Daar S. Pregnancy Outcomes in Women with Homozygous Beta Thalassaemia: A single-centre experience from Oman. Sultan Qaboos University medical journal 2014;14(3):e337–41.

26. Merchant R, Italia K, Ahmed J, et al. A successful twin pregnancy in a patient with HbE-beta-thalassemia in western India. Journal of postgraduate medicine 2015; 61(3):203–5.

27. Walker EH, Whelton MJ, Beaven GH. Successful pregnancy in a patient with thalassaemia major. J Obstet Gynaecol Br Commonw 1969;76(6):549–53.

28. Ansari S, Azarkeivan A, Tabaroki A. Pregnancy in patients treated for beta thalassemia major in two centers (Ali Asghar Children's Hospital and Thalassemia Clinic): outcome for mothers and newborn infants. Pediatr Hematol Oncol 2006;23(1):33–7.

29. Cassinerio E, Baldini IM, Alameddine RS, et al. Pregnancy in patients with thalassemia major: a cohort study and conclusions for an adequate care management approach. Ann Hematol 2017;96(6):1015–21.

30. Santarone S, Natale A, Olioso P, et al. Pregnancy outcome following hematopoietic cell transplantation for thalassemia major. Bone Marrow Transplant 2017; 52(3):388–93.

31. Toumba M, Kanaris C, Simamonian K, et al. Outcome and management of pregnancy in women with thalassaemia in Cyprus. East Mediterr Health J 2008;14(3): 628–35.

32. Skordis N, Petrikkos L, Toumba M, et al. Update on fertility in thalassaemia major. Pediatr Endocrinol Rev 2004;2(Suppl 2):296–302.

33. Tsironi M, Karagiorga M, Aessopos A. Iron overload, cardiac and other factors affecting pregnancy in thalassemia major. Hemoglobin 2010;34(3):240–50.

34. Lao TT. Obstetric care for women with thalassemia. Best Pract Res Clin Obstet Gynaecol 2017;39:89–100.

35. Meloni A. Changes of cardiac iron and function during pregnancy in transfusion-dependent thalassemia patients. J Cardiovasc Magn Reson 2016;18:270.

36. Thompson AA, Kim HY, Singer ST, et al. Pregnancy outcomes in women with thalassemia in North America and the United Kingdom. Am J Hematol 2013;88(9): 771–3.

37. Perniola R, Magliari F, Rosatelli MC, et al. High-risk pregnancy in beta-thalassemia major women. Report of three cases. Gynecol Obstet Invest 2000; 49(2):137–9.

38. Tuck SM. Fertility and pregnancy in thalassemia major. Ann N Y Acad Sci 2005; 1054:300–7.

39. Leung TY, Lao TT. Thalassaemia in pregnancy. Best Pract Res Clin Obstet Gynaecol 2012;26(1):37–51.

40. Ambroggio S, Peris C, Picardo E, et al. beta-thalassemia patients and gynecological approach: review and clinical experience. Gynecol Endocrinol 2016;32(3): 171–6.

41. Nassar AH, Usta IM, Rechdan JB, et al. Pregnancy in patients with beta-thalassemia intermedia: outcome of mothers and newborns. Am J Hematol 2006;81(7):499–502.
42. Petrakos G, Andriopoulos P, Tsironi M. Pregnancy in women with thalassemia: challenges and solutions. Int J Womens Health 2016;8:441–51.
43. Davies JM, Lewis MP, Wimperis J, et al. Review of guidelines for the prevention and treatment of infection in patients with an absent or dysfunctional spleen: prepared on behalf of the British Committee for Standards in Haematology by a working party of the Haemato-Oncology task force. Br J Haematol 2011;155(3): 308–17.
44. Taher A, Isma'eel H, Cappellini MD. Thalassemia intermedia: revisited. Blood Cells Mol Dis 2006;37(1):12–20.
45. Vogiatzi MG, Macklin EA, Fung EB, et al. Bone disease in thalassemia: a frequent and still unresolved problem. J Bone Miner Res 2009;24(3):543–57.
46. Triunfo S, Lanzone A, Lindqvist PG. Low maternal circulating levels of vitamin D as potential determinant in the development of gestational diabetes mellitus. J Endocrinol Invest 2017;40:1049–59.
47. Spencer DH, Grossman BJ, Scott MG. Red cell transfusion decreases hemoglobin A1c in patients with diabetes. Clin Chem 2011;57(2):344–6.
48. Ibba RM, Zoppi MA, Floris M, et al. Neural tube defects in the offspring of thalassemia carriers. Fetal Diagn Ther 2003;18(1):5–7.
49. Butwick A, Findley I, Wonke B. Management of pregnancy in a patient with beta thalassaemia major. Int J Obstet Anesth 2005;14(4):351–4.
50. Chatterjee R, Katz M, Cox TF, et al. Prospective study of the hypothalamic-pituitary axis in thalassaemic patients who developed secondary amenorrhoea. Clin Endocrinol 1993;39(3):287–96.
51. Bronspiegel-Weintrob N, Olivieri NF, Tyler B, et al. Effect of age at the start of iron chelation therapy on gonadal function in beta-thalassemia major. N Engl J Med 1990;323(11):713–9.
52. Skordis N, Gourni M, Kanaris C, et al. The impact of iron overload and genotype on gonadal function in women with thalassaemia major. Pediatr Endocrinol Rev 2004;2(Suppl 2):292–5.
53. Castaldi MA, Cobellis L. Thalassemia and infertility. Hum Fertil (Camb) 2016; 19(2):90–6.
54. Chung K, Donnez J, Ginsburg E, et al. Emergency IVF versus ovarian tissue cryopreservation: decision making in fertility preservation for female cancer patients. Fertil Steril 2013;99(6):1534–42.
55. Taylor DJ, Lind T. Red cell mass during and after normal pregnancy. Br J Obstet Gynaecol 1979;86(5):364–70.
56. Diamantidis MD, Neokleous N, Agapidou A, et al. Iron chelation therapy of transfusion-dependent beta-thalassemia during pregnancy in the era of novel drugs: is deferasirox toxic? Int J Hematol 2016;103(5):537–44.
57. Singer ST, Vichinsky EP. Deferoxamine treatment during pregnancy: is it harmful? Am J Hematol 1999;60(1):24–6.
58. Tsironi M, Ladis V, Margellis Z, et al. Impairment of cardiac function in a successful full-term pregnancy in a homozygous beta-thalassemia major: does chelation have a positive role? Eur J Obstet Gynecol Reprod Biol 2005;120(1):117–8.
59. Kumar RM, Rizk DE, Khuranna A. Beta-thalassemia major and successful pregnancy. J Reprod Med 1997;42(5):294–8.
60. Rachmilewitz EA, Giardina PJ. How I treat thalassemia. Blood 2011;118(13): 3479–88.

61. Voskaridou E, Kyrtsonis MC, Terpos E, et al. Bone resorption is increased in young adults with thalassaemia major. Br J Haematol 2001;112(1):36–41.
62. Cappellini MD, Robbiolo L, Bottasso BM, et al. Venous thromboembolism and hypercoagulability in splenectomized patients with thalassaemia intermedia. Br J Haematol 2000;111(2):467–73.
63. Nassar AH, Naja M, Cesaretti C, et al. Pregnancy outcome in patients with beta-thalassemia intermedia at two tertiary care centers, in Beirut and Milan. Haematologica 2008;93(10):1586–7.
64. Howard J, ST, Eissa A, et al. Hemoglobinopathies in pregnancy. In: Cohen H, O'Brien P, editors. Disorders of thrombosis and hemostasis in pregnancy. Cham (Switzerland): Springer; 2015. p. 343–63.
65. Skordis N. Fertility in pregnancy. In: Cappellini MD, Cohen A, Porter J, editors. Guidelines for the management of transfusion dependent thalassaemia (TDT). 3rd edition. 2014.
66. Modell B, Khan M, Darlison M, et al. Improved survival of thalassaemia major in the UK and relation to T2* cardiovascular magnetic resonance. J Cardiovasc Magn Reson 2008;10:42.
67. Kokkali G, Traeger-Synodinos J, Vrettou C, et al. Blastocyst biopsy versus cleavage stage biopsy and blastocyst transfer for preimplantation genetic diagnosis of beta-thalassaemia: a pilot study. Hum Reprod 2007;22(5):1443–9.
68. Cao A, Kan YW. The prevention of thalassemia. Cold Spring Harb Perspect Med 2013;3(2):a011775.
69. Rechitsky S, Pakhalchuk T, San Ramos G, et al. First systematic experience of preimplantation genetic diagnosis for single-gene disorders, and/or preimplantation human leukocyte antigen typing, combined with 24-chromosome aneuploidy testing. Fertil Steril 2015;103(2):503–12.
70. Gianaroli L, Ferraretti AP, Magli MC, et al. Current regulatory arrangements for assisted conception treatment in European countries. Eur J Obstet Gynecol Reprod Biol 2016;207:211–3.
71. Tabor A, Alfirevic Z. Update on procedure-related risks for prenatal diagnosis techniques. Fetal Diagn Ther 2010;27(1):1–7.
72. Meleti D, De Oliveira LG, Araujo Junior E, et al. Evaluation of passage of fetal erythrocytes into maternal circulation after invasive obstetric procedures. J Obstet Gynaecol Res 2013;39(9):1374–82.
73. Lo YM, Corbetta N, Chamberlain PF, et al. Presence of fetal DNA in maternal plasma and serum. Lancet 1997;350(9076):485–7.
74. Gregg AR, Skotko BG, Benkendorf JL, et al. Noninvasive prenatal screening for fetal aneuploidy, 2016 update: a position statement of the American College of Medical Genetics and Genomics. Genet Med 2016;18(10):1056–65.
75. Chan KC, Zhang J, Hui AB, et al. Size distributions of maternal and fetal DNA in maternal plasma. Clin Chem 2004;50(1):88–92.
76. Lun FM, Tsui NB, Chan KC, et al. Noninvasive prenatal diagnosis of monogenic diseases by digital size selection and relative mutation dosage on DNA in maternal plasma. Proc Natl Acad Sci U S A 2008;105(50):19920–5.
77. Li Y, Di Naro E, Vitucci A, et al. Detection of paternally inherited fetal point mutations for beta-thalassemia using size-fractionated cell-free DNA in maternal plasma. JAMA 2005;293(7):843–9.
78. Lench N, Barrett A, Fielding S, et al. The clinical implementation of non-invasive prenatal diagnosis for single-gene disorders: challenges and progress made. Prenat Diagn 2013;33(6):555–62.

79. Xiang Y, Zhang J, Li Q, et al. DNA methylome profiling of maternal peripheral blood and placentas reveal potential fetal DNA markers for non-invasive prenatal testing. Mol Hum Reprod 2014;20(9):875–84.

80. Parks M, Court S, Bowns B, et al. Non-invasive prenatal diagnosis of spinal muscular atrophy by relative haplotype dosage. Eur J Hum Genet 2017;25(4): 416–22.

81. Lam KW, Jiang P, Liao GJ, et al. Noninvasive prenatal diagnosis of monogenic diseases by targeted massively parallel sequencing of maternal plasma: application to beta-thalassemia. Clin Chem 2012;58(10):1467–75.

Hematopoietic Stem Cell Transplantation in Thalassemia

Luisa Strocchio, MD[a], Franco Locatelli, MD, PhD[a,b],*

KEYWORDS

- Thalassemia • Hematopoietic stem cell transplantation
- Sibling donor transplantation • Unrelated donor transplantation
- Haploidentical transplantation • Cord blood transplantation

KEY POINTS

- HLA-matched family donors are still considered the gold standard for hematopoietic stem cell transplantation (HSCT) in thalassemia major (TM), with excellent results after either bone marrow or cord blood transplantation.
- TM children with a suitable HLA-identical sibling donor should be offered HSCT at an early disease stage, before the development of significant iron overload-related complications.
- Using strict criteria of donor/recipient compatibility (ie, high-resolution molecular typing for HLA class I and II), outcomes after MUD-HSCT now approach those of HLA-identical sibling recipients.
- Unrelated cord blood transplantation appears to be a suboptimal option in TM patients and is not routinely advisable, unless it is performed in the context of clinical trials.
- Despite few data available to date, results after haploidentical HSCT in children with TM appear encouraging.

INTRODUCTION

The improvements achieved over the last decades in supportive care for transfusion-dependent thalassemia (thalassemia major, TM) have dramatically improved survival rates and quality of life of patients. This holds particularly true for high-income countries, where life expectancy may now achieve the fourth/fifth decade of life.[1] However, TM still represents a relevant cause of childhood mortality in countries where access to regular and safe transfusion programs and/or iron chelation therapy remains difficult.

Disclosure Statement: The authors declare no conflict of interest related to this work.
[a] Department of Pediatric Hematology and Oncology, IRCCS Bambino Gesù Children's Hospital, Piazza S Onofrio, 4, Roma 00165, Italy; [b] Department of Pediatric Science, University of Pavia, Viale Brambilla 74, Pavia, Italy
* Corresponding author. Dipartimento di Onco-Ematologia Pediatrica, IRCCS Ospedale Pediatrico Bambino Gesù, Piazza S Onofrio, 4, Roma 00165, Italy.
E-mail address: franco.locatelli@opbg.net

Allogeneic hematopoietic stem cell transplantation (HSCT), as a way to replace the ineffective endogenous erythropoiesis and correct the phenotypic expression of the disease, has represented a turning point in the treatment of TM, holding the potential to release patients from both a life-long demanding treatment and long-term disease-related and/or therapy-related complications.

Although recent advances in gene therapy are expected to increase the chance of curing TM, this therapeutic approach is currently performed only in the context of clinical trials, and many obstacles remain to be overcome before it becomes available as an effective and routinely accepted clinical practice. Strategies of genome editing, although promising, are still at the preclinical level.

Therefore, at the present time, HSCT is the only consolidated approach holding the potential to definitively cure TM.

PRETRANSPLANTATION RISK STRATIFICATION

Since the curative potential of allogeneic HSCT for TM was first demonstrated,[2] more than 3000 transplant procedures have been reported worldwide.[3]

Outcomes have been shown to depend on patient age and disease status at time of transplantation. Indeed, since earlier experiences with HSCT in the 1980s and early 1990s, better survival rates have been observed in children, compared with adults.[4,5]

A prognostic score predicting transplant outcome in the pediatric population (patients younger than 17 years) was developed by the Pesaro group (**Table 1**). The Pesaro score system identified 3 independent prognostic factors, representing indirect estimates of the degree and extent of iron overload, predicting the risk of transplant-related complications and the chance to benefit from HSCT. These factors allow the stratification of patients into 3 risk groups, as shown in **Table 1**.[4,5]

The extensive Pesaro experience showed a thalassemia-free survival (TFS) estimate of 85% to 90%, 80%, and 65% to 70% for patients belonging risk class 1, 2, and 3, respectively, with probability of transplant-related mortality (TRM) progressively increasing from Pesaro class 1 to class 3, being highest for adult patients.[4–7]

The Pesaro classification has been validated in children having received adequate medical care before HSCT. Limitations of this risk stratification approach become evident when it is applied to patients with a history of inadequate pretransplantation medical care, as commonly seen in developing countries. For such high-risk children, Mathews and colleagues[8] proposed a risk evaluation based on patient age (above or below 7 years) and liver size (more or <5 cm below the costal margin), identifying a very high-risk subset within the Pesaro class 3 group. This observation was confirmed by an analysis based on data reported to the Center for International Blood and Marrow Transplant Research (CIBMTR).[9]

Table 1
Pesaro risk classification for predicting outcome of hematopoietic stem cell transplantation for thalassemia major patients

Risk Factors	Class 1	Class 2 (1 or 2 Risk Factors)	Class 3
Hepatomegaly >2 cm	No	Yes/No	Yes
Portal fibrosis	No	Yes/No	Yes
History of inadequate iron-chelation therapy	No	Yes/No	Yes

Data from Refs.[4,5,56]

More recently, the European Society for Blood and Marrow Transplantation (EBMT) reported a retrospective study on 1493 consecutive TM patients given HSCT between 2000 and 2010, identifying a significant threshold age of 14 years for optimal results.[10]

CONDITIONING REGIMEN

Given TM disease-specific features (ie, hyperplastic bone marrow [BM] and allo-sensitization due to multiple transfusions), for years, a protocol combining busulfan (Bu) and cyclophosphamide (Cy) has been considered the gold standard in patients undergoing HSCT.[4]

Unfortunately, such regimen, although capable of eradicating thalassemia marrow and facilitating persistent engraftment, has been associated with a high incidence of hepatic toxicity, in particular sinusoidal obstruction syndrome, related to the administration of both oral and intravenous Bu, while the heart is the most relevant target of Cy-associated toxicity.

In an attempt to reduce conditioning-related toxicity, in more recently developed protocols Cy has been replaced by fludarabine (Flu) and thiotepa (TT).[11] Use of treosulfan, a structural analogue of Bu with strong myeloablative/immunosuppressive activity and low extramedullary toxicity, has been explored as an alternative to Bu, with encouraging results.[12]

Considering both the nonnegligible risk of graft rejection in TM patients and the detrimental effect of graft-versus-host disease (GvHD) in nonmalignant disorders, the benefit of either anti T-lymphocyte globulins (ATLG) or alemtuzumab has been investigated.[13] Goussetis and colleagues[14] reported a low incidence of both graft failure and GvHD in 75 children given HLA-matched family donor (MFD)-HSCT, with the addition of antithymocyte globulin (ATG) to a Bu/Cy conditioning regimen. Although the incidence of infectious complications was not increased, the need/utility of using ATLG remains debated.

DONOR-RECIPIENT CHIMERISM

A remarkable immunologic peculiarity of HSCT in TM is the possibility, reported in approximately 10% of patients, to observe a condition of stable coexistence of donor and recipient hematopoietic cells (persistent mixed chimerism, PMC) in the presence of a functional graft.

Indeed, several studies support the observation that full donor chimerism is not mandatory in TM for the clinical success of HSCT, as the persistence of even a small percentage of donor erythropoiesis may maintain the potential to correct the phenotypic expression of the disease, due to a competitive advantage of both donor peripheral erythrocytes and erythroid progenitors over their TM counterparts.[15]

The predictive value of mixed chimerism with respect to loss of donor hematopoiesis has been thoroughly studied. As documented by long-term analysis of 295 transplanted TM patients, the occurrence of transient mixed chimerism does not necessarily lead to graft rejection and evolve, in most cases, toward complete donor chimerism or toward a status of stable PMC.[15] In most reports, although the risk of rejection appears greatest in the first 2 months after transplantation, once PMC is established, patients seem to be no longer exposed to the risk of graft failure, showing a stable functional graft and not requiring additional red blood cell transfusion support.[15,16]

These considerations provide a rational basis for the use of reduced-intensity conditioning regimens in TM, with the aim of facilitating a sustained engraftment of at least a threshold fraction of donor cells, sufficient to correct the abnormal hemoglobin phenotype, while reducing conditioning regimen-related toxicity.

HLA-MATCHED FAMILY DONOR HEMATOPOIETIC STEM CELL TRANSPLANTATION IN THALASSEMIA MAJOR

The widest experience of HSCT in TM has been obtained using BM grafts harvested from an MFD.[3,4]

In 1990, the Italian experience on 222 TM patients aged less than 16 years, transplanted from an HLA-identical sibling (n = 212) or a phenotypically identical (for HLA-A, B, C and DR) parent (n = 10), was reported.[4] Overall survival (OS) and event-free survival (EFS) were 82% and 75%, respectively, for the whole cohort. Multivariate analysis identified hepatomegaly, portal fibrosis, and a history of inadequate iron chelation therapy as significant prognostic factors, laying the foundations for the Pesaro classification.

Continuous improvements in outcomes were successively observed, with recently published studies reporting OS and TFS probabilities of over 90% and 85%,[12,13,17–19] and a reduction of TRM to 5% or even lower in young low-risk children.[3]

The extent of pretransplantation tissue exposure to iron overload still negatively affects HSCT outcomes, with probabilities of TFS of 87%, 85%, and 80%, for Pesaro class I, II, and III recipients, respectively.[20]

The already mentioned EBMT retrospective analysis reported best results in patients given the allograft from an MFD, in which 2-year OS and EFS were 91% and 83%, respectively (compared with a 77% 2-year probability of both OS and EFS in recipients of matched unrelated donor (MUD)-HSCT).[10]

The use of alternative sources of hematopoietic stem cells (HSCs) in the MFD setting, including umbilical cord blood (UCB) and peripheral-blood stem cells (PBSCs) in lieu of bone-marrow HSC, has been investigated.

OS and TFS probabilities after HLA-matched sibling UCB transplantation (UCBT) in patients with TM, reported in the largest analysis published to date, approach survival rates obtained after sibling BM transplants, provided that the UCB unit contains an adequate number of total nucleated cells (TNCs; ie, >3.5 $\times$ 10^7/kg).[17,21] Related UCBT has been associated with a reduced risk of GvHD, and, notably, in this setting, the use of methotrexate as part of GvHD prophylaxis has been reported to negatively affect transplantation outcomes.

Good results have been observed after cotransplantation of a related UCB unit and BM cells harvested from the same MFD. The combined infusion, aimed at increasing the number of HSCs transplanted, resulted in a better hematopoietic recovery, while maintaining the cord blood-related protective effect on the occurrence of GvHD.[22]

Conversely, despite good results in terms of engraftment, the use of PBSCs from an MFD is not advisable for transplantation in patients with TM, due to an increased risk of both acute and chronic GvHD (aGvHD, cGvHD).[23]

HLA-MATCHED UNRELATED DONOR HEMATOPOIETIC STEM CELL TRANSPLANTATION

As for most TM patients a suitable healthy MFD is not available, alternative transplantation strategies are needed. Thanks to the introduction of high-resolution molecular techniques for HLA-typing, associated with the progressive increase in the number of volunteer donors worldwide, the use of MUD-HSCT has remarkably increased in the last decades. Currently, a MUD can be identified for 40% to 50% of patients of Caucasian origin, while the likelihood of finding a suitable donor for patients belonging to ethnic minorities is more limited, due the under-representation of non-Caucasian donors in the registries.[24]

In 2002, the outcomes of the first large series of 32 TM patients (aged 2–28 years) given MUD-HSCT were reported by the Italian cooperative group for bone marrow transplantation (GITMO).[25] A Bu/Cy protocol was administered as a conditioning regimen for the first 4 patients, while TT was added for the remaining patients due to lack of sustained engraftment. The OS and TFS estimates were 79% and 66%, with rejection and TRM rates of 12.5% and 19%, respectively. The incidences of grade II to IV aGvHD and cGvHD were 41% and 25%, respectively.

In 2005, the same group reported the results of 68 consecutive TM patients transplanted from an MUD selected by high-resolution HLA molecular typing, after a Bu-based conditioning regimen, combined with either Cy ± TT or TT and Flu. OS and EFS were 79.3% and 65.8%, with rates of TRM and graft failure of 20.7% and 14.4%, respectively.[26] Grade II to IV aGvHD and cGvHD occurred in 40% and 18% of patients, respectively. Better outcomes were observed in Pesaro class 1 and 2 patients (OS 96.7%, TFS 80%) compared with class 3 patients (OS 65.5%, TFS 54.5%).

Similar results were published in 2006 by Hongeng and colleagues,[27] who reported the outcomes of 49 TM children belonging to Pesaro class 2 or 3, given either MFD or MUD-HSCT after a conditioning regimen containing Bu combined with Cy or with Flu and total lymphoid irradiation. In the MUD-HSCT group, the 2-year OS and TFS probabilities were 82% and 71%, respectively, compared with 92% and 82%, respectively, for MFD-HSCT recipients (p=NS).

Encouraging results were reported by GITMO also in the adult setting (17–37 years), with OS, TFS, TRM, and rejection rate of 70%, 70%, 30%, and 4%, respectively, and an incidence of grade II-IV aGvHD and cGvHD of 37% and 27%, respectively.[26]

In 2012, Bernardo and colleagues[12] confirmed, in a large cohort of TM patients, the safety and efficacy of a combination of Treosulfan with TT and Flu, as conditioning regimen for 60 TM children given either MFD (n = 20) or MUD (n = 40)-HSCT. The Authors reported a 5-year OS and TFS of 93% and 84%, respectively, for the whole cohort, with a TFS probability of 78% in MUD recipients.

In the same year, Li and colleagues[28] reported the outcomes of 52 children given PBSC transplantation from MUDs, comparing this population with a cohort of 30 patients receiving MFD-HSCT. The preparative regimen included a combination of Cy, Flu, TT and Bu, all patients being also given azathioprine and hydroxyurea on days −45 to −11. Cyclosporine, mycophenolate mofetil, short-term methotrexate, and ATG were given as GvHD prophylaxis. No statistically significant difference was observed between the MFD- and the MUD-PBSCT groups in terms of 3-year OS (90.0% vs 92.3%), TFS (83.3% vs 90.4%), TRM (7.7% vs 10.0%), cumulative incidence of graft failure (6.9% vs 1.9%), and grade III-IV aGvHD (3.6% vs 9.6%).

In the previously mentioned EBMT retrospective study including 1493 consecutive TM patients, of whom 210 were transplanted from MUD, the 2-year probability of both OS and EFS in the MUD-HSCT subgroup was 77%.[10]

MUD-HSCT is hampered by an increased risk of acute and chronic GVHD, which accounts for a significant part of the morbidity and mortality occurring after allogeneic HSCT. Various factors (summarized in Fig. 1) have been considered to affect the incidence and/or severity of GVHD.[29–33]

Despite an increasingly growing number of HLA-typed volunteers in worldwide registries, the need to respect strict criteria for donor selection in order to reduce the risk of complications due to alloreactivity, still limits donor availability for TM patients.

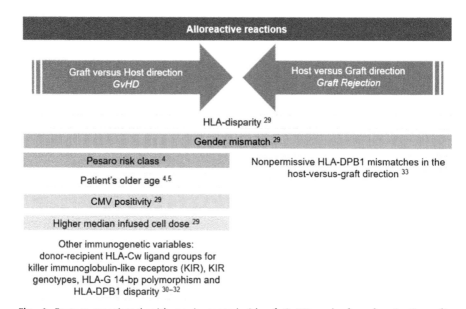

Fig. 1. Factors associated with an increased risk of GvHD and of graft rejection after MUD-HSCT for TM.

UNRELATED UMBILICAL CORD BLOOD TRANSPLANTATION IN THALASSEMIA MAJOR

For patients lacking MFD or MUD, unrelated UCBT holds the potential to broaden the access to HSCT and appears appealing in a nonmalignant disease by virtue of a supposed lower risk of GvHD.

Although outcomes after HLA-identical sibling UCBT in TM approach those obtained using BM cells from MFD,[17,21] the limited experience with unrelated UCBT has been hampered by high rates of graft failure and delayed hematopoietic recovery, mainly due to inadequate cell dose in the graft.[34]

In 2011, Ruggeri and colleagues[35] described the outcomes of 35 TM patients given unrelated UCBT, reporting OS and TFS estimates of 62% and 21%, respectively, with a cumulative incidence of grade II to IV aGvHD and cGvHD of 23% and 16%, respectively. Primary graft failure was the main cause of treatment failure (occurring in 20 out of 35 TM patient). A TNC dose of greater than or equal to 5×10^7/kg was associated with better outcomes.

Better results were observed by Jaing and colleagues[36] in 35 TM patients given unrelated UCBT employing a double UCBT approach when no single unit containing at least 2.5×10^7 TNC/kg was available. The 5-year OS and TFS were 88.3% and 73.9%, respectively, such good outcomes being ascribed to the high cell dose infused.

As the risk of graft failure and delayed hematopoietic recovery represent major obstacles to the success of unrelated UCBT, current recommendations for UCBT in nonmalignant disorders suggest using units containing at least 3.5×10^7 TNC/kg recipient body weight before cryopreservation, and having less than 2 HLA disparities.[37]

Strategies aimed at overcoming the cell dose limitation include cotransplantation of multiple units,[38] cotransplantation of UCB and either T-cell depleted (TCD) HLA-haploidentical CD34 + cells or mesenchymal stromal cells,[39,40] direct intrabone injection of UCB,[41] ex vivo expansion of UCB-derived stem and progenitor cells,[42–46] or pre-modulation of the unit to enhance the homing to the BM niche of the UCB-derived HSC.[47,48]

HLA-HAPLOIDENTICAL HEMATOPOIETIC STEM CELL TRANSPLANTATION (HAPLO- HSCT) IN THALASSEMIA MAJOR

Since the probability of finding a suitable MUD is conditioned by the patient's ethnic background and HLA-genotype frequency, and considering that many countries lack appropriate registries or the resources for extensive donor screening and search, transplantation from a haploidentical relative can represent a response to the unmet need for HSCT in patients lacking a matched donor.

Thanks to the optimization of transplantation techniques, the haploidentical approach can now be considered a valuable alternative also in the treatment of nonmalignant hematological disorders.

Due to the previously mentioned TM disease-specific features, haplo-HSCT, especially TCD, is associated with a significant risk of graft failure.[49]

The first series of TM patients transplanted from related donors other than HLA-identical siblings was reported by the Pesaro group in 2000.[50] Donors were HLA-phenotypically identical relatives in 6 cases and mismatched relatives in 23 cases. In an attempt to facilitate engraftment, ATG or irradiation was associated, in most patients, with a Bu/Cy protocol. OS and EFS probabilities were 65% and 21%, respectively, with a high incidence of graft failure (55%) and an incidence of grade II to IV aGvHD and cGvHD of 47.3% and 37.5%, respectively.

In 2010, the same group reported the outcomes of 22 children given a TCD allograft from a haploidentical relative.[49] TCD was achieved either by means of CD34+ cell positive selection or through CD3+/CD19+ depletion. The pretransplantation strategies designed with the aim of reducing the risk of graft failure are summarized in **Fig. 2**. Six patients experienced graft rejection (cumulative incidence, CI 29%), while 2 patients died of transplantation-related complications (CI 14%), leading to a TFS of 61%. In a recent update including 31 patients, cumulative incidences of graft rejection and TRM were 23% and 7%, respectively, with TFS improved to 70%.[51]

A new method of ex vivo graft manipulation, consisting in negative depletion of T-cell receptor (TCR) $\alpha\beta$ T-lymphocytes and CD19 B-cells from PBSC grafts has been recently described. Leaving in the final product large numbers of mature NK cells and TCR$\gamma\delta$+ T-cells, this approach potentially contributes to infection control. In a pilot study, including 23 patients affected by nonmalignant disorders, the feasibility and efficacy of this strategy were demonstrated, with a low TRM (9.3%).[52] One of the patients was affected by TM and autoimmune hemolytic anemia, and was successfully transplanted from his haploidentical mother. In order to further improve post-transplantation immune reconstitution, a new study protocol based on the add-back of donor T-lymphocytes transduced with the new suicide gene-inducible Caspase 9 after TCR$\alpha\beta$-CD19 depleted HSCT was developed.[53] Through this new approach, 9 TM patients were successfully transplanted.[54]

Recently, Anurathapan and colleagues[55] explored the use of T-cell replete PBSC haplo-HSCT in 31 TM patients, using an immunosuppressive/lymphodepleting approach, summarized in **Fig. 1**. Twenty-nine patients achieved engraftment with 100% donor chimerism, while 2 patients experienced primary graft failure. Two-year OS and EFS were 95% and 94%, respectively. Nine patients developed grade II aGvHD, and 5 patients developed limited-severity cGvHD.

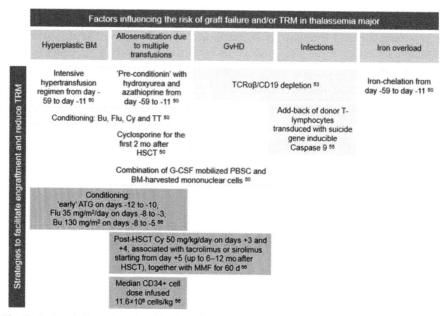

Fig. 2. Factors influencing the risk of graft failure and/or of TRM in haplo-HSCT for TM and strategies adopted to overcome them.

SUMMARY/DISCUSSION

Although the clinical application of gene therapy approaches is currently confined to the context of experimental protocols, at present HSCT represents the only consolidated curative option for TM.

Best results have been obtained using BM cells from an MFD, with OS and TFS probabilities of over 90% and 80%, respectively. Outcomes after related UCBT are at least as good as those of patients receiving BM MFD allografts, provided the UCB unit contains an adequate cell dose.

The combined infusion of BM and UCB cells from the same HLA-identical donor can be pursued in case of low numbers (ie, <3.5 x 10^7/kg) of stem cells per kg of recipient body weight in the stored unit, in order to increase the number of cells infused.

Considering such good results, TM children with a suitable, unaffected, HLA-identical sibling should be offered HSCT at an early disease stage.

For patients lacking such a donor, alternative transplantation strategies include MUD-HSCT, unrelated UCBT, and haploidentical HSCT. However, the option to offer an alternative-donor allograft in a disease with an estimated average life-expectancy now achieving the fourth/fifth decade of life[1] needs to be carefully weighted.

Thanks to the advances in the field of allogeneic HSCT, outcomes after MUD-HSCT now approach those obtained in the MFD setting, provided that the donor selection is performed using high-resolution molecular typing for HLA class I and II loci and according to strict criteria of donor/recipient compatibility (ie, full match or single allelic disparity for HLA-A, B, C, DRB1, and DQB1 loci).

Less successful results have been reported after unrelated UCBT, mainly because of high rates of graft failure, associated with low hematopoietic progenitors/stem cells content in UCB units.[35] Based on currently available data, unrelated UCBT appears to be a suboptimal option in TM patients, unless it is performed in the context of clinical trials.

Experience with haplo-HSCT in children with TM is still limited. Currently explored platforms hold the potential to extend the access to HSCT to the proportion of TM patients lacking an HLA-matched either related or unrelated donor, offering also the advantage of immediate accessibility to the transplant procedure.

REFERENCES

1. Borgna-Pignatti C, Rugolotto S, De Stefano P, et al. Survival and complications in patients with thalassemia major treated with transfusion and deferoxamine. Haematologica 2004;89(10):1187–93.
2. Thomas ED, Buckner CD, Sanders JE, et al. Marrow transplantation for thalassaemia. Lancet 1982;2(8292):227–9.
3. Angelucci E, Matthes-Martin S, Baronciani D, et al. Hematopoietic stem cell transplantation in thalassemia major and sickle cell disease: indications and management recommendations from an international expert panel. Haematologica 2014; 99(5):811–20.
4. Lucarelli G, Galimberti M, Polchi P, et al. Bone marrow transplantation in patients with thalassemia. N Engl J Med 1990;322(7):417–21.
5. Giardini C, Lucarelli G. Bone marrow transplantation for beta-thalassemia. Hematol Oncol Clin North Am 1999;13(5):1059–64.
6. Lucarelli G, Clift RA, Galimberti M, et al. Marrow transplantation for patients with thalassemia: results in class 3 patients. Blood 1996;87(5):2082–8.
7. Lucarelli G, Galimberti M, Giardini C, et al. Bone marrow transplantation in thalassemia. The experience of Pesaro. Ann New York Acad Sci 1998;850:270–5.
8. Mathews V, George B, Deotare U, et al. A new stratification strategy that identifies a subset of class III patients with an adverse prognosis among children with beta thalassemia major undergoing a matched related allogeneic stem cell transplantation. Biol Blood Marrow Transplant 2007;13(8):889–94.
9. Sabloff M, Chandy M, Wang Z, et al. HLA-matched sibling bone marrow transplantation for beta-thalassemia major. Blood 2011;117(5):1745–50.
10. Baronciani D, Angelucci E, Potschger U, et al. Hemopoietic stem cell transplantation in thalassemia: a report from the European Society for Blood and Bone Marrow Transplantation Hemoglobinopathy Registry, 2000-2010. Bone Marrow Transplant 2016;51(4):536–41.
11. Locatelli F, Rocha V, Reed W, et al. Related umbilical cord blood transplantation in patients with thalassemia and sickle cell disease. Blood 2003;101(6):2137–43.
12. Bernardo ME, Piras E, Vacca A, et al. Allogeneic hematopoietic stem cell transplantation in thalassemia major: results of a reduced-toxicity conditioning regimen based on the use of treosulfan. Blood 2012;120(2):473–6.
13. Lawson SE, Roberts IA, Amrolia P, et al. Bone marrow transplantation for beta-thalassaemia major: the UK experience in two paediatric centres. Br J Haematol 2003;120(2):289–95.
14. Goussetis E, Peristeri I, Kitra V, et al. HLA-matched sibling stem cell transplantation in children with beta-thalassemia with anti-thymocyte globulin as part of the preparative regimen: the Greek experience. Bone Marrow Transpl 2012;47(8):1061–6.
15. Andreani M, Nesci S, Lucarelli G, et al. Long-term survival of ex-thalassemic patients with persistent mixed chimerism after bone marrow transplantation. Bone Marrow Transplant 2000;25(4):401–4.
16. Andreani M, Testi M, Battarra M, et al. Relationship between mixed chimerism and rejection after bone marrow transplantation in thalassaemia. Blood Transfus 2008;6(3):143–9.

17. Locatelli F, Kabbara N, Ruggeri A, et al. Outcome of patients with hemoglobinopathies given either cord blood or bone marrow transplantation from an HLA-identical sibling. Blood 2013;122(6):1072–8.

18. Hussein AA, Al-Zaben A, Ghatasheh L, et al. Risk adopted allogeneic hematopoietic stem cell transplantation using a reduced intensity regimen for children with thalassemia major. Pediatr Blood Cancer 2013;60(8):1345–9.

19. Di Bartolomeo P, Santarone S, Di Bartolomeo E, et al. Long-term results of survival in patients with thalassemia major treated with bone marrow transplantation. Am J Hematol 2008;83(7):528–30.

20. Gaziev J, Sodani P, Polchi P, et al. Bone marrow transplantation in adults with thalassemia: treatment and long-term follow-up. Ann N Y Acad Sci 2005;1054: 196–205.

21. Kabbara N, Locatelli F, Rocha V, et al. A multicentric comparative analysis of outcomes of HLA identical related cord blood and bone marrow transplantation in patients with beta-thalassemia or sickle cell disease. Bone Marrow Transplant 2008;41:S29.

22. Tucunduva L, Volt F, Cunha R, et al. Combined cord blood and bone marrow transplantation from the same human leucocyte antigen-identical sibling donor for children with malignant and non-malignant diseases. Br J Haematol 2015; 169(1):103–10.

23. Ghavamzadeh A, Iravani M, Ashouri A, et al. Peripheral blood versus bone marrow as a source of hematopoietic stem cells for allogeneic transplantation in children with class I and II beta thalassemia major. Biol Blood Marrow Transpl 2008;14(3):301–8.

24. Rocha V, Locatelli F. Searching for alternative hematopoietic stem cell donors for pediatric patients. Bone Marrow Transplant 2008;41(2):207–14.

25. La Nasa G, Giardini C, Argiolu F, et al. Unrelated donor bone marrow transplantation for thalassemia: the effect of extended haplotypes. Blood 2002;99(12): 4350–6.

26. La Nasa G, Caocci G, Argiolu F, et al. Unrelated donor stem cell transplantation in adult patients with thalassemia. Bone Marrow Transplant 2005;36(11):971–5.

27. Hongeng S, Pakakasama S, Chuansumrit A, et al. Outcomes of transplantation with related- and unrelated-donor stem cells in children with severe thalassemia. Biol Blood Marrow Transplant 2006;12(6):683–7.

28. Li C, Wu X, Feng X, et al. A novel conditioning regimen improves outcomes in beta-thalassemia major patients using unrelated donor peripheral blood stem cell transplantation. Blood 2012;120(19):3875–81.

29. Lucarelli G, Giardini C, Angelucci E. Bone marrow transplantation in thalassemia. In: Winter J, editor. Blood stem cell transplantation. Boston: Kluwer Academic; 1997. p. 305–15.

30. La Nasa G, Littera R, Locatelli F, et al. Status of donor-recipient HLA class I ligands and not the KIR genotype is predictive for the outcome of unrelated hematopoietic stem cell transplantation in beta-thalassemia patients. Biol Blood Marrow Transplant 2007;13(11):1358–68.

31. La Nasa G, Littera R, Locatelli F, et al. The human leucocyte antigen-G 14-basepair polymorphism correlates with graft-versus-host disease in unrelated bone marrow transplantation for thalassaemia. Br J Haematol 2007;139(2):284–8.

32. Littera R, Orru N, Vacca A, et al. The role of killer immunoglobulin-like receptor haplotypes on the outcome of unrelated donor haematopoietic SCT for thalassaemia. Bone Marrow Transplant 2010;45(11):1618–24.

33. Fleischhauer K, Locatelli F, Zecca M, et al. Graft rejection after unrelated donor hematopoietic stem cell transplantation for thalassemia is associated with nonpermissive HLA-DPB1 disparity in host-versus-graft direction. Blood 2006; 107(7):2984–92.
34. Strocchio L, Romano M, Cefalo MG, et al. Cord blood transplantation in children with hemoglobinopathies. Expert Opin Orphan Drugs 2015;3(10):1125–36.
35. Ruggeri A, Eapen M, Scaravadou A, et al. Umbilical cord blood transplantation for children with thalassemia and sickle cell disease. Biol Blood Marrow Transplant 2011;17(9):1375–82.
36. Jaing TH, Hung IJ, Yang CP, et al. Unrelated cord blood transplantation for thalassaemia: a single-institution experience of 35 patients. Bone Marrow Transplant 2012;47(1):33–9.
37. Gluckman E. Milestones in umbilical cord blood transplantation. Blood Rev 2011; 25(6):255–9.
38. Sideri A, Neokleous N, Brunet De La Grange P, et al. An overview of the progress on double umbilical cord blood transplantation. Haematologica 2011;96(8): 1213–20.
39. Kwon M, Bautista G, Balsalobre P, et al. Haplo-cord transplantation using CD34+ cells from a third-party donor to speed engraftment in high-risk patients with hematologic disorders. Biol Blood Marrow Transplant 2014;20(12):2015–22.
40. Kim DW, Chung YJ, Kim TG, et al. Cotransplantation of third-party mesenchymal stromal cells can alleviate single-donor predominance and increase engraftment from double cord transplantation. Blood 2004;103(5):1941–8.
41. Frassoni F, Gualandi F, Podesta M, et al. Direct intrabone transplant of unrelated cord-blood cells in acute leukaemia: a phase I/II study. Lancet Oncol 2008;9(9): 831–9.
42. Delaney C, Heimfeld S, Brashem-Stein C, et al. Notch-mediated expansion of human cord blood progenitor cells capable of rapid myeloid reconstitution. Nat Med 2010;16(2):232–6.
43. de Lima M, McNiece I, Robinson SN, et al. Cord-blood engraftment with ex vivo mesenchymal-cell coculture. N Engl J Med 2012;367(24):2305–15.
44. Horwitz ME, Chao NJ, Rizzieri DA, et al. Umbilical cord blood expansion with nicotinamide provides long-term multilineage engraftment. J Clin Invest 2014; 124(7):3121–8.
45. Stiff PJ, Montesinos P, Peled T, et al. StemEx (R)(Copper Chelation Based) ex vivo expanded umbilical cord blood stem cell transplantation (UCBT) accelerates engraftment and improves 100 day survival in myeloablated patients compared to a registry cohort undergoing double unit UCBT: results of a multicenter study of 101 patients with hematologic malignancies. Blood 2013;122(21):295.
46. Wagner JE, Brunstein C, McKenna D, et al. Acceleration of Umbilical Cord Blood (UCB) stem engraftment: results of a phase i clinical trial with Stemregenin-1 (SR1) expansion culture. Biol Blood Marrow Transplant 2015;21(2):S48–9.
47. Cutler C, Multani P, Robbins D, et al. Prostaglandin-modulated umbilical cord blood hematopoietic stem cell transplantation. Blood 2013;122(17):3074–81.
48. Robinson SN, Simmons PJ, Thomas MW, et al. Ex vivo fucosylation improves human cord blood engraftment in NOD-SCID IL-2R gamma(null) mice. Exp Hematol 2012;40(6):445–56.
49. Sodani P, Isgro A, Gaziev J, et al. Purified T-depleted, CD34+ peripheral blood and bone marrow cell transplantation from haploidentical mother to child with thalassemia. Blood 2010;115(6):1296–302.

50. Gaziev D, Galimberti M, Lucarelli G, et al. Bone marrow transplantation from alternative donors for thalassemia: HLA-phenotypically identical relative and HLA-nonidentical sibling or parent transplants. Bone Marrow Transplant 2000; 25(8):815–21.

51. Sodani P, Isgro A, Gaziev J, et al. T cell-depleted hLA-haploidentical stem cell transplantation in thalassemia young patients. Pediatr Rep 2011;3(Suppl 2):e13.

52. Bertaina A, Merli P, Rutella S, et al. HLA-haploidentical stem cell transplantation after removal of alphabeta+ T and B cells in children with nonmalignant disorders. Blood 2014;124(5):822–6.

53. Di Stasi A, Tey SK, Dotti G, et al. Inducible apoptosis as a safety switch for adoptive cell therapy. N Engl J Med 2011;365(18):1673–83.

54. Bertaina A, Merli P, Mahadeo K, et al. The use of BPX-501 donor T cell infusion (with inducible caspase 9 gene) together with HLA-haploidentical stem cell transplant to treat children with hemoglobinopathies and erythroid disorders. Haematologica 2017;102:130–1.

55. Anurathapan U, Hongeng S, Pakakasama S, et al. Hematopoietic stem cell transplantation for homozygous beta-thalassemia and beta-thalassemia/hemoglobin E patients from haploidentical donors. Bone Marrow Transplant 2016;51(6): 813–8.

56. Lucarelli G, Andreani M, Angelucci E. The cure of thalassemia with bone marrow transplantation. Blood Rev 2002;16(2):81–5.

Gene Therapy and Genome Editing

Farid Boulad, MD[a,b,]*, Jorge Mansilla-Soto, PhD[a], Annalisa Cabriolu, PhD[a],
Isabelle Rivière, PhD[a], Michel Sadelain, MD, PhD[a]

KEYWORDS

- Thalassemia • Gene transfer • Gene editing • Lentivirus • CRISPR/Cas9

KEY POINTS

- The β-thalassemias are inherited blood disorders that result from the insufficient production of the β-chain of hemoglobin. β-thalassemia major is characterized by transfusion-dependence.
- The only means to cure severe β-thalassemia is to provide patients with hematopoietic stem cells that harbor functional globin genes.
- Successful allogeneic hematopoietic stem cell transplantation is potentially curative, but this option is not available to most patients with thalassemia because a suitably matched donor cannot be found.
- Globin gene therapy offers the promise of a curative autologous stem cell transplantation without incurring the risks of the immunologic complications of allogeneic transplantation.
- Future directions of gene therapy include the enhancement of the lentiviral vector-based approaches, fine tuning of the conditioning regimen, and the design of safer vectors.

INTRODUCTION

Of course, a gene therapy cure is still some time away and when it comes will be expensive; in the meantime, I believe that the richer countries should do all they can through developing partnerships with the poorer countries to try to help them establish some kind of services for the control and management of thalassemia.
—Sir David Weatherall (Interview with the Cooley's Anemia Foundation December 3, 2009)

The β-thalassemias are among the most common inherited blood disorders worldwide. They are recessive genetic disorders that are caused by mutations in, or near, the β-globin gene. More than 200 mutations have been described that reduce or abolish the synthesis

No conflicts of interest for all authors.
a Center for Cell Engineering, Memorial Sloan Kettering Cancer Center, 1275 York Avenue, New York, NY 10065, USA; b Department of Pediatrics, Memorial Sloan Kettering Cancer Center, 1275 York Avenue, New York, NY 10065, USA
* Corresponding author. 1275 York Avenue, New York, NY 10065.
E-mail address: bouladf@mskcc.org

Hematol Oncol Clin N Am 32 (2018) 329–342
https://doi.org/10.1016/j.hoc.2017.11.007
0889-8588/18/© 2018 Elsevier Inc. All rights reserved.

hemonc.theclinics.com

of the β-globin chain of adult hemoglobin (HbA, $\alpha_2\beta_2$).[1] Homozygotes and compound heterozygotes may develop thalassemia intermedia or β-thalassemia major. Absent β-globin chains (β^0/β^0) or profound decrease in the synthesis of β-globin (β^0/β^E or β^0/β^+) trigger the precipitation of unpaired α-globin chains in erythroid cell precursors, resulting in intramedullary hemolysis, dyserythropoiesis with increased expansion of erythroid cell precursors but decreased production of mature red cells, and increased production of erythropoietin.[2]

The standard of care treatment modalities for β-thalassemia major consist of palliative care with transfusion of red blood cells and chelation of the iron overload, or curative treatment with allogeneic hematopoietic stem cell transplantation when an HLA-matched related donor is available.[3] Despite the considerable improvement in the life expectancy of transfusion-dependent individuals in the last decades,[4–6] the risk of serious complications arising over the long term from viral infections, iron toxicity, and liver cirrhosis remain.[7]

Hematopoietic stem cell transplantation has been performed in more than 1 thousand patients from matched related donors worldwide with very good results. At our center, we have performed allogeneic stem cell transplantation in 32 patients with β-thalassemia major from HLA-matched related donors, with an overall 95% survival and 91% disease-free survival (Boulad F, unpublished results, 2017). A number of trials of allogeneic hematopoietic stem cell transplantation from matched unrelated or mismatched related donors have occurred or are in progress.[8,9] However, there remains to date an increased risk for complications, including graft rejection, graft-versus-host disease, and mortality.[8–12]

For patients lacking a matched related donor, globin gene therapy offers the promise of a curative autologous stem cell transplantation without incurring the risks of graft-versus-host disease.[3]

RATIONALE FOR GLOBIN GENE TRANSFER TO CURE β-THALASSEMIA

Since the foundational report by May and colleagues[13] in 2000, which opened a path for therapeutic globin gene transfer by demonstrating erythroid-specific expression of the human β-globin gene at therapeutic levels in thalassemic bone marrow (BM) transplanted recipient mice, several studies have confirmed the efficacy of lentiviral-mediated globin gene transfer and extended these results to additional mouse models of β-thalassemia, paving the way for the clinical application of globin gene transfer.

The goal of globin gene transfer is to restore the capacity of the hematopoietic stem cells of the patient with thalassemia to generate red blood cells with a normal hemoglobin content[14,15]

Only transduced HSCs can provide long-term clinical benefits through productive erythropoiesis based on a normalized α/β globin chain synthesis ratio. The goal of curative therapy for thalassemia is to achieve transfusion independence without exposing patients to the risks of HSCT from a suboptimally matched donor. For patients who lack an HLA-matched donor and thus have a higher risk of mortality after allogeneic HSCT, globin gene transfer in autologous stem cells offers the prospect of a curative stem cell-based therapy.[3]

GLOBIN GENE TRANSFER
How It All Started: The First 10 Years (–2000): Preclinical Proof-of-Principle and Safety Studies

The human β-globin gene (*HBB*), which spans less than 5 Kb on the short arm of chromosome 11, contains 3 exons and 2 introns, one of which at least is required for high-level globin expression. A major regulatory region containing powerful erythroid enhancers maps 50 Kb upstream off *HBB*. This region, termed the locus control region, contains 4 erythroid specific DNAse hypersensitive sites (HS1 to HS4), that all contribute to HBB regulation.[16] These hypersensitive sites comprise multiple DNA motifs interacting with transcription factors and assemble into a chromatin hub.[17]

The implementation of globin gene transfer for the treatment of severe β-thalassemia requires the efficient introduction of a regulated human β- (or β-like) globin gene in HSCs. The β-globin gene must be expressed in erythroid-specific fashion and at high level, especially for the treatment of transfusion-dependent $β^0$-thalassemias. After an exhaustive and systematic testing of numerous lentiviral vector designs that took approximately 10 years of experiments, we at Memorial Sloan Kettering identified in the late 1990s several combinations of genomic sequences that could be stably transferred at high efficiency in murine HSCs and express in their erythroid progeny the human β-globin gene at therapeutic levels.[13]

The TNS9 vector (**Fig. 1**) encodes more than 5 kb of genetic material, most of which are regulatory sequences intended to direct the high-level, erythroid-specific expression of the therapeutic globin transgene. Globin vectors, thus, differ from the more common lentiviral vectors, including those designed for the treatment of inherited immunodeficiencies or metabolic disorders, which typically encode a simple constitutive enhancer promoter driving expression of a cDNA.[18]

This study conducted by May and colleagues[13] in a murine model of β-thalassemia opened up a field that, for well over a decade, had eluded all international groups despite best efforts. The vector termed TNS9 encodes a particularly potent combination of promoter, intron, enhancer, and locus control region elements, sufficient to effectively correct the thalassemia syndrome in mice with β-thalassemia. In this and subsequent studies,[13,19,20] we demonstrated that mice with thalassemia and engrafted with TNS9-transduced BM cells corrected their anemia, extramedullary hematopoiesis, and iron accumulation in peripheral tissues and organs.[19] In a lethal model of $β^0$-thalassemia major, wherein mice succumb within 60 days of birth to

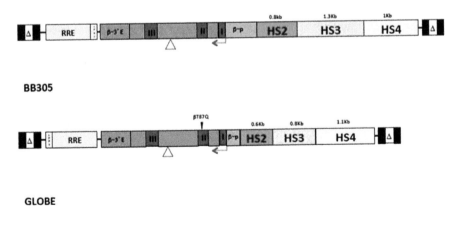

Fig. 1. Structure of integrated SIN LV.

severe anemia, massive splenomegaly, extramedullary hematopoiesis, and hepatic iron overload, we showed rescue and long-term survival after TNS9 transfer in fetal liver HSCs.[20] In large cohorts of mice, we did not observe evidence of vector silencing over time, neither in primary, secondary, or even tertiary chimeras, indicating that the TNS9 vector functioned continuously for 26 months (study duration).

Several groups subsequently generated variants of the TNS9 vector and also reported curative responses in similarly treated mice presenting with β-thalassemia or sickle/β-thalassemia (reviewed in[3,14,15,21]). These vectors differed slightly in the length of the promoter and hypersensitive site elements, but none expressed more β-globin chain than TNS9.

Multiple studies in different animal models established that correction of anemia and secondary organ damage owing to iron accumulation was feasible using lentiviral vectors encoding a regulated human β- or β-like globin gene (β-like chains include the γ−chain and mutant β-chains) and strongly supported the merit of transferring a human globin gene in autologous HSCs as a rational alternative to high-risk, nonmatched related donor transplantation in patients with severe β-thalassemia.

The first vector to be tested in patients was a βA-T87Q globin vector, developed by Philippe Leboulch[22] and later acquired by Blue Bird Bio (BBB), which was used in a clinical trial at Necker Hospital in France (Trial LG001). Soonafter, TNS9 was the first globin vector to be evaluated in the United States.

The Following 10 Years

The Memorial Sloan Kettering Cancer Center (MSKCC) group submitted a clinical gene therapy protocol proposal to the Recombinant DNA Advisory Committee in the United States in 2007 (protocol# 0704-852). The initial protocol included the use of peripheral blood stem cells to be collected after granulocyte colony stimulating factor (G-CSF) mobilization. The plan was to obtain approximately 6 to 8 × 10⁶ CD34 hematopoietic progenitor cells (HPCs) and 2 × 10⁶ CD34$^+$ HPCs for backup. The HPCs would be transduced and cryopreserved. Patients would then receive a reduced intensity conditioning regimen followed by the infusion of the CD34$^+$TNS9.3$^+$ cells.

Before proceeding to clinical studies, we decided to first assess the safety and feasibility of harvesting HPCs from patients with thalassemia and further use these CD34$^+$ cells from patients with thalassemia to optimize globin gene transfer under current Good Manufacturing Practice conditions. We conducted a pilot trial to investigate the safety and effectiveness of mobilizing CD34$^+$ HSCs in adults with β-thalassemia major.[23]

A secondary objective of this clinical study was to assess whether these CD34$^+$ HPCs could be transduced under current Good Manufacturing Practice conditions at levels sufficient for proceeding to a therapeutic clinical trial, using the TNS9.3.55 lentiviral vector. All 5 patients enrolled tolerated G-CSF well with minimal side effects, confirming prior mobilization studies in pediatric[24] and adult[25] patients with thalassemia. All CD34$^+$ cell collections achieved the minimum targeted dose of 8 × 10⁶ CD34$^+$ cells/kg after leukapheresis on days 5 and 6. Using clinical grade TNS9.3.55 vector stock, we demonstrated gene transfer in the range of 1 vector copy per cell in small-scale patient CD34$^+$ cell transduction studies. Transduction efficiency was, however, less in scaled-up validation runs performed under current Good Manufacturing Practice conditions, in the range of 0.2 to 0.6. The transduced CD34$^+$ cells maintained their potential to engraft NOD/scid-γ$_c$^{null} mice, maintaining a stable vector copy number 6 months after transplantation.[23] This validated procedure for stem cell collection and globin gene transduction was approved by the US Food and Drug Administration and implemented in the first US trial to evaluate globin gene transfer in patients with severe inherited globin disorders (NCT01639690 at clinicaltrials.gov).

In 2010, the group of Cavazzana-Calvo and Leboulch in Paris published the first result of the lentiviral β-globin gene transfer in an 18-year-old male patient with transfusion-dependent β^E/β^0-thalassemia (NCT01745120).[26] This group used a myeloablative conditioning regimen followed by BM–derived HPCs transduced with a βA-T87Q vector named HPV569. The patient was 33 months after lentiviral β-globin gene transfer at the time of writing, and had become transfusion independent for 21 months. Blood hemoglobin was maintained between 9 and 10 g dL^{-1}, of which one-third contains vector-encoded β-globin. Of note, most of the therapeutic benefit resulted from a dominant, myeloid-biased cell clone, in which the integrated vector caused transcriptional activation of HMGA2 in erythroid cells, with further increased expression of a truncated HMGA2 mRNA insensitive to degradation by let-7 microRNAs. The clonal dominance that accompanied therapeutic efficacy resulted from a benign cell expansion caused by dysregulation of the HMGA2 gene in stem and progenitor cells.[27]

This initial trial was sponsored by Genetix Pharmaceuticals (Cambridge, MA). This company renamed Blue Bird Bio (BBB; Cambridge, MA) subsequently bought the β87 vector, now termed BB305 (see **Fig. 1**). BBB removed the double copy cHS4 core insulator of the βA-T87Q vector, which had been found to rearrange upon integration,[27] as is typically the case for repeat sequences of this size in retroviral vectors.[28]

The TNS9 trial and Northstar BBB trial are overall similar in design, except for one fundamental difference in the conditioning regimen. The TNS9 trial, conducted between MSKCC, Ospedale Cervello in Palermo, and the Microcitemico in Cagliari used a reduced intensity conditioning (8–10 mg/kg busulfan), whereas the Northstar trial used upfront myeloablative conditioning consisting of 12.8 mg/kg of busulfan. The purpose of the reduced intensity conditioning chosen by our center was for 2 reasons: It was primarily for ethical concerns, that is, to avoid excessive and possibly life-threatening toxicity in a first trial in human, in patients who do not have an immediately life-threatening disease, and to allow for autologous reconstitution should the transduced stem cells fail to engraft. In addition, at the time of the "first" trials for hemoglobinopathies, the depth and degree of myelosuppression required for the engraftment of genetically engineered HPCs were not clear.

A third trial opened more recently using the globin vector termed Globe[29] (see **Fig. 1**). This vector is also similar to TNS9, but for the removal of the HS4 locus control region element. We previously found that globin vectors lacking this element produce significantly less β-globin,[30] but this deficiency may be compensated for by a higher titer, enabling the transduction of a higher vector copy number in patient CD34$^+$ cells.[30,31] Other differences in this protocol included the inclusion of younger patients, the use of Plerixafor plus G-CSF for HPC mobilization, and the administration route of the transduced CD34$^+$ cells, intraosseously (under light general anesthesia).

The present state of affairs: Gene therapy trials

The past and present gene therapy trials are summarized in **Table 1**. The trials include the following.

- The first trial was started in France in 2006 by the Cavazzana-Calvo and Leboulch group and sponsored by Genetix Pharmaceuticals (later acquired by BBB). This trial used a myeloablative regimen including high-dose busulfan at 12.8 mg/kg, BM–derived stem cells, and transduction with the HPV569 vector. Three patients were treated. Two patients required the reinfusion of backup stem cells, presumably because of graft failure. One patient with the β^0/β^E genotype as mentioned

Table 1
Lentiviral beta thalassemia trials

Sponsor	City	Trial	Dates	Vector	Gene	Phase	Patient Age	Conditioning	HPCs	N
Genetix (BlueBird Bio)	Paris	LG001	2006–2011	HPV569	β-A T87Q globin	I/II	NA	BU 12.8 mg/kg	BM	10 patients (3 treated)
MSKCC	New York	MSKCC 10-164 NCT01639690	2011–2014	TNS0.3.55	β-globin	I/II	>18 y	BU 8 mg/kg BU 14 mg/kg	G-CSF mobilized PBSC	10 patients (4 treated)
Bluebird Bio	Los Angeles Oakland Chicago Philadelphia Sydney Bangkok	NORTHSTAR HGB-204 NCT01745120	2013–2018	BB305	β-A T87Q globin	I/II	12–17 y	BU 12.8 mg/kg	G-CSF mobilized PBSC	18 patients (18 treated)
Bluebird Bio	Paris	HGB-205 NCT02151526	2013–2019	BB305	β-A T87Q globin	I/II	5–35 y	BU 12.8 mg/kg	BM or PBSC	7 patients (4 treated)
Telethon	Milan	TIGET-BTHAL NCT02453477	2015–2019	GLOBE	β-globin	I/II	18 y n = 3 / 8–17 y n = 3 / 3–7 y N = 4	TREO 42 mg/m^2 + THIO 8 mg/kg	G-CSF Plerixafor mobilized PBSC	10 patients (7 treated)
Bluebird Bio	Oakland Chicago Philadelphia Marseille Hannover London Rome Thessaloniki Bangkok	NORTHSTAR2 HGB-207 NCT02906202	2016–2020	BB305	β-A T87Q globin	III	12–50 y	BU 12.8 mg/kg	PBSC	15 patients (excluding β0/β0 genotype)
Bluebird Bio	Chicago	NCT03207009	2017–2021	BB305	β-A T87Q globin	III	12–50 y	BU 12.8 mg/kg	PBSC	15 patients only β0/β0 Genotype

Abbreviations: BM, bone marrow; BU, busulfan; G-CSF, granulocyte colony stimulating factor; PBSC, peripheral blood stem cells; TREO, treosulfan; THIO, thiotepa.

engrafted with evidence of transfusion independence. However, this outcome was associated with the HMGA2 clone dominance. The patient is now 10 years post transplant. The benign clonal dominance persisted for almost 9 years; it has started to decrease and now currently contributes to less than 10% of the circulating nucleated cells. The patient now has lower levels of therapeutic hemoglobin and requires occasional transfusions.

- The MSKCC trial was the first gene therapy trial approved in the United States in 2010. It was also the first academic-only trial for gene therapy for thalassemia, conducted in collaboration with Dr Aurelio Maggio in Palermo and Drs Galanello and Moi in Cagliari. This phase I and II trial at MSKCC included the treatment of 4 adult patients to date. Three patients had β^0/β^+-thalassemia and 1 patient had β^0/β^0-thalassemia. The first 3 patients received busulfan at a dose of 8 mg/kg, and the fourth patient received busulfan at a dose of 14 mg/kg. The patients received 8.3 to 12.0 CD34$^+$ TNS9.3.55 cells/kg. The transduction in the final CD34$^+$ cell product had a vector copy number (VCN) of 0.25 on average. There was no toxicity greater than grade 3. All patients showed durable and stable gene marking. There was no evidence of clonal dominance. One subject experienced a significant decrease in transfusion requirements lasting 5 years and still ongoing.

- BBB sponsored 4 trials thereafter, and completed 2 trials. They all use the BB305 vector. Transducer enhancers have been mentioned for the 2 most recent trials.
  - The NorthStar–HGB 204 trial included the treatment of patients 12 to 35 years of age in Los Angeles, Oakland, Chicago, Philadelphia, Sydney, and Bangkok. Eighteen patients with transfusion-dependent thalassemia were treated to date; they had β^0/β^0 (n = 8), β^0/β^E (n = 6), β^+/β^+ (n = 2), β^0/β^+ (n = 1), and β^0/β^x genotypes. They were 12 to 35 years of age (median, 20). They received myeloablative busulfan at 12.8 mg/kg followed by 5.2 to 18.1 CD34$^+$ BB305$^+$ cells/kg. The transduction VCN was 0.7 copies (range, 0.3–1.5). As of the December 2016 American Society of Hematology meeting, with at least 6 months of follow-up, the following results were published: There was no toxicity of grade 3 or higher. The median posttransplant VCN in peripheral blood was 0.4 (range, 0.2–1.0) for 13 patients. Five patients with the non-β^0/β^0 genotypes were transfusion independent, whereas 5 patients with the β^0/β^0 genotype remained transfusion dependent. There was no evidence of clonal dominance.
  - The HGB 205 trial was open in Paris for patients with thalassemia and sickle cell disease. Five patients were treated, including 4 patients with thalassemia. Partial results by Negre and colleagues[26] stated that all 4 patients with thalassemia were transfusion independent.
  - The HGB 206 and HGB 207 trials are the most recently opened trials. They are phase III trials using the BB305 vector for non-β^0/β^0 and β^0/β^0 genotypes, respectively. The use of transducer enhancers have been mentioned for these 2 most recent trials.

- The Gene Therapy for Transfusion Dependent Beta-thalassemia (TIGET-BTHAL) is a trial sponsored by Telethon Institute of Genetics and Medicine (TIGEM). The Telethon Foundation is a leading Italian charitable organization investing in the research of rare genetic diseases and includes the TIGEM. This trial is led by Dr Giuliana Ferrari and uses the GLOBE vector. This trial uses plerixafor plus G-CSF mobilized peripheral blood stem cells. It also uses a myeloablative conditioning regimen including treosulfan and thiotepa. It has 3 patient groups: 3 adult patients aged greater than 18 years, 3 adolescent patients aged 8 to 17 years, and 4 patients aged 3 to 7 years. Patients included in this trial have the β^0/β^0, the β^0/β^+, or β^+/β^+ genotypes. The other elegant aspect of the study includes the intraosseous infusion of the transduced cells into the iliac crests to improve homing and engraftment, bypassing the splanchnic system and preventing the engineered HPCs to be trapped in the liver and spleen. As of June 2017, 7 patients have received 16.3 to 19.5 $\times$ 10^6 CD34$^+$GLOBE$^+$ cells with a prior VCN of 0.7 to 1.5 copies. The procedure was well-tolerated, with no product-related adverse events. There was evidence of multilineage engraftment in all patients, without any clonal expansion. The clinical outcome indicates so far a significant decrease in transfusion requirements, an improved quality of life in adult patients, and greater clinical benefit in younger patients (G. Ferrari, unpublished results, 2017).

Essential features of globin gene therapy trials
The summary of these trials, which are ongoing, provides several important insights into some features of the host, the conditioning, and the transduction (**Fig. 2**).

The host Host selection plays an important role in the success of gene therapy for thalassemia. As seen in the results presented, patients with the severe β^0/β^0 genotype did not do as well as patients with the milder β^0/β^+, β^+/β^+, or β^0/β^E genotypes. This finding shows that the investigators will need better transduction to make a therapeutic impact in the former group.

The impact of age is not clear from these preliminary results of the trials, as has been suggested in some trials for immunodeficiency disorders. However, it remains possible that CD34$^+$ cell collection, transduction, and engraftment may be superior in younger patients.

Last, from our MSKCC trial, the patient with the best gene marking and the better hematologic response was the one patient who was previously splenectomized. It is not clear whether this played a role in the success of gene transfer. If it is true that the reinfused genetically engineered cells may undergo some degree of entrapment

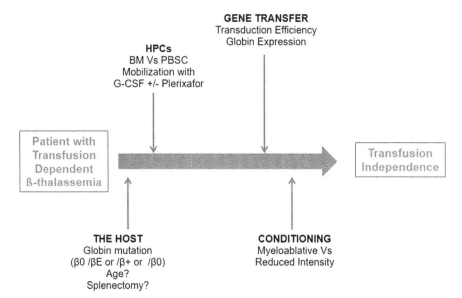

Fig. 2. Factors influencing gene therapy outcome in patients with β-thalassemias. BM, bone marrow; HPC, hematopoietic progenitor cells; PBSC, peripheral blood stem cells.

in the liver and spleen, the selection of splenectomized patients may yield better results. CD34$^+$ cell infusion into the marrow cavity may alleviate this effect, although HSCs still need to circulate to the vascular system to reach other hematopoietic sites.

The hematopoietic progenitor cells Current HPC collection sites include nonmobilized BM HPCs as used in the first Paris trial, G-CSF mobilized peripheral blood HPCs as used in the New York trial and the BBB trials, or the plerixafor plus G-CSF mobilized peripheral blood HPCs as used in the Milano trial. The overall results have suggested that "more is better," giving the advantage to the peripheral blood HPCs versus the marrow HPCs, which have become the standard of care for gene transfer in patients with thalassemia. A question is whether the addition of plerixafor to G-CSF select not necessarily "more" but maybe also "better" stem cells with superior biological characteristics, homing capacity, and repopulation potential and would lead to better results. This finding will need to be studied in later trials that should include not only overall results but also costs of a procedure that are already high.

Another eventual potential source of HPCs is umbilical cord blood. Once current trials have provided more clarity on the safety and efficacy of globin gene transfer, a next step would be to cryopreserve the umbilical cord blood of patients affected with thalassemia and use these, once the patient is at an age where transplantation and the use of chemotherapy for cytoreduction is safer, for transduction with or without stem cell expansion.

The cytoreduction As stated, the MSKCC trial started with the use of reduced intensity conditioning for the ethical reasons stated before. However, the transduction efficiency as seen in the pre-transplant VCN studies and the post transplant peripheral blood VCN studies was insufficient to achieve complete transfusion independence. This outcome does not necessarily prove the inadequacy of the reduced intensity conditioning. One may argue that as the transduction efficiency improves, one could reassess the de-escalation of the intensity of the conditioning regimen. In addition, it is possible that the use of a "pre-conditioning" regimen as pioneered by the Gaziev and Lucarelli group for allogeneic transplantation may also improve outcomes by further decreasing BM cellularity and ineffective erythropoiesis.

The transduction efficiency The therapeutic level of transduction of HPCs and transgene expression in erythroid progenitors are critical factors in the effectiveness of globin gene therapy for patients with thalassemia. In aggregate, the results of the Memorial Sloan Kettering, BBB, and Milano trials show that a higher VCN pretransplantation with a VCN of 0.5 to 1.0 copy per cell were associated with good outcomes in patients with the milder β-thalassemia genotypes. However, the transduction level required to achieve a durable therapeutic benefit depends on the level of expression afforded by the vector. Thus, vectors expressing lower levels of expression per vector copy will require higher transduction levels, which in turn may pose greater genotoxic risks.

The risks of globin gene therapy

The major risks of globin gene therapy include the risk of transplant-related morbidity associated with autologous transplantation, and the risks associated with lentiviral-mediated globin gene transfer with insertional oncogenesis and the generation of a replication-competent lentivirus.

Some level of recipient conditioning is required to facilitate hematopoietic engraftment of genetically modified HSCs. Busulfan used at 4 mg/kg has been sufficient to enhance engraftment of autologous CD34$^+$ cells in patients with ADA deficiency.[32]

This dose, however, may not be sufficient in disorders other than immune deficiencies, in which corrected lymphocytes acquire a substantial proliferative advantage. The dose of 8 mg was well-tolerated in 2 patients with chronic granulomatous disease treated with genetically modified, autologous CD34[+] cells,[33] as well as in patients with thalassemia treated with reduced intensity conditioning.[34,35]

These data supported the use of 8 mg/kg busulfan, the dosage we used in our initial phase I/II clinical trial. As stated, once the efficiency of transduction is maximized and able to produce sufficient engraftment of genetically engineered HPCs in patients with the severe genotype of β-thalassemia, we should consider deescalating the intensity of the conditioning regimen, especially in older patients, with or without the addition of a preconditioning agent such as hydroxyurea.

The risk of leukemia owing to insertional oncogenesis is difficult to estimate, but it is widely thought to be considerably less than that associated with the use of long terminal repeat-driven γ-retroviral vectors, which were used in patients with severe combined immune deficiency and chronic granulomatous disease. Insertional oncogenesis has been observed initially in 3 of these 22 patients in a single trial.[36] This number has increased since that report, including the recent EBMT presentation of the onset of leukemia in an SCID patient 15 years after gene therapy. The potential risk of transformation in thalassemic patients treated with an erythroid-specific lentiviral vector such as TNS9 should be less by virtue of the restricted expression of the globin vector,[20,37] the innocuous properties of the β-chain of hemoglobin, and the more favorable integration site distribution of lentiviral vectors compared with γ-retroviral vectors.[38] Nonetheless, a case of major clonal expansion has occurred in a patient treated with the β87 vector.[27]

The probability of replication-competent lentivirus generation is unknown, but there is no reason to expect it to be greater than for γ-retroviral vectors, because the vector and cell manufacturing processes are closely related. Importantly, no replication-competent retrovirus has been reported to date in trials using γ-retroviral or lentiviral-mediated gene transfer.

GENE EDITING

New genetic technologies are emerging in the laboratory. Thus, an expanding set of genome editing tools is creating novel prospects for impacting directly on disease mutations and targeting genes or regulatory sequences.[39] Several approaches have been used to restore hemoglobin production in preclinical models.[40] Of these, the reversal of the globin switching, which consists in the silencing of mutated β-globin gene with concurrent expression of the γ−globin gene, is a promising approach because it can be potentially applied to all β-thalassemia mutations. The discovery of Bcl11a as a central regulator of the γ-globin silencing, as well as its erythroid-specific intronic enhancer, provides compelling argument to knock out its erythroid expression to reverse globin switching.[41] Using gene editing technologies, 2 independent groups have determined that an intron 2 region, located 58 kilobases (+58) downstream from the transcription start site of the human Bcl11a gene, plays a major role in controlling Bcl11a expression.[42,43] Zinc-finger nucleases designed to target 5 DNAse I hypersensitive sites located in the +58 region were used to induce mutations at these sites in human CD34[+] cells. Mutations induced by a zinc-finger nuclease targeting a GATA1 motif resulted in marked increase of the γ-globin transcripts, which was associated with a decrease of the Bcl11a transcript levels in the CD34[+] HSC-derived erythroid cells.[43] In the other study, Canver and colleagues[42] used in situ saturating

CRISPR/Cas9-based mutagenesis of the Bcl11a enhancer region in human erythroblasts. After selecting for high HbF-expressing cells, guide RNA sequences targeting mainly the +58 region were enriched in these cells. The top guide RNA sequences targeted either the predicted GATA1 motif or a region containing predicted motifs for RXRA, EHF, ELF1, and STAT1. Further support for the role of the GATAA motif in regulating Bcl11a gene expression and β- to γ–globin switching came from studies using zinc-finger nuclease–edited healthy BM CD34[+] cells. Clonal erythroid cells obtained from edited BM CD34[+] cells showed increased expression of fetal globin. In addition, edited BM CD34[+] cells bearing targeted gene deletions showed stable engraftment over 16 weeks in NSG mice, and genotyping of BFU-E colonies derived from BM cells at this time point showed significant editing of the GATAA motif (26% KO/KO and 14% WT/KO).[44] Although promising, the introduction of genome-editing approaches in the clinic requires better definition of the genotoxicity (off-target activity) of the targeted nucleases. The clinical applicability of targeted gene delivery approaches is currently limited by the difficulty to efficiently target genomic DNA in true HSCs.[45–47]

SUMMARY AND PERSPECTIVES

Lentiviral vector transduction of human CD34[+] cells is by now a mature technology that has resulted in curative responses in some patients with severe combined immune deficiency or metabolic disorders.[48] Although the follow-up time is still limited (<5 years in a majority of patients), this approach, using relatively weak enhancers and promoters in comparison with globin vectors,[28] has so far proven to be safe. The case of patient 1003 treated in the Necker trial invites continued caution and circumspection with current globin vectors.

One approach to increase the safety of semi-randomly integrating vectors is the incorporation of insulators into the vector.[49,50] Another is to pursue alternative approaches that do not rely on semi-random vector integration, but on targeted gene editing. An expanding set of available genome editing tools will create novel prospects for impacting directly on disease mutations and targeting genes or regulatory sequences.[39] Several experimental approaches have already been reported to restore hemoglobin production in preclinical models,[40] but their introduction in the clinic requires better definition of the off-target activity of these targeted nucleases. The clinical applicability of these exciting technologies is further limited by the present difficulty to efficiently target genomic DNA in true HSCs.[42–47]

Globin lentiviral vectors are thus at present the most advanced approach for treating globin disorders. Encouraging preliminary results point to their efficacy in at least some patients. Their safety still remains to be ascertained. What is certain is that the prospects for finding a genetic cure for the severe thalassemias, whether using lentiviral vectors or gene editing, have greatly improved and continue to make progress.

REFERENCES

1. Giardine B, Borg J, Viennas E, et al. Updates of the HbVar database of human hemoglobin variants and thalassemia mutations. Nucleic Acids Res 2014; 42(Database issue):D1063–9.
2. Galanello R, Origa R. Beta-thalassemia. Orphanet J Rare Dis 2010;5:11.
3. Sadelain M, Boulad F, Galanello R, et al. Therapeutic options for patients with severe beta-thalassemia: the need for globin gene therapy. Hum Gene Ther 2007; 18(1):1–9.

4. Borgna-Pignatti C, Rugolotto S, De Stefano P, et al. Survival and complications in patients with thalassemia major treated with transfusion and deferoxamine. Haematologica 2004;89(10):1187–93.

5. Telfer PT, Warburton F, Christou S, et al. Improved survival in thalassemia major patients on switching from desferrioxamine to combined chelation therapy with desferrioxamine and deferiprone. Haematologica 2009;94(12):1777–8.

6. Ladis V, Chouliaras G, Berdoukas V, et al. Survival in a large cohort of Greek patients with transfusion-dependent beta thalassaemia and mortality ratios compared to the general population. Eur J Haematol 2011;86(4):332–8.

7. Mancuso A, Sciarrino E, Renda MC, et al. A prospective study of hepatocellular carcinoma incidence in thalassemia. Hemoglobin 2006;30(1):119–24.

8. Lucarelli G, Andreani M, Angelucci E. The cure of thalassemia by bone marrow transplantation. Blood Rev 2002;16(2):81–5.

9. Thomas ED, Buckner CD, Sanders JE, et al. Marrow transplantation for thalassaemia. Lancet 1982;2(8292):227–9.

10. La Nasa G, Giardini C, Argiolu F, et al. Unrelated donor bone marrow transplantation for thalassemia: the effect of extended haplotypes. Blood 2002;99(12):4350–6.

11. La Nasa G, Argiolu F, Giardini C, et al. Unrelated bone marrow transplantation for beta-thalassemia patients: the experience of the Italian Bone Marrow Transplant Group. Ann N Y Acad Sci 2005;1054:186–95.

12. Gaziev D, Galimberti M, Lucarelli G, et al. Bone marrow transplantation from alternative donors for thalassemia: HLA-phenotypically identical relative and HLA-nonidentical sibling or parent transplants. Bone Marrow Transplant 2000;25(8):815–21.

13. May C, Rivella S, Callegari J, et al. Therapeutic haemoglobin synthesis in beta-thalassaemic mice expressing lentivirus-encoded human beta-globin. Nature 2000;406(6791):82–6.

14. Persons DA, Tisdale JF. Gene therapy for the hemoglobin disorders. Semin Hematol 2004;41(4):279–86.

15. Sadelain M. Recent advances in globin gene transfer for the treatment of beta-thalassemia and sickle cell anemia. Curr Opin Hematol 2006;13(3):142–8.

16. Li Q, Peterson KR, Fang X, et al. Locus control regions. Blood 2002;100(9):3077–86.

17. Patrinos GP, de Krom M, de Boer E, et al. Multiple interactions between regulatory regions are required to stabilize an active chromatin hub. Genes Dev 2004;18(12):1495–509.

18. Chang AH, Sadelain M. The genetic engineering of hematopoietic stem cells: the rise of lentiviral vectors, the conundrum of the ltr, and the promise of lineage-restricted vectors. Mol Ther 2007;15(3):445–56.

19. May C, Rivella S, Chadburn A, et al. Successful treatment of murine beta-thalassemia intermedia by transfer of the human beta-globin gene. Blood 2002;99(6):1902–8.

20. Rivella S, May C, Chadburn A, et al. A novel murine model of Cooley anemia and its rescue by lentiviral-mediated human beta-globin gene transfer. Blood 2003;101(8):2932–9.

21. Sadelain M, Boulad F, Lisowki L, et al. Stem cell engineering for the treatment of severe hemoglobinopathies. Curr Mol Med 2008;8(7):690–7.

22. Bank A, Dorazio R, Leboulch P. A phase I/II clinical trial of beta-globin gene therapy for beta-thalassemia. Ann N Y Acad Sci 2005;1054:308–16.

23. Boulad F, Wang X, Qu J, et al. Safe mobilization of CD34+ cells in adults with beta-thalassemia and validation of effective globin gene transfer for clinical investigation. Blood 2014;123(10):1483–6.
24. Li K, Wong A, Li CK, et al. Granulocyte colony-stimulating factor-mobilized peripheral blood stem cells in beta-thalassemia patients: kinetics of mobilization and composition of apheresis product. Exp Hematol 1999;27(3):526–32.
25. Yannaki E, Papayannopoulou T, Jonlin E, et al. Hematopoietic stem cell mobilization for gene therapy of adult patients with severe beta-thalassemia: results of clinical trials using G-CSF or plerixafor in splenectomized and nonsplenectomized subjects. Mol Ther 2012;20(1):230–8.
26. Negre O, Eggimann AV, Beuzard Y, et al. Gene therapy of the beta-hemoglobinopathies by lentiviral transfer of the beta(A(T87Q))-globin gene. Hum Gene Ther 2016;27(2):148–65.
27. Cavazzana-Calvo M, Payen E, Negre O, et al. Transfusion independence and HMGA2 activation after gene therapy of human beta-thalassaemia. Nature 2010;467(7313):318–22.
28. Rhode BW, Emerman M, Temin HM. Instability of large direct repeats in retrovirus vectors. J Virol 1987;61(3):925–7.
29. Miccio A, Cesari R, Lotti F, et al. In vivo selection of genetically modified erythroblastic progenitors leads to long-term correction of beta-thalassemia. Proc Natl Acad Sci U S A 2008;105(30):10547–52.
30. Lisowski L, Sadelain M. Locus control region elements HS1 and HS4 enhance the therapeutic efficacy of globin gene transfer in beta-thalassemic mice. Blood 2007;110(13):4175–8.
31. Roselli EA, Mezzadra R, Frittoli MC, et al. Correction of beta-thalassemia major by gene transfer in haematopoietic progenitors of pediatric patients. EMBO Mol Med 2010;2(8):315–28.
32. Aiuti A, Slavin S, Aker M, et al. Correction of ADA-SCID by stem cell gene therapy combined with nonmyeloablative conditioning. Science 2002;296(5577):2410–3.
33. Ott MG, Schmidt M, Schwarzwaelder K, et al. Correction of X-linked chronic granulomatous disease by gene therapy, augmented by insertional activation of MDS1-EVI1, PRDM16 or SETBP1. Nat Med 2006;12(4):401–9.
34. Slavin S, Nagler A, Naparstek E, et al. Nonmyeloablative stem cell transplantation and cell therapy as an alternative to conventional bone marrow transplantation with lethal cytoreduction for the treatment of malignant and nonmalignant hematologic diseases. Blood 1998;91(3):756–63.
35. Iannone R, Casella JF, Fuchs EJ, et al. Results of minimally toxic nonmyeloablative transplantation in patients with sickle cell anemia and beta-thalassemia. Biol Blood Marrow Transplant 2003;9(8):519–28.
36. Fischer A, Hacein-Bey-Abina S, Lagresle C, et al. Gene therapy of severe combined immunodeficiency disease: proof of principle of efficiency and safety issues. Gene therapy, primary immunodeficiencies, retrovirus, lentivirus, genome. Bull Acad Natl Med 2005;189(5):779–85 [discussion: 786–8]. [in French].
37. Baum C, Dullmann J, Li Z, et al. Side effects of retroviral gene transfer into hematopoietic stem cells. Blood 2003;101(6):2099–114.
38. Dunbar CE. Stem cell gene transfer: insights into integration and hematopoiesis from primate genetic marking studies. Ann N Y Acad Sci 2005;1044:178–82.
39. Maeder ML, Gersbach CA. Genome-editing technologies for gene and cell therapy. Mol Ther 2016;24(3):430–46.
40. Mansilla-Soto J, Riviere I, Boulad F, et al. Cell and gene therapy for the beta-thalassemias: advances and prospects. Hum Gene Ther 2016;27(4):295–304.

41. Sankaran VG, Orkin SH. The switch from fetal to adult hemoglobin. Cold Spring Harb Perspect Med 2013;3(1):a011643.
42. Canver MC, Smith EC, Sher F, et al. BCL11A enhancer dissection by Cas9-mediated in situ saturating mutagenesis. Nature 2015;527(7577):192–7.
43. Vierstra J, Reik A, Chang KH, et al. Functional footprinting of regulatory DNA. Nat Methods 2015;12(10):927–30.
44. Chang KH, Smith SE, Sullivan T, et al. Long-term engraftment and fetal globin induction upon BCL11A gene editing in bone-marrow-derived CD34+ hematopoietic stem and progenitor cells. Mol Ther Methods Clin Dev 2017;4:137–48.
45. Dever DP, Bak RO, Reinisch A, et al. CRISPR/Cas9 beta-globin gene targeting in human haematopoietic stem cells. Nature 2016;539(7629):384–9.
46. Genovese P, Schiroli G, Escobar G, et al. Targeted genome editing in human re-populating haematopoietic stem cells. Nature 2014;510(7504):235–40.
47. Wang J, Exline CM, DeClercq JJ, et al. Homology-driven genome editing in he-matopoietic stem and progenitor cells using ZFN mRNA and AAV6 donors. Nat Biotechnol 2015;33(12):1256–63.
48. Naldini L, Trono D, Verma IM. Lentiviral vectors, two decades later. Science 2016; 353(6304):1101–2.
49. Rivella S, Callegari JA, May C, et al. The cHS4 insulator increases the probability of retroviral expression at random chromosomal integration sites. J Virol 2000; 74(10):4679–87.
50. Emery DW, Yannaki E, Tubb J, et al. A chromatin insulator protects retrovirus vec-tors from chromosomal position effects. Proc Natl Acad Sci U S A 2000;97(16): 9150–5.

Emerging Therapies

Amaliris Guerra, PhD[a], Khaled M. Musallam, MD, PhD[b],
Ali T. Taher, MD, PhD, FRCP[c], Stefano Rivella, PhD[a,d],*

KEYWORDS

- β-Thalassemia • β-Globin • Gene transfer • Hemichromes • New therapies
- Trap ligands

KEY POINTS

- At present, the only definitive cure for β-thalassemia is a bone marrow transplant (BMT); however, HLA–blood-matched donors are scarcely available.
- Current therapies undergoing clinical investigation with most potential for therapeutic benefit are the β-globin gene transfer of patient-specific hematopoietic stem cells followed by autologous BMT.
- Other emerging therapies deliver exogenous regulators of several key modulators of erythropoiesis or iron homeostasis.
- This review focuses on current approaches for the treatment of hemoglobinopathies caused by disruptions of β-globin.

INTRODUCTION

Hemoglobinopathies arise from genetic mutations in HBA1, HBA2, and HBB that compromise the structure-function of the α-globin and β-globin chains of hemoglobin (Hb). Collectively, mutations in the β-globin gene are referred to as β-thalassemia (BT).[1] Mutations in the HBB are remarkably heterogeneous at the molecular level with more than 300 variations identified (http://globin.cse.psu.edu/). Despite the diversity of mutations, most cause disruption in the α-globulin, β-globin balance, resulting

Conflict-of-interest statement: K.M. Musallam received honoraria from Novartis, Celgene, and CRISPR Therapeutics. A.T. Taher received honoraria and research support from Novartis and Celgene. S. Rivella is a member of scientific advisory board of Ionis Pharmaceuticals. S. Rivella has received grants from Ionis and NIH. A. Gonzalez declares no conflict of interest. Work related to this article was funded by grants from the NIH-NIDDK- R01 DK095112 and R01 DK090554 (S. Rivella).

[a] Department of Pediatrics, Division of Hematology, Children's Hospital of Philadelphia (CHOP), Philadelphia, PA, USA; [b] International Network of Hematology, 31-33 High Holborn, London WC1V 6AX, UK; [c] Department of Internal Medicine, American University of Beirut Medical Center, PO Box: 11-0236, Cairo Street, Hamra, Raid E Solh, Beirut 1107 2020, Lebanon; [d] Cell and Molecular Biology Graduate Group (CAMB), University of Pennsylvania, 421 Curie Boulevard/6064 160 Biomedical Research Building (BRB) 2/3, Philadelphia, PA 19104-6064, USA
* Corresponding author. 3615 Civic Center Boulevard, Philadelphia, PA 19104.
E-mail address: rivellas@email.chop.edu

in long-term ineffective erythropoiesis (IE) and extramedullary hematopoiesis of the spleen and liver. IE leads to various degrees of chronic hemolytic anemia and transfusion dependence as well as upregulation of iron absorption. Strategies to treat BT are based on gene therapy strategies as well as pharmacologic treatments to target pathways that modulate erythropoiesis and iron homeostasis. Here, the authors review emerging therapies in clinical trials and preclinical stages of development.

EMERGING THERAPIES IN CLINICAL TRIALS

Sotatercept (ACE-011) and luspatercept (ACE-536) are 2 compounds that showed success in clinical trials (**Table 1**). Sotatercept was originally developed to treat bone-loss disorders, but clinical studies unexpectedly revealed increased hematocrit and Hb levels in treated patients.[2] Structurally designed to compete with the extracellular domains of Activin Receptor A Type 2A (ACVR2A) or 2B, these peptides act as ligand traps for transforming growth factor-β (TGF-β)–like molecules.[3,4] Growth differentiation factor 11 (GDF11), a member of TGF-β superfamily, is the identified ligand target for luspatercept. Treatment with luspatercept is thought to remove GDF11 from circulation and cause subsequent increases of Hb levels.[5] GDF11 is well established as a ligand capable of activating the SMAD2/3 pathway through ACVR2A or 2B.[6] Administration of the luspatercept mouse analogue, RAP-536, to BT mice ameliorates intracellular accumulation of hemichromes (HCMs), oxidative stress, and splenomegaly, while also inducing late-stage erythroid progenitor differentiation.[7] In phase 1 studies of healthy volunteers, luspatercept and sotatercept showed a dose-dependent and sustainable increase in Hb level and were well tolerated.[8,9] Luspatercept subsequently entered a phase 2, open-label, dose-ranging study in adults with BT (NCT01749540, completed) including an ongoing 2-year extension (NCT02268409). Patients received luspatercept at doses of 0.2 to 1.25 mg/kg administered subcutaneously every 3 weeks. Available data indicate that luspatercept was generally well tolerated and had a favorable safety profile. Luspatercept reduced transfusion requirements and liver iron concentration among patients with transfusion-dependent (TD) BT and increased Hb levels, reduced liver iron concentration, and improved patient-reported outcomes among those with non-transfusion-dependent (NTD) BT.[10,11] A double-blind, randomized, placebo-controlled phase 3 study (BELIEVE) has begun to evaluate the efficacy and safety of luspatercept among adults with TD BT. Demonstration of efficacy will require at least a 33% improvement in the number of transfused red blood cell (RBC) units from baseline (NCT02604433). In the phase 2a study of sotatercept among adults with TD or NTD BT (NCT01571635, completed), data indicated an increase in Hb levels, a reduced transfusion burden, and a favorable safety profile,[12] but no phase 3 studies are publicly announced.

The JAK2 pathway has been long thought of as a potential link between erythropoiesis and iron metabolism.[13] Negating effects of erythropoietin (EPO) overstimulation in BT by inhibiting the JAK2/STAT3 pathway has been an attractive area of therapy exploration. One of the first agents to be approved by the US Food and Drug Administration as a JAK2 inhibitor was ruxolitinib.[14] Studies on mice models of BT show that the JAK2 inhibitor reduces IE and splenomegaly.[13,15] A single-arm, phase 2 study (NCT02049450, completed) to evaluate the efficacy and safety of ruxolitinib administered orally at a starting dose of 10 mg twice daily among adults (n = 30) with TD BT and splenomegaly has been completed.[16] Ruxolitinib was associated with a slight increase in pretransfusional Hb levels (by 0.5 g/L increase) and a trend toward reduced transfusion requirements (by 45 mL of hematocrit-adjusted RBC volume per 4 weeks) following 30 weeks of treatment. Mean spleen volume also decreased during ruxolitinib treatment. No major adverse effects were reported.

The only cure available for patients suffering from BT is a bone marrow transplant (BMT) with cells harboring a functional HBB gene; however, finding a donor source is challenging. Gene transfer (GT) technology and autologous BMT provide an alternative with potential to reach more patients. The development of safe lentiviral vectors and discovery of the β-globin's locus control region (LCR) has made GT a possibility for BT. The first clinical study (LG001) in a BT patient tested the HPV569 vector[17–20] harboring a critical amino acid modification (T87Q) that allowed researchers to successfully identify modified cells and accurately measure viral integration and chimerism.[21] The patient became transfusion independent 1 year after GT, exhibiting increased levels of several Hb variants, including HbF with equal proportions of HbA containing the T87Q mutation. New vectors are currently in various stages of clinical trials (NCT02633943, NCT02453477, NCT03275051, NCT02453477, NCT01745120, NCT02151526, NCT03207009, NCT02906202, NCT01639690) (see **Table 1**). Interim data from a phase 1/2 study of autologous hematopoietic stem cells transduced ex vivo with a lentiviral vector among patients with TD BT (NCT01745120) suggest increased levels of HbA and reduced transfusion requirements.[22] New strategies for allogenic BMT and reduced intensity conditioning (RIC) are also in clinical trials (NCT00408447, NCT02038478, NCT02165007), which could eventually also aid the success of GT (see **Table 1**).

INNOVATIVE THERAPIES IN PRECLINICAL STAGES

Patients with high levels of endogenous HbF do not exhibit the symptoms associated with BT. Chemical agents such as hydroxyurea are used to induce HbF in BT patients[23]; however, these agents are not effective in all patients.[24,25] Genome-wide associated studies[26] identified BCL11a as a regulator of HbF. Knock-down studies of BCL11a using RNA interference (RNAi)[24,27,28] proved it to be rheostat for silencing of the γ-globin gene. One novel approach to induce HbF by silencing BCL11a uses an erythroid-specific promoter to drive a microRNA-adapted short hairpin (shRNA).[29,30] By using erythroid-specific HS2 and HS3 regions of the β-globin LCR alongside its promoter, the toxicity and engraftment impairments characteristic of Pol III/II–driven shRNA and microRNAs are circumvented while simultaneously inducing HbF in erythroid cells.[30]

Other strategies for BCL11a inhibition in preclinical stages use gene-editing (GE) strategies: zinc finger nucleases (ZFNs), transcription activator-like effector nucleases (TALENS), and clustered regularly interspaced palindromic repeats (CRISP) in association with Cas 9 (CRISP/Cas9). All GE strategies have successfully targeted BCL11a[31–34] decreasing protein expression of BCL11a and causing expression of γ-globin. Several studies using ZFNs, TALENS, and CRISP/Cas9 systems have also shown the potential of editing HBB in both patient-derived CD34+ cells and induce pluripotent stem cells (iPSC).[35–38] Although questions concerning off-target events remain, latest studies show GE as a strategy with clinical potential.[34,39]

By targeting iron regulation by direct action on the main iron transporter, transferrin has had promising results. Studies on BT mice treated with exogenous apotransferrin resulted in a net decrease of iron uptake by RBC precursors through TfR1 and subsequent reduction of HMCs.[40] As HMCs were reduced, the lifespan of RBCs and total amount of Hb in circulation increased. In addition, haplo-insufficient TfR1 mice also resulted in improved erythropoiesis with results closely mirroring findings of exogenous apotransferrin treatment.[41] Increasing circulating hepcidin and manipulating the hepcidin pathway by targeting its regulators may provide patients with more effective options for iron overload management. Preclinical studies of administration of

Table 1
Emerging therapies in clinical trials for treatment of β-thalassemia

Strategy	Phase	National Clinical Number (NCT)	Study Title	Interventions	Status
Trap-ligand targeting TGF-β ligands	Phase 2	NCT01571635	Study to determine the safety and tolerability of sotatercept (ACE-011) in adults with BT	Sotatercept	Active, not recruiting
	Phase 2	NCT02268409	ACE-536 extension study, BT	Luspatercept	Active, not recruiting
	Phase 3	NCT02604433	An efficacy and safety study of luspatercept (ACE-536) vs placebo in adults who require regular RBC transfusions due to BT	Luspatercept	Active, not recruiting
HbF induction	Early phase 1	NCT02981329	Fetal Hb induction treatment metformin	Metformin	Recruiting
RIC	Phase 2	NCT00408447	Stem cell transplant in sickle cell disease and thalassemia	Busulfan, fludarabine, alemtuzumab	Recruiting
	Phase 2	NCT02038478	Allograft for sickle cell disease and thalassemia	Donor stem cell transplantation	Recruiting
	Phase 1	NCT02165007	Haploidentical hematopoietic stem cell transplantation for children with sickle cell disease and thalassemia using CD34$^+$ positive selected grafts	Peripheral blood stem cell graft that are CD34$^+$ selected	Recruiting
JAK2 inhibition	Phase 2	NCT02049450	Study of efficacy and safety of INC424 in regularly transfused patients with thalassemia	Ruxolitinib	Completed

	Phase	NCT	Description	Name / Assessment	Status
GT	Early phase 1	NCT02633943	Long-term follow-up of subjects with hemoglobinopathies treated with ex vivo gene therapy	Safety and efficacy assessments	Enrolling by invitation
	Phase 2	NCT03275051	Long-term safety and efficacy follow-up of subjects treated with GSK2696277 for TDBT in San Raffaele Telethon Institute of Gene Therapy-Beta Thalassemia (TIGET-BTHAL) Study	Safety and efficacy assessments	Not yet recruiting
	Phase 1/phase 2	NCT02453477	Gene therapy for TD BT	GLOBE	Recruiting
	Phase 1	NCT01639690	BT major with autologous CD34$^+$ hematopoietic progenitor cells transduced with TNS9.3.55 a lentiviral vector encoding the normal human β-globin gene	TNS9.3.55	Active, not recruiting
	Phase 1/phase 2	NCT02453477	Gene therapy for TD BT	LentiGlobin BB305	Recruiting
	Phase 1/phase 2	NCT01745120	A study evaluating the safety and efficacy of the LentiGlobin BB305 drug product in BT major subjects		Active, not recruiting
	Phase 1/phase 2	NCT02151526	A study evaluating the safety and efficacy of the LentiGlobin BB305 drug product in BT major and sickle cell disease		Active, not recruiting
	Phase 3	NCT03207009	A study evaluating the efficacy and safety of the LentiGlobin BB305 drug product in subjects with TD BT, who have a β_0/β_0 genotype		Recruiting
	Phase 3	NCT02906202	A study evaluating the efficacy and safety of the LentiGlobin BB305 drug product in subjects with TD BT		Recruiting

exogenous sources of hepcidin, such as minihepcidins and other hepcidin agonists, as well as inhibiting negative regulators of *Hamp* (TMPRSS6) expression are shown to successfully prevent iron overload, improve anemia, and ameliorate IE in mice models of BT.[42–46]

NOVEL TOOLS FOR DRUG DEVELOPMENT AND THERAPY DISCOVER

Novel therapeutics are not possible without innovation at the bench side. New animal models, in vitro systems with potential to more closely mimic in vivo conditions and tools for gathering in vivo data in mice models, are necessary for the advancement of BT therapies. A Thal-Biobank has been established with goals to supply researchers with the samples of the same cells for studies aimed at solving the plethora of biological and biomedical issues involved in using patient cell cultures.[47] Erythroid precursors collected from 72 BT patients were expanded, cryopreserved, characterized with respects their individual Hb profile, and tested for abilities to produce HbF by hydroxyurea. Furthermore, several laboratories characterized samples from the same donors, showing that data were reproducible using protocols developed by the Thal-Biobank.

In the last decade, immortalizing human progenitor cells has become possible. Two cell lines in particular stand out, human immortalized erythroid progenitor cell lines (HUDEPs)[48] and the newly established Mui009.[49] HUDEPs were generated from human umbilical cord blood and immortalized with conditional (doxycycline-inducible) expression of human papilloma virus (HPV)-derived E6/E7 proteins. The cells can be expanded infinitely, and characterization shows them to be arrested at the proerythroblast stage. The line has several clones available, each with its own unique gene expression fingerprint of erythroid-specific markers. These cells can be differentiated into enucleated RBCs, providing a useful tool to study erythropoiesis. The Mui009 cell lines were generated from a 32-year-old man with homozygous β-globin deletion and heterozygous α-thalassemia. Peripheral blood mononuclear cells were enriched for CD34$^+$ cells and reprogrammed into iPSC cells. Resultant cells exhibited embryonic stem cell characteristics, including the capability of differentiating into the endodermal, ectodermal, and mesodermal germinal layers. However, work is still needed to determine if the cells are suitable for studies requiring RBC differentiation.

Measuring potential therapeutics for inhibition of iron overload has been limited by the inability to measure iron loading on live animal models. The use of MRI offers a clinically relevant assessment tool to measure the presence of iron loading in humans and recently has been optimized for the use on small animal models.[50] Tissue resonance relaxation rates, spleen volume, and cardiac function are now quantifiable in live BT mouse models during treatment course.

DISCUSSION

Despite the success of GT in the last decade, improvements of both the transduction efficiency of lentiviruses and the HSC expression of the β-globin transgene are needed. Patients treated with GT display a spectrum of phenotypic heterogeneity in endogenous and GT-delivered β-globin variants. Although some patients treated reach therapeutic HbA thresholds, a majority are left TD.[17,21,51] The potential of GE and reactivation of HbF production awaits future data from human studies.

Therapeutic strategies aiming to modulate iron metabolism are also showing promise in reducing IE, reactive oxygen species (ROS), and ameliorating anemia. Exogenous administration of apotransferrin ascertains to be a therapeutic with much potential. The safety profile and Hb increasing abilities in clinical trials have been previously reported in treating hypotransferrinemia.[52] RNAi technology has been used in innovative ways to target modulators of both erythropoiesis. Activating HbF by using RNAi is pushing the bounds of discovery by creating new molecules capable of intervening at the level of transcriptional regulation.

Sotatercept and luspatercept are frontrunners as emerging therapies for BT management. Although they were designed to target different TGF-β ligands, results of clinical studies show similar outcomes. The unknown role of the TGF-β ligands family on erythropoiesis and their potential contributions of BT treatment make the initial serendipitous sotatercept and luspatercept findings especially exciting. As very little is known about the role the activin pathways play on normal hematopoietic function, current mechanisms suggested do not completely explain the effects of sotatercept and luspatercept.[5,7,8,53] Further characterization of the TGF-β ligands will undoubtedly lead to new insights into both fundamental hematological mechanisms and therapies.

ACKNOWLEDGMENTS

The authors extend special thanks to Ping La (Children's Hospital of Philadelphia) for helpful discussion and support.

REFERENCES

1. Weatherall DJ, Clegg JB. Inherited haemoglobin disorders: an increasing global health problem. Bull World Health Organ 2001;79(8):704–12.
2. Carrancio S, Markovics J, Wong P, et al. An activin receptor IIA ligand trap promotes erythropoiesis resulting in a rapid induction of red blood cells and haemoglobin. Br J Haematol 2014;165(6):870–82.
3. Pearsall RS, Canalis E, Cornwall-Brady M, et al. A soluble activin type IIA receptor induces bone formation and improves skeletal integrity. Proc Natl Acad Sci U S A 2008;105(19):7082–7.
4. Sako D, Grinberg AV, Liu J, et al. Characterization of the ligand binding functionality of the extracellular domain of activin receptor type IIb. J Biol Chem 2010; 285(27):21037–48.
5. Suragani RN, Cadena SM, Cawley SM, et al. Transforming growth factor-beta superfamily ligand trap ACE-536 corrects anemia by promoting late-stage erythropoiesis. Nat Med 2014;20(4):408–14.
6. Oh SP, Yeo CY, Lee Y, et al. Activin type IIA and IIB receptors mediate Gdf11 signaling in axial vertebral patterning. Genes Dev 2002;16(21):2749–54.
7. Suragani RN, Cawley SM, Li R, et al. Modified activin receptor IIB ligand trap mitigates ineffective erythropoiesis and disease complications in murine beta-thalassemia. Blood 2014;123(25):3864–72.
8. Attie KM, Allison MJ, McClure T, et al. A phase 1 study of ACE-536, a regulator of erythroid differentiation, in healthy volunteers. Am J Hematol 2014;89(7):766–70.
9. Sherman ML, Borgstein NG, Mook L, et al. Multiple-dose, safety, pharmacokinetic, and pharmacodynamic study of sotatercept (ActRIIA-IgG1), a novel erythropoietic agent, in healthy postmenopausal women. J Clin Pharmacol 2013; 53(11):1121–30.
10. Antonio Piga SP, Melpignano A, Borgna-Pignatti C, et al. Luspatercept decreases transfusion burden and liver iron concentration in regularly transfused adults with beta-thalassemia (S836). Haematologica 2016;101(s1):338–9.
11. Antonio G, Piga IT, Gamberini R, et al. Luspatercept increases hemoglobin, decreases transfusion burden and improves iron overload in adults with beta-thalassemia. Blood 2016;128:851.

12. Cappellini MD, Porter J, Origa R, et al. Interim results from a phase 2a, open-label, dose-finding study of sotatercept (ACE-011) in adult patients with beta-thalassemia. Haematologica 2015;100(s1):17–8.

13. Rivella S. Ineffective erythropoiesis and thalassemias. Curr Opin Hematol 2009; 16(3):187–94.

14. Ostojic A, Vrhovac R, Verstovsek S. Ruxolitinib: a new JAK1/2 inhibitor that offers promising options for treatment of myelofibrosis. Future Oncol 2011;7(9): 1035–43.

15. Casu C, Rivella S. Iron age: novel targets for iron overload. Hematology Am Soc Hematol Educ Program 2014;2014(1):216–21.

16. Aydinok Y, Karakas Z, Cassinerio E, Siritanaratkul N, et al. Efficacy and safety of ruxolitinib in regularly transfused patients with thalassemia: results from single-arm, multicenter, phase 2a truth study. Blood 2016;128:852.

17. Negre O, Eggimann AV, Beuzard Y, et al. Gene therapy of the beta-hemoglobinopathies by lentiviral transfer of the beta(A(T87Q))-globin gene. Hum Gene Ther 2016;27(2):148–65.

18. Negre O, Bartholomae C, Beuzard Y, et al. Preclinical evaluation of efficacy and safety of an improved lentiviral vector for the treatment of beta-thalassemia and sickle cell disease. Curr Gene Ther 2015;15(1):64–81.

19. Cavazzana-Calvo M, Payen E, Negre O, et al. Transfusion independence and HMGA2 activation after gene therapy of human beta-thalassaemia. Nature 2010;467(7313):318–22.

20. Ribeil JA, Hacein-Bey-Abina S, Payen E, et al. Gene therapy in a patient with sickle cell disease. N Engl J Med 2017;376(9):848–55.

21. Bank A, Dorazio R, Leboulch P. A phase I/II clinical trial of beta-globin gene therapy for beta-thalassemia. Ann N Y Acad Sci 2005;1054:308–16.

22. Thompson AA, Kwiatkowski J, Rasko J, et al. Lentiglobin gene therapy for transfusion-dependent β-thalassemia: update from the Northstar Hgb-204 phase 1/2 clinical study. Blood 2016;128(22):1175.

23. Arruda VR, Lima CS, Saad ST, et al. Successful use of hydroxyurea in beta-thalassemia major. N Engl J Med 1997;336(13):964.

24. Basak A, Hancarova M, Ulirsch JC, et al. BCL11A deletions result in fetal hemoglobin persistence and neurodevelopmental alterations. J Clin Invest 2015; 125(6):2363–8.

25. Musallam KM, Taher AT, Cappellini MD, et al. Clinical experience with fetal hemoglobin induction therapy in patients with beta-thalassemia. Blood 2013;121(12): 2199–212 [quiz:2372].

26. Uda M, Galanello R, Sanna S, et al. Genome-wide association study shows BCL11A associated with persistent fetal hemoglobin and amelioration of the phenotype of beta-thalassemia. Proc Natl Acad Sci U S A 2008;105(5):1620–5.

27. Giani FC, Fiorini C, Wakabayashi A, et al. Targeted application of human genetic variation can improve red blood cell production from stem cells. Cell Stem Cell 2016;18(1):73–8.

28. Sankaran VG, Menne TF, Xu J, et al. Human fetal hemoglobin expression is regulated by the developmental stage-specific repressor BCL11A. Science 2008; 322(5909):1839–42.

29. Guda S, Brendel C, Renella R, et al. miRNA-embedded shRNAs for lineage-specific BCL11A knockdown and hemoglobin F induction. Mol Ther 2015;23(9):1465–74.

30. Brendel C, Guda S, Renella R, et al. Lineage-specific BCL11A knockdown circumvents toxicities and reverses sickle phenotype. J Clin Invest 2016;126(10): 3868–78.

31. Bjurstrom CF, Mojadidi M, Phillips J, et al. Reactivating fetal hemoglobin expression in human adult erythroblasts through BCL11A knockdown using targeted endonucleases. Mol Ther Nucleic Acids 2016;5:e351.

32. Cavazzana M, Antoniani C, Miccio A. Gene therapy for beta-hemoglobinopathies. Mol Ther 2017;25(5):1142–54.

33. Makis A, Hatzimichael E, Papassotiriou I, et al. 2017 Clinical trials update in new treatments of beta-thalassemia. Am J Hematol 2016;91(11):1135–45.

34. Genovese P, Schiroli G, Escobar G, et al. Targeted genome editing in human repopulating haematopoietic stem cells. Nature 2014;510(7504):235–40.

35. Xu P, Tong Y, Liu XZ, et al. Both TALENs and CRISPR/Cas9 directly target the HBB IVS2-654 (C > T) mutation in beta-thalassemia-derived iPSCs. Sci Rep 2015;5: 12065.

36. Finotti A, Borgatti M, Gambari R. Ground state naive pluripotent stem cells and CRISPR/Cas9 gene correction for beta-thalassemia. Stem Cell Investig 2016;3:66.

37. Chattong S, Ruangwattanasuk O, Yindeedej W, et al. CD34+ cells from dental pulp stem cells with a ZFN-mediated and homology-driven repair-mediated locus-specific knock-in of an artificial beta-globin gene. Gene Ther 2017;24(7): 425–32.

38. DeWitt MA, Magis W, Bray NL, et al. Selection-free genome editing of the sickle mutation in human adult hematopoietic stem/progenitor cells. Sci Transl Med 2016;8(360):360ra134.

39. Dever DP, Bak RO, Reinisch A, et al. CRISPR/Cas9 beta-globin gene targeting in human haematopoietic stem cells. Nature 2016;539(7629):384–9.

40. Li H, Rybicki AC, Suzuka SM, et al. Transferrin therapy ameliorates disease in beta-thalassemic mice. Nat Med 2010;16(2):177–82.

41. Li H, Choesang T, Bao W, et al. Decreasing TfR1 expression reverses anemia and hepcidin suppression in beta-thalassemic mice. Blood 2017;129(11):1514–26.

42. Casu C, Oikonomidou PR, Chen H, et al. Minihepcidin peptides as disease modifiers in mice affected by beta-thalassemia and polycythemia vera. Blood 2016; 128(2):265–76.

43. Liu J, Sun B, Yin H, et al. Hepcidin: a promising therapeutic target for iron disorders: a systematic review. Medicine (Baltimore) 2016;95(14):e3150.

44. Nai A, Rubio A, Campanella A, et al. Limiting hepatic Bmp-Smad signaling by matriptase-2 is required for erythropoietin-mediated hepcidin suppression in mice. Blood 2016;127(19):2327–36.

45. Schmidt PJ, Toudjarska I, Sendamarai AK, et al. An RNAi therapeutic targeting Tmprss6 decreases iron overload in Hfe(-/-) mice and ameliorates anemia and iron overload in murine beta-thalassemia intermedia. Blood 2013;121(7):1200–8.

46. Casu C, Aghajan M, Oikonomidou PR, et al. Combination of Tmprss6- ASO and the iron chelator deferiprone improves erythropoiesis and reduces iron overload in a mouse model of beta-thalassemia intermedia. Haematologica 2016;101(1): e8–11.

47. Cosenza LC, Breda L, Breveglieri G, et al. A validated cellular biobank for beta-thalassemia. J Transl Med 2016;14:255.

48. Kurita R, Suda N, Sudo K, et al. Establishment of immortalized human erythroid progenitor cell lines able to produce enucleated red blood cells. PLoS One 2013;8(3):e59890.

49. Wongkummool W, Maneepitasut W, Tong-Ngam P, et al. Establishment of MUi009—a human induced pluripotent stem cells from a 32year old male with

homozygous beta degrees -thalassemia coinherited with heterozygous alpha-thalassemia 2. Stem Cell Res 2017;20:80–3.

50. Jackson LH, Vlachodimitropoulou E, Shangaris P, et al. Non-invasive MRI biomarkers for the early assessment of iron overload in a humanized mouse model of beta-thalassemia. Sci Rep 2017;7:43439.

51. Mansilla-Soto J, Riviere I, Boulad F, et al. Cell and gene therapy for the beta-thalassemias: advances and prospects. Hum Gene Ther 2016;27(4):295–304.

52. Boshuizen M, van der Ploeg K, von Bonsdorff L, et al. Therapeutic use of transferrin to modulate anemia and conditions of iron toxicity. Blood Rev 2017;31(6): 400–5.

53. Zhang YH, Cheng F, Du XT, et al. GDF11/BMP11 activates both smad1/5/8 and smad2/3 signals but shows no significant effect on proliferation and migration of human umbilical vein endothelial cells. Oncotarget 2016;7(11):12063–74.

Moving?

Make sure your subscription moves with you!

To notify us of your new address, find your **Clinics Account Number** (located on your mailing label above your name), and contact customer service at:

Email: journalscustomerservice-usa@elsevier.com

800-654-2452 (subscribers in the U.S. & Canada)
314-447-8871 (subscribers outside of the U.S. & Canada)

Fax number: 314-447-8029

**Elsevier Health Sciences Division
Subscription Customer Service
3251 Riverport Lane
Maryland Heights, MO 63043**

*To ensure uninterrupted delivery of your subscription,
please notify us at least 4 weeks in advance of move.

Printed and bound by CPI Group (UK) Ltd, Croydon, CR0 4YY

07/10/2024

01040505-0017